Soundtrack of a Misfit
Adventures in ADD & Addiction

By Rachel Leigh Wills
www.Rachelleighwills
Rachel.lwills13@gmail.com
202.579.1144 (Google Voice)
April 21, 2021

Contents

FOREWORD

You're a misfit. So am I. But this is the book that finally, at long last, gives us permission to own it. Fully, boldly, ferociously, and unapologetically, through Rachel's adventure that will set your senses ablaze.

Being a misfit has always been woven into my DNA (which is why my outlet has been stand-up comedy since the Clinton years, and Sweet Jesus, was that era the gift that kept on giving…), but rarely have I seen a work of literature that captures its essence quite like this one. Because each one of us has some level of misfit woven in. Rachel's journey encapsulates it to the very last detail.

Over the past decade, I've had the privilege of writing for some of the most famous people I'm not allowed to mention, or I'll break our confidentiality agreements and get sued, but one thing I've learned from working with them is this—whether they were NFL hall-of-famers, U.S. Senators who were in front of the cameras all day or award-winning neurosurgeons, they were all misfits. There was a part of them that wasn't "quite right." Even the most accomplished, most impressive superstars among them.

The label of "misfit" has been one I've also been proud to own myself, ever since I was a child, and, like Rachel, was cast aside for being different. For having a brain that didn't quite fit with the rest. For having the attention span of a drunken gnat. And for daring to not find boring, mundane things as interesting as I was told they needed to be.

Rachel's journey through the world of addiction, fractured relationships, self-loss, and self-discovery is one that every misfit can relate to on a visceral level. It illustrates a life on the edges as well as any book possibly could and gets into the gritty details of an existence spent searching.

So often in life, we're told to sit down, shut up and blend in. But for so many of us, and I suspect, you as well, that simply wasn't an option. There was more to see. More to experience. More to enjoy. And a different perception around each one of those life checkmarks that enriched

1

the experience beyond our wildest dreams. But only if we accepted that we were different. And that's a difficult road to travel for most.

Rachel's memoir is the road that each of us will take to heart in a singular way. It's misfitting 101. It's the blueprint for how to come full circle and embrace the crazy, make love to the divergent and become one with the offbeat.

If this book leaves you half as inspired as it left me, you will still be buzzing for days after you've finished it.

Geoff Woliner, Founder, Winning Wit
www.Facebook.com/WinningWit
www.GeoffWoliner.com
@WinningWit

Dedication

Soundtrack Of A Misfit is dedicated to the rugged, wildflowers among us who show the full spectrum of their riotous beauty. We are not misfits. We break the molds, color outside the lines, and dance to the beat of our own inner soundtracks. Rock on!

INTRODUCTION

Reading and writing have been woven into the fibers of my being from birth. My mom read aloud to me nightly from my favorite books, until I could read them myself at the early age of three and a half. Writing was more difficult for me to master. It was already evident by age five that I didn't have the same degree of eye-hand coordination as other kids my age. I was taught cursive writing in the first grade because my teachers believed it would be easier for me to write if I didn't have to constantly pick up my pen to make the different parts of the printed alphabet. Take that, *Leo the Late Bloomer!*

Leo was a late blooming tiger in a childhood book I adored because I related to him. Despite being young, I identified with the concept of *otherness*. I was different from others. I used cursive, whereas everyone else used print.

I absentmindedly made careless errors on schoolwork and acted impulsively, heedless of the potential consequences. Most kids I knew were able to demonstrate restraint when they got ideas and they weren't sure about their consequences. Not me. The moment I had an idea, I acted on it. My impulse usually led to significant albeit unintended consequences.

I accidentally set off our home smoke detector, ruined landscaping, and made a mess in the kitchen. One time for Valentine's Day, I wanted to surprise my mom and stepdad with a homemade cake. I baked a pretty yummy cake, but the entire kitchen was covered in a thick film of flour and frosting. It took my mom weeks to clean it from the nooks and crannies of the kitchen. She was mostly furious with me and only slightly touched by my intended act of kindness. I coined the most overused acronym in my household – IDDIOP - "I Didn't Do It On Purpose!"

Like a first grader, I asked "*Why?*" so often when given instructions that my mom and stepdad yelled at me for being stubborn and argumentative (how's that for irony?). I sought to understand the meaning behind others' suggestions or instructions when I asked "*why.*" I wouldn't agree to anything unless I understood the "*why*" of it. I never outgrew this type of questioning.

3

I became more impulsive and unintentionally divisive the older I became. I longed for my parents (I refer to my mom and stepdad as my parents) to praise me for my brave ambitions, such as becoming a punk rocker but all I ever heard was, "Rach, your head is in the clouds. Put your feet on the ground." I knew I had it in me to become a scuba-diving paleontologist who sang in a rock band, but my parents saw me as unfocused and "all over the place." I longed to be bold and rebellious like those I literally, as well as physically, looked up to.

I was also smaller than everyone else in my classes—always. In junior high school my mom took me to Children's Hospital in Washington, DC, to be tested for a possible genetic growth disorder. Even though everyone on both sides of my family was small except for my mom and her brother, I was the shortest.

My younger sister was taller than me by that time and she was just ten years old. At the hospital, Dr. Well Hung (yes, that was his name) informed my mom and me that I was fine. I was just "constitutionally" short. My mom and I broke out in tears. We weren't crying out of relief or sadness but from the insinuated irony of the doctor's name.

I grew proportionately, meaning that I didn't have any features that are common among individuals with dwarfism. But I'm all of 4'10.5", technically a half-inch taller than a "Little Person." At age 49, I will not accept that I will soon start shrinking. I'm afraid I'll become like Lily Tomlin's character in the movie, *The Incredible Shrinking Woman*.

As I matured, my otherness revealed itself in other ways. I didn't get sarcasm. I was a literal thinker. And I often struggled to get my point across to others even when I knew exactly what I was trying to say. My sense of timing was also different from everyone else I knew. I knew how to tell time at the age of six because the Roto-Rooter man at our house taught me. He was at our house (for what seemed like an eternity) trying to fix something in our basement. He got tired of my not knowing how to answer him whenever he asked me what time it was.

I can tell time but time as a construct, at being fixed at a certain point, baffles me. Albert Einstein once said that *time is the thing that keeps everything from happening at once.* But in my inner world, everything felt like it did happen at once. I didn't get how I could get into bed at 8:30 p.m. to read my book and the next time I looked up it was "suddenly" 11 p.m. My mom would stride down the hallway and kindly but firmly say, "Rach, close your book. It's time to go to bed. You have school in the morning." I also didn't get time management despite understanding the benefit of and need for it.

My stepdad, David, moved in when I was nine. He was a mechanical engineer with a specialty in electronics packaging. I already liked him, but I thought he was the most anal-retentive man ever. He didn't understand, for the life of him, why I couldn't get myself out the door on time when I was old enough to be able to. We had yelling matches, "One minute, DP (my nickname for him as his last name is Perlmutter), I have to go back inside. I forgot my coat." I grabbed my coat and pulled the door locked behind me and started walking to the bus stop.

Two minutes later I'd walk back into the house. "I forgot my lunch." David would cry in exasperation, "Rach, you missed the bus. Let's go now. In the car. I'll drive you on my way to work." Being uber-sensitive, I'd get into the passenger seat and snivel all the way to school. I cried if my sister, named Stacey, looked at me "wrong." I cried often at our nightly family dinners. In fact, my mom, DP, and Stacey placed bets on who would make me cry before we sat down to eat. Their teasing wasn't malicious. It was intended to get me to laugh at myself or at least to get me to laugh along with them. I however, felt like I'd been roughly exfoliated from head to toe. I was constantly told to "grow a thicker skin" and I didn't know how to.

At school, the ribbing was worse. I was taunted about being the shortest one in school. In the eighties, there was no shortage of short comparisons: "Monchichi," "Chia Pet," "Shrinky Dink," "Smurfette." I was also teased for the hump in the middle of my "witchy, Jewish nose" from the time I was in elementary school until I had it cosmetically altered at the age of 16. I also experienced less overt forms of anti-Semitism. After I got my nose fixed, people who hadn't known about my pre-nose job made remarks like "I didn't know you were Jewish," "You don't look Jewish; your hair is blond and straight." Years later, I would feel like a misfit even among my own people because I was "the one with the tattoos."

My otherness wasn't all bad. I tended to be more reflective and empathetic than others. I had more vivid dreams than anyone I knew. Some-

5

times I even had lucid dreams. Other times, I was able to influence the content of my dreams by purposefully telling myself what I would dream about that night. My family was amazed by the feature-length film quality of them. As I got older, I wrote them down in my journals and entertained family and friends by reading them aloud to them.

I was also very imaginative. I could amuse myself for hours by writing poems and turning creeks and woods into magical worlds well into my teens when most girls my age had outgrown play and were deep into play-adulting. I was curious, spontaneous, and brave! And I always had good intentions even when things went awry. My mom used to counter all my IDDIOPs by saying, "The road to Hell is paved with good intentions."

I had a highly developed sense of right and wrong, but I lacked what most people refer to as common sense. My mom often asked, "Rach, what did you think would happen when you did x, y, or z?" I answered, "I don't know. I didn't think about it." And it wasn't that I didn't think. I thought all the time —so much so, that it took me hours to fall asleep at night because I couldn't stop thinking. I was furious with myself whenever I got into trouble for my apparent lack of thinking. "Thinking" and "timing" are integrally linked for many people, but they don't logically go together for me.

In the book *Is It You, Is It Me, Or Is It Adult ADD*, author Gina Pera explains that individuals with ADD experience time as being "'now' or 'not now.'" This is how my impulsiveness manifested itself. I did think about things, but I couldn't wait for "now." I needed instant gratification because I couldn't stand the feeling of self-explosion, the degree of anxiety I experienced if I were made to wait for anything. I couldn't wait because waiting meant not thinking, which I couldn't stop doing.

I wasn't intentionally a *bad* daughter, student, friend, or employee—I was a curious and confused one. A lot of life went over my head. Sadly, the older I got, the more self-destructive my behaviors became and the more urgently I needed a means of escaping from both myself and reality. When I was younger, I was able to escape the heaviness of reality through listening to music and playing outdoors. Music and nature were my ideas of sheer bliss. My mom calls me her "flower child" because of this.

Even when I was two, I literally danced to the downbeats of music and the "Beat of my own drum." I could listen to music or play at the neighborhood creek for hours and all by myself. Playing outdoors made me feel less small because everything was small in comparison to the trees and the sky. Nature gave me a sense of peace and made me feel less alone. Aloneness has always been a mixed bag for me. I'm introverted and crave peace and solitude as sources of refuge and recharge. I like to be alone—not feel alone. I hate *feeling* alone. I always felt alone when I was growing up —even with my family.

It became even harder to balance the scales of belonging and aloneness once I hit puberty. In junior high, I shut myself in my room for hours at a time. I turned my stereo/cassette player on and listened to Duran Duran, Howard Jones, and OMD. I sang along with the heady and often overwrought lyrics and wrote and wrote and wrote in my journals.

After college, I added alcohol and marijuana to the things I did alone in my room. In keeping with my late bloomer ways, I began drinking at 19 but began partying hard at 25, an age when most others slowed down and gave up their evil ways. I was just getting into counterculture when most had already conformed to society's standards of adulthood. They were done with their personal rebellions but mine had just begun.

I wasn't embattled simply because I wanted to wage war against my parents, friends, and society or because it simply felt good. I did so because I was lost within. I couldn't see any other way to get "through" or "by" in life. Euphoric nights of chemical escape turned into "euphoric mourning," to paraphrase and pay homage to one of my musical heroes, Chris Cornell.

This book is equal parts wreckage and resurrection. It's my personal anthem. It tells the story of how I discovered that my *otherness* was due to my having Attention Deficit Hyperactivity Disorder (ADHD [or more commonly called ADD]). I didn't learn to embrace my being different until I was 36 —nine years after my ADHD diagnosis —when I entered recovery.

Today, I take a certain sense of pride in being a rogue, disorderly dandelion among a battalion of neatly planted roses. Today, I own who I am. I'm bisexual. I'm a writer and a mental health therapist. I'm a wife and a mom (to an adorable black cat and an aging beagle-dachshund).

I'm a Jewish, badass earth mother, punkish, ADHD wildflower. I hope my story will help you if you're wrestling with ADHD or chemical dependency, have a love of adventure, are sexually fluid, or are kindred wandering Jew.

Note: I've changed some names and places to protect individual and workplace anonymity.

Spoiler alert: my paragraphs might seem disjointed in some places, but my editor and book coach suggested leaving my work as is. He argued, and rightfully so, that it gives a truer representation of who I am, being an individual with ADD.

CHAPTER 1 – FAMILY PORTRAIT

The morning my dad moved out of our house, both my mom and my dad took Stacey and me to school to tell our teachers the news. It was the worst day of my life. Stacey's stupid teacher made it worse because she got the two of us mixed up.

What is worse than being mistaken for a first grader when you're in the third grade? Our dad's moving out. The double dose of evil was like pouring salt on a festering wound.

I wish I could say that my dad had no part in my stepdad David's moving in with us. It would've made my mom's newfound happiness with him easier to stomach. My mom and DP's love would've been more like a fairy tale if my dad wasn't THE key factor in their getting together. But what Disney story begins with the king introducing the queen to a better man? What fairy tale ends with its two young heroines being neither truly abandoned nor rescued by the voluntarily ousted king? That story doesn't exist because its plot is too confusing.

How DP came to live with us depended upon whether my mom or dad told the story. If you wanted to remain in the castle, it was important to believe my mom's version. It was truly only a matter of semantics anyways. My dad's version went like this:

> Rach *I'm not the type of husband who takes out the trash or does chores without being nagged. I'm never going to be the dad who remembers dance recitals and horse shows. But David is that guy. I want that for you girls, and I want your mom to be happy, too, so I'm going to step aside and let David take care of the three of you. I can't think of a better man for you girls.*

My mom's version went like this:

> *One day your dad pulled David aside and confidentially but likely not too quietly declared, "You should fuck Cookie.*

9

She's a good lay. Anyways, she's made it clear that she doesn't want me around anymore."

I think my dad's version of the story was a PG equivalent of his inner monologue. It was important to him that he saw himself as the hero in this docudrama. I also believe that my mom's recounting is closer to reality. My dad left one day, and DP moved in the next. It didn't take any of us long to realize the irony of the new order. My dad was the consolation prize —not DP. If Stacey and I were desert saguaros that reached skyward with prickly limbs outstretched, then DP was rain sent from heaven. The skies opened to herald his arrival and our home smelled as fragrant and as wonderful as petrichor.

Don't get me wrong; things were awkward at first. Stacey desperately wanted to sit on DP's lap. She lived life either bouncing around like Tigger or glued to my mom or my dad's legs but she was too shy to accept DP's overtures. And I didn't take well to being corrected by him every time I wanted his help to reach a cup from high kitchen cabinets that I needed a stepstool to reach. I'd ask for a cup and he would say, "Oh, you mean a glass. Cups are plastic." It was infuriating.

When our dad lived with us, their bedroom door was always open. We climbed into bed with them when we had bad dreams and hopped on the bed to snuggle every morning upon awakening. My dad especially loved to snuggle. Afterward, he got up and made us pancakes and ham. My mom insists that it was turkey bacon but I'm sticking with my memory.

With DP's arrival, the bedroom door was perpetually closed. He required privacy. Many of my memories before he moved in were blocked by my brain. The clinical term for this is dissociation. It's how our brains protect our bodies from experiencing intense physical and emotional pain. To try to make sense of things, Stacey and I had to adapt. Since time as a construct was muddled and raucous, we learned to measure it differently. We would often remark "Was that before or after we got DP?"

DP hates my description of how we "got" him. He says it makes him feel like we bought him from a used parts store but it's how Stacey and I mentally document our family chronology. DP made me realize and grudgingly accept that structure isn't synonymous with torture. He also helped me to see how I benefited from adding order to my life. My natural structure free soundtrack sounded like this:

I need to do my homework but, look, a squirrel! OK. I need to finish this task. But wait, look what I found! What was I supposed to be doing? Right, I'm supposed to be doing a load of laundry. Wait, I'm hungry. I better grab a snack. Ooh, what are you doing, DP?

My music sounded like a gently flowing stream, interrupted here and there by chirping. While I flitted from one thing to another like a songbird, Stacey never stopped moving! I got distracted by movement, whereas she lost her mind when made to sit still. We dubbed her the "whirling dervish." Stacey was vibrant and graceful, always engaged in a complexly choreographed ballet. She's the rhythm to my melody. In music, these opposites make for either harmony or discordance.

By the time our dad left, my mom was a weary composer. She basically raised us as a single mom until DP's arrival because my dad wasn't what my mom considered to be "consistently reliable." When DP moved in, our mom finally had the choreographic partner she needed. DP helped raise his own kids, Mike, and Debbie, at least until he came to live with us. It saddened me to think about how much they must've missed him, but I was more grateful that we got him.

DP and my mom were on the same page when it came to parenting. There was no more good cop-bad cop shtick now that my mom had back-up. If my mom and DP got hung up on discipline or guidance, Stacey and I never knew it because it seemed like they effortlessly co-parented and orchestrated things.

Everyone flourished and floundered together under this new conductorship. No one was a lone instrument. The walls no longer echoed with our dad's thunderous voice. And the house no longer felt devoid of a male's presence. I truly don't know how we would've survived without our stepdad. There were times when our parents were our life rafts. Since DP entered our lives, there's been no doubt about who I'm referring to when I say, "my parents."

Our dad wasted no time moving in with a new family. I don't remember the kids because they were older than we were, but I know they existed. The other woman, Annie, was a close second to Cruella De Vil. She had the longest nails I ever saw. She once accidentally scratched Stacey's bottom with them when she was helping to dry her off after a shower.

Annie became just one of the many women who vied for my dad's affection over the years. Before my mom and dad separated, it didn't seem like such a big deal that my dad was sometimes gone for weeks at a time. We knew he would always come back. Even living with Annie, he wasn't but a mile or two away from us. But on the day, he announced his move out of town, the time and space continuum sealed. I struggled to grasp why, when he was already out of the house, did he need to move even further away? Did he still love Stacey and me? Did I do something wrong? Am I the reason my parents' marriage didn't work? Did I require too much attention? I know my dad was often frustrated with the slow pace at which I moved.

Our dad moved to Philadelphia shortly after moving in with Annie, or so it seemed. His relocation brought on a new line of questioning: Where is Philadelphia? How far away is it? Are you ever coming back? My dad moved out, moved in with another family, and then moved to another state in rapid succession. It literally made me sick.

I got horrible staph infections on my tush, legs, and sides. It was DP who tended to me. He microwaved wet washcloths until they were hotter than I could stand. I had to burn myself by placing them on the infected spot until the ugly green head of the boils softened up enough to pop. My mom took over then, squeezing the life out of the greenish-yellow oozing bubbles until no pus was left in them. I wailed in pain each time she performed this ritual.

My tush was so sore that I had to bring a plastic yellow, smiley-face cushion to school so I could sit without too much pain. It was embarrassing. One pus-filled monstrosity was on my left calf just a short distance below the circular scar I still bear from being hit by fireworks the year prior. That staph infection was so bad it had to be lanced by a doctor who I accidentally kicked in the face due to the pain.

Then there were the women. In my mind, that is the exact sequence of events. I got staph infections and then, my dad dated. There was Bon-

12

nie, a blond, pixie-haired teacher. She was nice, but my dad thought she was too normal. Then there was Rosie, who was anything but ordinary. I adored her because she was both a bohemian and a Valkyrie. She had thick, long, unruly dirty-blond curls and was the tallest, most fulsome woman I ever saw or have seen since. Rosie was an artist. She made funky necklaces out of teeny plastic animals, amulets, and other random miniature objects. I often wondered what my dad's life would look like had he stayed with her.

Then there was Ellen. She ended my dad's dating habit because they got married. Ellen came with two children, Robbie, and Marci. Robbie was a couple years older than I was and Marci was the same age as my sister. Ellen lived in a big house in a suburb of Philly. Her downstairs furniture was oddly and eerily all covered in plastic. It was clear that a messy young girl like me who liked to play in the dirt wasn't welcome. Easy-breezy Stacey had no problems making friends with Marci. Sometimes I'd join them in whatever it was they did together. And sometimes I'd hang out with Robbie who I thought was cute and cool because he listened to Billy Idol.

I honestly don't remember much from this period of my life. It wasn't a happy one. The only happy memory I have from the Ellen Period involves their maid, Susan. She was from the Caribbean. I don't know how old she was, but she was comfort. Ellen didn't cook at all but Susan made tasty homemade meals. She always had her Christian Bible radio programs on. Sometimes I'd sit and listen with her just to be near someone warm.

Exchange Weekends

Before my dad got remarried, Stacey and I often took a Greyhound bus up to see him —or we did until a perverted old man tried to get one of us to sit with him and not next to him but on his lap. The "exchange weekend" was the result. These were weekends when my mom and DP drove Stacey and me two hours into Delaware, where our dad was *supposed* to pick us up at Christiana Mall. When he showed up for these weekends, he would then drive us the remaining hour-and-a-half to his bachelor pad in Center City Philadelphia.

Some weekends, he arrived hours late. Our mom and DP would try to make things easier by treating us to ice cream and shopping. But there were also numerous times when our dad just never showed. I don't remember these times, as they were too painful for my nine-year-old brain to acknowledge and process. I wish my mom and David could've forgotten these times too. It made it harder for them to hear about any quality time Stacey, and I had with our dad. My parents sadly remember all too clearly how they were left to console two distraught young girls on so many occasions.

There was the time when our dad drove Stacey and me back home to Gaithersburg two days earlier than he, my mom, and DP agreed upon. This would've been somewhat okay had she and DP been home or even in the country. They were on some island scuba diving. My dad didn't stay with us in our house until they returned like a responsible parent but deposited us like we were luggage. He left us at a family friend's home unannounced.

If my dad always stood us up, it would've been easier to turn him into a villain. But Stacey and I also had lots of fun times with him. He lived downtown near the Free Library near two tall towers or office buildings. Somewhere near there was a city park where we'd go roller-skating while my dad smoked a cigar and watched us from a bench. Sometimes, he took us to the Franklin Institute or the Philadelphia Zoo. Once, my dad had me come up by myself for a weekend and surprised me by taking me to see a stage performance of the musical *Annie*.

I came back home singing "Tomorrow" and "Hard Knock Life"and I especially loved to belt them out emphatically whenever I was pissed at my parents and missed my dad. Every time my dad drove Stacey and I back from Philly to "Gaitherspatch," our condescending nickname for Gaithersburg, we sang our favorite rendition of Kenny Rogers' song "Lucille." The original song referenced four hungry children and a crop in the field, but we changed the lyrics to "You picked a fine time to leave me, Cookie. Two hungry children and a kick in the rear."

Our dad also gave Stacey and me cursing minutes when he timed one minute and allowed us to scream as many curse words as we knew. My mom was more proper when it came to language. She got angry with us for saying "mad" instead of "angry." She always said, "Horses get mad; people get angry." Whenever we came back from visiting with our dad, she remarked, "You two sound just like your father. You curse like sailors!" I smiled inside whenever she said that. I didn't think there was anything wrong with sailors —especially if they got to curse for a living.

1981 was one of the most traumatic years of my life but the years before that were like living in Disney's *Fantasia*. It was a musically miasmic era. The Dad Days and David Days blurred, as did the sounds of good days and bad ones. Basically, life sounded like an out-of-tune marching band going back and forth in time.

CHAPTER 2 – SOUND OF SMALLNESS

In 1974, I was three years old. I was given a red plastic record player that year as a Hanukkah gift. "Band on the Run" by Paul McCartney and Wings was just released. It was my favorite song. I played it daily on that record player along with my age-appropriate Disney favorites. I didn't know any other kids my age who collected records, but I was obsessed. I recall that my mom taught me to delicately hold them on their sides so that I wouldn't get them dirty or break them. I tried to be careful, but even 45s were too large for my tiny hands. I loved studying the record's concentric circles and watching them get all wavy as the player's needle meandered around them.

Two years later, I was listening to the newest musical genre: disco. People in Fort Lauderdale (where we lived at the time) were high on marijuana, cocaine, and "Disco Fever." I was in kindergarten then, so I alternated between listening to Hooked on Phonics and Disco. I was a mimic of my dad and uncles Jon and David. Every sentence they uttered began with "groovy this" and "jive turkey that." "Disco Duck," "Car Wash," "Bohemian Rhapsody," and "Fly Like an Eagle" were in constant rotation on the radio and on my red record player. I remember driving around with Uncle Jon listening to the Bee Gees and feeling that all was right with the world.

Listening to music was my primary means of refuge. I used music, even at the age of five, to help me to figure out how I felt and to better express myself. It was hard for me to figure out how I felt inside. I struggled to find the right words to describe my emotions because they were more complex than my vocabulary. Music provided me with a safe space to help me listen to myself and to calmly figure out what to say and how to say it. Music has always helped me to clearly delineate the chapters of my life. Whenever I replay scenes in my mind, I'm transported back through time to them via the songs I listened to "back when …."

The upbeat melodies of Barry Manilow and Neil Diamond evoke nostalgia for Sunday chore day in my household in the days after we "got" DP. I love thinking back to the happiness of those days. We were in our individual rooms or tidying up different parts of the house but united through our stereo's eight-track deck blaring "Jewish music" throughout our home. My mom, Stacey and I sang along and tone-deaf DP whistled along to "Copacabana" by Barry Manilow and "Kentucky Woman" by Neil Diamond. We called "Kentucky Woman" my song because I was born in Louisville, Kentucky.

By the time I was in high school, I practically locked myself in my bedroom 24/7 and just "was." I didn't do anything except listen to music. I was a lovelorn teenager who swore that the cure to heartache was through listening to the entire collections of Depeche Mode and The Cure. Later still, adult me (still prone to melancholia) gravitated towards the heartbreaking lyrics of Sarah McLachlan's album *Surfacing* and, later still, the nostalgic ballads on No Doubt's *Return of Saturn* album. I endured dark days sitting alone in my bedroom singing along to "Good Enough" and "Ex-Girlfriend." Music has always been the gospel by which I live. It helps me cope with minutiae and malady.

Kindergarten

There's a newspaper article my mom saved that features me for some reason. I keep asking her to sit with me and find it, but she doesn't relish going through reminders of her time married to my father. The last time I accidentally uncovered it, my stomach sank to my feet like it does whenever I fly, and the plane hits a patch of turbulence. I ache for my five-year-old self who wore a smock and stood in front of an easel that was easily twice my size. At the age of five, I still wore clothes designed to fit toddlers.

My ash brown hair was long again (my best friend Nonnie, who was overzealous in playing hairdresser, had accidentally given me a crewcut not that long before) and I wore it in a disheveled ponytail held fast with rubber bands that had colored plastic baubles on either end of them. My eyes were pained, my mouth was askew, my right hand held a paintbrush tightly, and my left pointer finger pressed hard against my upper lip. I felt frustrated and hopeless. I knew exactly what I was supposed to be painting but I couldn't do it.

I should have been carefree, but I was the farthest thing from it. I was forlorn and had heart-palpitating anxiety. I clearly remember how all the other kids in my kindergarten class were praised for how well they drew and colored within the lines. I tried to copy the kids on either side of me who took their time and colored neatly. I know that I took the same amount of time and applied the same degree of effort. At some point, however, I must've opted for scribbling because it didn't matter that I had given it my all. The teacher praised the "normal kids'" work; when she got to my seat, I nervously chewed the insides of my cheeks. It's funny how typing this memory triggers the recall and I find myself unconsciously chewing on my cheeks.

"Rachel, take your time and try to stay within the lines," she said. I didn't even get, "Nice try or Good effort." I was five, but I was already indirectly told that I wasn't worthy of praise or positive attention. I readily concluded that my classmates' work was better than mine, that they were better than me. My kindergarten classmates towered over me and were physically frightening. I was still the same size I'd been in nursery school. I was the only one who wasn't noticeably taller.

I didn't play much with the other kids in my class. I liked them, but they were able to play on different play structures than I was because they were taller. I couldn't reach the first bar of the jungle gym. I was too short to climb onto the see-saw. And regardless of my lack of height, I thought that everyone else ran around and shrieked too much. I didn't do Loud or Fast. Loud scared me and Fast wasn't safe for me.

Every time I ran around to keep up with the bigger kids, I fell and got scraped up. I was too clumsy to go as fast as they did. I was safer doing my own thing and I preferred it that way. I was a shy, introverted kid. One day, I was on the top of a climbing structure on the school's playground. I have a hazy memory of sitting on top of the slide. I was daydreaming like I always did. My mom called this "spacing out." I was so engrossed in my own thoughts that I didn't notice that my classmates went back inside. We must've been outside at the same time as the nursery schoolers because why else would my teacher not have noticed that she left me behind?

I remember another teacher called the remaining kids to line up. Somehow, I got lumped in with them. What's weirder than my teacher not noticing I was gone was that this other teacher didn't notice that I wasn't supposed to be in her class. I was too stunned to say anything on the playground. I simply followed the rest of the flock inside. The other teacher (not mine) informed everyone that it was nap time. She walked around the classroom, ensuring everyone lay down on their mats like they were told. I was the only one who stayed in a seated position. One thing I never did was nap. The preschool teacher got to my mat and barked, "Lay down!" I insisted that I was five and that I didn't nap.

The "other" teacher called over to the kindergarten class on the black, plastic rotary phone. Sure enough, they were down a student. Suddenly, my real teacher appeared and took my tiny hand in hers and escorted me back to our classroom. I recall being so angry that I burst into tears. I knew that this embarrassing ordeal only happened to me because I was the same size as the nursery school kids.

My mom laughed when she learned of this latest travail. My mom lets you know when she thinks something's funny or odd and she's quick to let you know exactly what she's thinking.

Unfortunately, I mistook her laughter as further invalidation. At five years old, I didn't have a protective shield of armor like hers. I needed her to tell me how sorry she was that I was mistaken for a nursery schooler. The moment my mom laughed; my brain filed the memory away as being harrowing. It haunted me like Pink Floyd's discordant song "Run Like Hell." I needed the soothing balm that only music provided for me. There was no other refuge from my teachers' cruelty or my mom's laughter.

"The playground incident" stands out as being the first time I struggled to make my voice heard. No one listened to me. No one trusted that I was a big kid. From that day on, my being small largely factored into the way I moved through my world: feeling different, unseen, not big or brave enough to stand my ground. To give an indication of just how small I was from the get-go, I wore doll's clothes when I was born. There weren't any baby clothes small enough to fit me. I wasn't born prematurely, and I didn't have a congenital birth defect or dwarfism. I simply inherited my ancestors' genetic shortness. My dad loves to recount how in love with me he was precisely because I was so teeny. He carried me around nestled into the crook of his forearm. When he held my head in the palm of his hand, I didn't even come close to his elbow.

In 1976, the year I started kindergarten, I couldn't climb the school bus steps by myself. I needed my mom to lift me up and pass me off to the bus driver, Mr. Green. No other kindergartner needed help boarding the bus. But every day, Mr. Green scooped me out of my mom's arms and gently set me down at the top of the stairs next to his seat. And on the ride back home, this routine reversed itself: Mr. Green handed me back down to my mom, who smiled at me with her startling blue eyes and her soft hair, streaked gold by sunlight, or possibly a frosting kit.

The only person who treated me like I wasn't small, or a baby was my kindergarten P.E. teacher, Mr. White. I adored him just as much as I adored Mr. Green. Mr. White was merciful enough to overlook my poor eye-hand coordination and he gave me good marks for effort. He's a fuzzy memory to me at this point, but I do remember that he was patient and encouraging. Unlike my dad, he never yelled at me to move faster whenever I couldn't do something as fast as he wanted me to.Everyone deserves to have a gym teacher as kind as Mr. White was.

The funniest thing about my affinity for Mr. Green and Mr. White was that I was fixated on their names. I thought about how funny their names were daily and I distinctly remember asking my mom why their names were so silly? She tried to stifle her amusement as she replied, "Rach, sweetie, their last names aren't connected to the color of their skin." I didn't get it. I couldn't fathom why they were named after different colors when they were both black.

In writing this memoir, I've gone through five drafts because it's hard for me to separate out my smallness from my life's events. Others defined me and referred to me as the "small," "short," and "teeny" one, so unsurprisingly, the constant references to my smallness greatly impacted the way I saw myself. Where others saw me as being physically small, I saw myself as being emotionally stunted.

I also tried separating out pre-divorce and post-divorce of my parents, but that didn't work either as my dad has always been either in the middle or on the periphery. His fluctuating presence and absence has always impacted me. Present Dad was Dr. Jekyll and Absent Dad-cum-Mr. Hyde influenced the way I viewed masculinity and related to men later in my life, as well as led to possibly obvious feelings of abandonment. I tried to place him in the chapters that deal more with relationships but part of the schema of this memoir is that my life, while not horrible, was chaotic and disorganized.

I have always struggled with organization because it involves the use of the prefrontal cortex, the part of our brains that oversees executive functioning such as chronology, time management, higher order logic and sound decision making, the management of emotions, and the prediction of consequences. It essentially rules the parts of ourselves that others judge us by —our actions. By continuing this book journey with me, you might find yourself smack in the folds of Calamity Jane, otherwise known as me. Consider this your trigger warning.

Circle Game

My family lived in a gated community in Fort Lauderdale called The Tennis Club. It was Everglade swamp land that had been filled in to make way for the city's burgeoning development. One of its sides abutted the state's intracoastal canal. It was an amazing place to play as a small kid because I could crawl into the belly of the banyan trees. They had massive trunks and labyrinthine root systems. I got to swing from their long, ropy vines like one of my heroes of the day, Tarzan, minus his grace.

My best friend Nonnie and I were inseparable. She was a few years older than I was and spent her time shuffling between her mom's house and her dad's (one of our neighbors). If Nonnie skinned her knee, I cried because I felt her pain as keenly as if it were my own. I don't know if I ever met her mother, Destiny, because she was something called a "hippie." It makes me chuckle to think that I thought that was a "dirty word" because my parents always whispered it when talking about Destiny. Nonnie's dad, Chuck, wasn't a hippie, but a businessman like my dad and my uncles.

Nonnie and I spent most of our days playing outdoors. You could usually find us in the banyan trees at the gatekeeper's station but sometimes we took to the cobblestoned streets of the Club on the lookout for this cool teenager who wore a boa constrictor named Thor draped around his shoulders. Other times, we'd be playing with my Scottish Terrier, Scotty (named for the Scotsman on *Star Trek*). We walked him up and down the cobblestones and along the canal encountering toads, lizards, and land crabs that crawled up the canal's embankment. The Fourth of July usually coincided with their mass exodus from the canal. Nonnie and I were terrified of these crustaceans because they found their way into our elevators, stairwells, and apartments.

We lived on the third floor of one of the apartment buildings. I knew my address and I knew how to find my way to our building within the Club. I wasn't too small or young to ride the elevator by myself because it was a safe community, as the adults looked out for one another's children. The problem was that I wasn't tall enough to press the elevator's buttons. My mom found a creative solution. She posted signs within the stairwell of our building that said my name because I could read it and then she drew one sign that had my name with an arrow facing toward our apartment.

Girls Just Want to Have Fun

I don't have many memories of how my small stature impacted me from my elementary school days, and it's not because I've blocked out memories from this period of my life. Elementary school was a happy time for me because it represented a change in the way I was schooled, which I'll talk about in a later chapter.

I only remember being angry about my diminutiveness once in elementary school and that's because it was a very public moment. It happened either during a sixth-grade production of a play called *How the West Was Won* or at my sixth-grade graduation ceremony. My mom and I are of different minds on this one, but we agree about what happened.

My tall, pale freckled-faced friend Brian decided to be funny while we were standing next to one another on stage. He dramatically demonstrated that he was bored by leaning his forearm against the crown of my head. I didn't think it was funny at all and I let him know it by using my right elbow as a battering ram. I elbowed him hard enough to make him wince and say, "Oomph!" According to my mom and DP, who were seated in the middle of the audience, a woman behind them exclaimed, "That little girl just punched my kid!" and she and DP sank a bit lower in their seats. They were equal parts mortified by and proud of my actions.

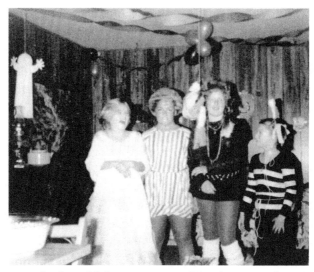

I am the one in the bumblebee costume. That's me at the age of 11.

The photo of the four costumed girls is the only one in this book, and I've added it for you to see just how small I was in relation to others my age. The photo was taken by my parents the night of my sixth grade Halloween party. The year was 1983. My friends were 12 already and were nearly a full year older than I was. I wouldn't turn 12 until we entered Gaithersburg Junior High the following fall. The song lyrics referenced above, popularized by Cyndi Lauper, played on our local radio station, Q107.3. Other songs that were popular around that time include "Mr. Roboto" by Styx, "Maniac" from the movie *Flashdance*, "Every Breath You Take" by The Police, and "Billie Jean" by Michael Jackson.

Stacey and all our friends were into sticker books, roller skates, and cute boys. We got together every Friday to swap stickers from our collections and go roller skating. We had every type of sticker imaginable: puffy, fuzzy, and smelly ones. We put neon-colored laces on our skates and wore black, shiny parachute pants like Michael Jackson's. At 11 and 12 years old, we were confident and giggly and thought we were "the bomb."

We skated forwards to "Get Down On It" by Kool & The Gang and backwards to "Rapper's Delight" by The Sugar Hill Gang. Whenever a slow song came on, we wistfully wished that a cute boy would ask us to slow skate. But if one did and we thought he was ugly, we'd politely say,

"No, thank you," then mimic gagging ourselves and say, "Grody to the max!" It was the era of Valley Girls made famous by the movie of the more-or-less same name and *Fast Times at Ridgemont High.*

When we entered Gaithersburg Junior High, I felt like I was the only one without parachute pants. My mom and I searched everywhere to find a pair, but none of them were small enough to fit me. I was embarrassed whenever I ran into friends while out shopping with my mom. I didn't want them to see me trying on clothes in the children's department while they browsed for theirs in the Juniors' section. My mom finally ended up finding a pair of Juniors' black nylon capris with buckles and side pockets. I adored them and had no clue that they weren't meant to fit girls my age as full-length pants. They were close enough to be MJ's and that's all that mattered.

I was the smallest student at GJHS, a krill swimming against a pod of baleen whales. My smallness endeared me to others and made them protective of me. But I was a teenager and I wanted to be considered anything but "cute." I wasn't bullied for being smaller than everyone else, but I was teased because of it. It was intended to be good fun, but I was overly sensitive. In fact, I cried my way through three-fourths of junior high.

There was just one incident that scared me but, for once, the taunting didn't have anything to do with my height or my "Jewish" nose, a humped protuberance I was very much aware of.

Ironically, I inadvertently prompted a verbal assault because I was a white girl who was gaga over Michael Jackson. I listened to his *Thriller* album so many times that I memorized the lyrics to nearly every song. I went so far as to have "P.Y.T." ironed onto the back of a neon pink T-shirt in black bubble letters. Like the "smooth criminal" that I was, I proudly wore my newly decaled T-shirt to school.

Five angry teenage black girls from my P.E. class whom I hardly knew were unimpressed by my fashion tastes. They circled around me and got right in my face. The biggest among them yelled, "You think you're a Pretty Young Thing. Hmmm, are you now?" I confidently stood my ground, but a lightbulb went off: *So that's what P.Y.T. means! How did I not know that?* I was so scared of those girls. Were they going to beat me up for wearing a T-shirt that I didn't even know the meaning of?

The thinnest girl among them was nothing more than a mimic. "Look y'all. She thinks she's a P.Y.T."

Before the incident could escalate, I was saved by our gym teacher, Mrs. Johnson. (In an odd coincidence, she died in her early fifties of a heart attack while in possession of my *Thriller* cassette.). I adored her because she gave me a B in her class based on my effort as opposed to my aptitude.

I nearly wet my pants every time I was made to play dodgeball —or any kind of ball. I was stuck in a hellhole of a small, graceless body and I honestly believed that the world was out to get me. I was an easy target. I was the one picking dandelions in the outfield whenever we played softball. Everyone else was astute and primed to catch the ball should it come near them. Not only was I the least coordinated student in gym class, but I was also the shortest. I was *that* kid, the one who got picked last for any team.

I couldn't even reach the classroom pencil sharpeners. I had to stand on a chair anytime I needed to sharpen one. No one else in the entire school had to do that.

Mrs. Johnson was caught totally off-guard by my parents' arrival on Parent-Teacher night. She remarked, "Oh my G—d, you must be Rachel's mom. She's your spitting image. But I had no idea you'd be so tall!" My mom doubled over laughing and explained that she and her brother were tall, but that everyone else on both sides of my family were short. And of course, she had to add that even my little sister, who Mrs. Johnson would have in her class next year, was taller than I was.

Even still, I was and am a mini replica of my mom. Whenever she showed up at school, kids helped her locate me without needing to ask who she was. They just said, "Hi, Rachel's mom! I'll show you where she is!"

The oversized textbooks I needed for classes weighed my backpack down. I wasn't big enough or strong enough to carry them all. Creative as always, my mom requested that I be given two lockers—one on either end of the school. I stashed books in both lockers, organized by the proximity of my classes. This gave me time to get to class without speed walking or straining under the weight of my books.

My mom also had the school loan me a set of books to keep at home, so I didn't need to lug a backpack bigger than when I was back and forth to school. These accommodations were written into my Independent Education Plan (IEP) that all students with learning disabilities had. At the time, I was no longer in special education classes (as I had been in past years), but I still met weekly with a resource specialist.

I was the last one out of the cafeteria one day. I was lost in a daydream and didn't realize that everyone else had finished their lunches and headed back to classes. The janitor just finished cleaning and didn't see me next to him at the entryway doors where the trash cans were stationed. He set the upturned trash can he had just emptied right on top of my head. I was mortified. I broke into tears and ran to the health room to call my mom to come pick me up. She chuckled upon hearing my sob story which was just as good as taking the janitor's side.

Yet the next week found me calling my mom from the nurse's office again. A dodgeball had hit me full on my "witchy Jewish" schnoz. Classmates called me "Witchy Woman" after the Eagles' song of this same title. My mom took one look at me and blithely replied, "Looks like you're going to get that nose job you've been begging me about after all, Rach." My nose wasn't broken but I did get a nose job—just not that day.

I was fed up with the constant teasing. The day my sister Stacey called me ugly for the umpteenth time, I totally lost it. I screamed, "That does it! I'm getting my nose fixed!" Luckily for me, my parents were on board with my decision. They knew that all the teasing had been detrimental to my self-esteem. And what Jewish mom doesn't want her daughter to be future dating material? Let's face it: I was going to have a hard time on that front with my nose—or so I was told and therefore believed.

I was told that my nose collapsed during surgery and that my septum was badly deviated. They had to mold the tip of my nose with hard cartilage, which made it immobile. I lost the ability to rub my nose around when it's cold outside, but it was a small price to pay for self-confidence. After my nose was fixed, I received more attention in school. I wouldn't say that I was popular, but I had more friends. Youth is brutal that way.

I wasn't prepared for guys to think I was cooler simply because my nose changed its shape, but one day a cute boy named Jonathan, who later became a good friend and Hebrew school carpool companion, teased me on our entire bus ride home. I ran off the bus crying. I know I hadn't done anything to provoke him. I called my mom at work looking for sympathy.

"Somebody called me a bad word and I don't even know what it means," I wailed into the phone! My mom asked what it was that I'd been called. "A Lilliputian!" I cried. A pregnant pause followed by cackling ensued. I'd never heard my mom laugh so hard. I couldn't see her, as there wasn't anything like FaceTime back then. Our phone was affixed to the wall and had a long cord that coiled, but suffice it to say that it was the kind of laugh that left my mom with tears streaming down her face; so much for sympathy. I mistakenly thought that she was laughing at my expense, too.

My size became less of an issue the older I got primarily because people tend to mature with age. In college, I was known less for being short and more for my extensive hat collection. I never wore baseball caps. I wore fedoras, floppy sunhats, and feathered hats. The quirkier the hat, the more likely I was to wear it.

I did have some issues relative to my size that other students didn't have. I had to sit up front or in the second row if the person in front of me was short enough to see over. My sitting in the first two rows didn't earn me many friends.

Also, my knees started to hurt a lot in college because my feet couldn't reach the floor when I was seated at either a table or an old-fashioned school desk. I asked DP if he could make me a footstool that was small enough and lightweight enough to fit in my backpack. I didn't want to be judged by anyone if they saw me walking around campus with a funny-looking metal contraption, so his invention was a lifesaver.

As an adult, being short has continued to endear me to others. However, my small size has also been mistaken as an invitation to take me less seriously and to treat me pejoratively. I hated (and still hate) being called "sweetie" or "honey" or any other pet names. My size has certainly never afforded me the experience of being called last for group photos. I'm always placed front and center. I automatically stand aside while everyone else organizes themselves by height and then I lead myself where I know I'm going to be placed anyways.

CHAPTER 3 – BIG FISH

My dad, Dan, has been one of the major influences in my life. We've always been close, no matter how present or absent he's been. It's hard for me to write about him because I have so many mixed emotions about his dualistic nature. Depending on the day and surrounding circumstances, he is either mellow and philosophical or grandiose and crass. He is "chill" and down-to-earth when he's not drinking. He got sober in 2008 and was allegedly abstinent from alcohol for a few years before he returned to drinking.

Depressed Dad is the worst because his behavior is singularly compensatory in nature. There is no getting through to him when he's in full-on narcissist mode. (Those are his sentiments —not mine; he is the first to admit that he's a textbook narcissist.) It's heartbreaking to hear him parrot phrases that he's been using since I was a kid, such as "living large" and "I'm feeling like a million dollars." I feel sorry for Depressed Dad, but I feel sorrier for myself when he's depressed because he rarely calls and doesn't listen to a word I say when he does.

He also is so into whatever his business venture du jour is that he doesn't pause to reflect that I might want to share with him what I'm doing or to hear him talk about me the way he talks about whomever is the coolest, brightest business partner, young kid, writer, etc. My dad has always been mercurial so I'm never sure which version of him I'm going to get.

If my dad were a record, Fun Dad cut would be the best take of him. Think of the persona of Hawkeye in *M.A.S.H.* or Chris Rock's zany zebra in *Madagascar*. He is raunchy and funny and fun loving. Today, he would be what's called my "ride or die." Fun Dad was the first version of himself I knew. He was the center of my world growing up and he made me feel genuinely loved and safe.

When I was young, he would lay on his back in our living room with his arms and legs straight in the air, and there I'd be — lying over his arms and feet, suspended, and flying just like I was Superman. Other times, I'd stand with my feet on top of his and we'd walk all over so I could see what it was like to be big. At bedtime, he told Stacey and me the most outrageous tales. I drifted off to sleep envisioning Señor Pepe, the talking frog who sang from his lily pad, and Flato, the farting field mouse. I begged him nightly for his stories because he never told any of them the same way twice.

My dad is average in height (about 5'8" or 5'9"), but his big personality fools everyone into thinking he's over six feet tall. He also has perfect posture which, depending on his mood, makes him seem domineering. I think this is a holdover from his days in the Army. He has always been big on posture —something I often forget to pay attention to and have not been so gently reminded to focus on.

He's also classically handsome. Even now, at 79 and with now-saggy jowls, you can tell my dad was a looker. This, too, has always been odd for me to deal with not due to any Freudian reasons, but because other women have used talking Stacey and me up to get closer to him. I once asked my paternal grandmother Harriett (his mom) who the hot guy in a photo was. I was embarrassed to learn it was my dad at 16 or 17.

Apart from his posture and sturdy build, my dad's hazel eyes also set him apart. They are as intense as a hawk's. If you saw and remember the father figure in the movie, *Big Fish*, and then make him better looking — that's my dad. I know exactly how Billy Crudup's character felt in that movie because my dad is so convincing in his stories and beliefs that he could sell you the world's deadliest snake and you'd buy it and cuddle it if he told you to.

He grew up in Larchmont, New York, and came of age in the late 1950s and early 1960s. He grew up in a traditional but nonreligious Jewish household. My dad is the oldest of four children. My aunt Carolyn died at 52 of breast cancer that metastasized to her ovaries. She was the one who informed my sister about the likelihood that she and I inherited the genetic mutation that many Jewish women and men of Ashkenazi or European Jewish descent are prone to inheriting.

My dad has two surviving brothers, my uncles David and Jonathan. My dad, aunt, and uncles grew up in a household with means. They owned a large home and had a yacht. I never got to meet my namesake, my Grandpa Ralph, because he died a couple of years before I was born, also at the age of 52 and also from cancer.

From the stories I've heard about him, he was a no-nonsense braini-ac. He made anyone who wanted to be on their yacht pass a rigorous, self-devised swim test in the Atlantic first. And he had no tolerance for lying or cursing. My Grandma Harriett told me that she used to walk into a closet and bang pans together if she wanted to curse so he wouldn't hear her.

His world had no margin for error because he was one of the nucle-ar engineers who worked on the Manhattan Project. It's not the kind of thing I brag about, but I'm proud of him nonetheless. In fact, his cancer was caused by his exposure to uranium during atomic testing. On his deathbed, he made the family swear that they wouldn't sue the federal government for wrongful death. My dad recently told me that, in 1927 or thereabouts, my grandpa had a seat at the Algonquin Round Table, where the cerebral greats of the day gathered at New York City's famous Algonquin Hotel.

My dad loves to have heart-to-heart conversations with me in which he imparts all the things he wished his dad had told him. He never heard his dad say, "I'm proud of you" because my dad was a hellion when he was a teenager and young man. He grew up believing he was stupid because he couldn't read until he was in the fourth grade and he didn't really care about it until he was older. My Grandpa did send my dad off to college in New Mexico, but his entrance into adulthood wasn't a cause for celebration; he initially went to dodge the draft. My dad said, "Rach, your Grandpa Ralph was one strict dude. He sent me away to university with two Brooks Brothers suits and a wad of cash. He said, 'Good luck, kid. Sink or swim.' Then he walked away."

My dad didn't last long at UNM, but he loved his time in Albuquer-que. My dad loves to recount how he used to get high on mezcal with his roommate and ride motorcycles through their house. But the good times quickly came to an end. My dad's draft number got called and he went into the Army and served in Vietnam for two years.

Despite my dad's time in the war being relatively short, I know he was greatly changed by it as many were. He lived in a village called Da-lat, which is a ritzy tourist attraction today. My dad never talked about the war no matter how much I cajoled him. I recently learned from Uncle Jon that my dad was trained with an elite group of soldiers under the

101st Airborne in jungle warfare and ambush tactics.

I wish I had a straight story. All soldiers were trained to kill. One thing both my uncles (Uncle David is essentially a clone of my Dad) agree on is that my dad was fearless and that they never wanted to mess with him. I have seen my dad enraged on numerous occasions and, while he never took his anger out on me physically, I have seen my dad turn into the Incredible Hulk and it is scary.

(A quick sidebar: My dad spanked me once when I was eight because I lied to him about something. I cried because he frightened me, and it hurt. I wet my pants all over his lap. He visited me in my room a few minutes later and profusely apologized. Apart from one other incident where he lifted me out of a pool by my bathing suit straps, he never laid a finger on me).

The only other things I know about my dad's days in Vietnam are that he carried the telecommunications radio that his father had a hand in designing years earlier and that his platoon was in an ambush once where everyone but him and another soldier died. They only survived because their tank flipped over, and they were hidden out of sight underneath it. Coincidentally, this was on Thanksgiving and Grandma Harriett via telepathy knew that something bad happened, but that my dad was alive. She broke down crying into her turkey.

According to my mom, my dad returned from the war (this was before they even met) and had so much bottled-up anger inside him. I imagine his anger as a living entity bubbling just under the surface, like magma inside the Earth's core.

He expected to return home to a hero's welcome and wasn't prepared to be regarded as an abomination. When he returned from fighting, it was 1968. Most people in the States opposed the war and supported peaceful protests, sit-ins, equality, and psychedelics.

My dad stepped back onto American soil and got lost in this conflict. The Kent State shootings were just two years away. With so much turmoil going on at home, not many cared that my dad had been fighting, so much for a hero's welcome. He didn't get a welcome home of any kind. His family didn't know he was back on American soil, so he hitchhiked home. Sadly, he couldn't thumb a ride dressed in his Army uniform. Most passersby honked at him and shouted insults. He said that

31

once he swapped into normal clothes, he didn't have any problem getting a ride. For someone who is usually so puffed-up about his abilities and interests, this was a humble way of acknowledging that he knew he cut a dashing figure in his civvies.

My dad came home only to find that his parents had moved to Florida while he was off fighting. They were no longer as wealthy and had to adjust to a new standard of living. My dad enrolled at Florida State University under the G.I. Bill then met and fell in love with my mom ostensibly because she was a good note-taker in classes.

I know my dad (and obviously my mom) were devastated by going through the experience of having a stillborn son who was carried full-term and birthed. I was born a couple years later and was supposedly conceived to "Running Against the Wind" by my dad's favorite, Bob Seger. I'm convinced I heard and fell in love with music in utero.

As I grew up, I heard plenty of stories from my mom about my dad's drinking, his anger, and his infidelity (before and after their marriage), as well as how my Grandma Harriett tried to discourage them from marrying because my mom didn't come from money and was "plainer" than other girls my dad dated.

I don't know what my grandma was thinking because my mom was beautiful. She wore her hair in a short-almost-pixie-cut blond bob. She had dazzling blue eyes and, at 5 '7", was as rail thin as a heroin-chic model.

There's an unwritten memoir crafted within the confines of my parents' marriage. I don't know half of what transpired between them and despite my curiosity, it isn't my business to pry. I do know from my own misadventures in love that just because something is shiny on the outside doesn't mean there aren't cracks and imperfections within. Nothing is as pure and simple as we think it will be when we lovingly whisper, "I do."

Despite my dad's extracurricular activities, he was crazy about my mom and loved her dearly. I know this is a lot of back story on my father, but having this knowledge informs my sense of and experiences with him.

Bottles of Beer on The Wall

My earliest memory of my dad involves us drinking beer. I was three years old, and we were sitting outside in our backyard on a warm, sunny day in Atlanta. He was the coolest person I knew, and I was fiercely attached to him. If he drank beer, then I did, too. I watched him as he took big sips of beer from a crinkly, aluminum can. I pestered him to try it. He hesitated and then said, "Here you go, kid."

Sometimes we were at restaurants together, just he and I. I cherished alone time with him away from my mom and sister. I loved pretending I was a grownup who got to "drink" beer. I remember the precise way the beer's froth sat atop his chilled beer mug. It reminded me of the big, fat marshmallow globs that floated on top of my hot chocolates. My nose and tongue were tickled by the bubbly, white foam. Whenever my dad drank beer, he loudly and proudly belched. Without missing a beat, I mimicked him and belched too. He'd loudly and proudly proclaim, "That's my girl," and so began one of our shared rituals.

When I was nine, I lost interest in taking sips of my dad's drinks and turned my nose up at alcohol until I went to college. I saw how it often impacted my dad's moods. Besides, my need to be my mom's "good girl" overrode my desire to be "exactly like my dad."

That phrase became something my mom often hurled at me like a lance. "You're just like your father" had a different meaning for her than it did for me. I idolized my dad. We have many shared interests, including a love of adventure, a thirst for knowledge, and a zeal for reading. We also crave the peace that comes from digging in the dirt and being outside surrounded by nature. My fondest memories of my dad involve gardening together. I might've been short, but I took pride in the fact that I was strong. My dad knew this too because like a fellow soldier, he always enlisted my help to complete his most difficult projects. I thought if he chose me to help him, that must mean I'm special.

He did hard, manual labor with his Paul Bunyan-like strength and I played in the mud alongside him. I felt safe and loved when I spent mellow time out in the garden with my dad. I was also less aware of my "otherness" then—especially when he praised me for helping him. Sometimes, this was just a few minutes after he reprimanded me for being too slow or inattentive in bringing him garden tools. I'd start to retrieve them from the last patch of dirt we worked, but I ended up lost somewhere deep in thought. My dad's mixed messages were confusing, but I shrugged my shoulders and basked in the sun and warmth of his praise. My mom fought battles about my disability at school and made sure I had resource teachers, but Fun Dad played the role of hero.

I was amazed by how adept my dad was with a hammer, some nails, and a "can-do" MacGyver-like attitude. I marveled that his powerful hands could demonstrate both brute strength and exacting delicateness. I remember wondering how it was possible for him to be so strong yet so gentle. He could separate a plant's roots without damaging one. How could he work for hours without tiring or napping? Maybe smoking cigars was his way to take breaks while remaining in constant motion. In stark contrast, I took plenty of time to literally smell the roses and everything else that was fragrant in the garden we planted together.

Doing "Daddy-Daughter shit" together (what he's always referred to these special times of ours) were major productions. He pretended to be strict. He barked orders at me. "Yo, kid, hand me that rake," or "Yo, Rach, no talking! We talk after we rake," or "Kid, gently tamp down the soil after you plant anything so as not to compact it. The plants won't grow if you're too rough with them."

My dad had his agenda and I had mine. Mine was less overt: I knew that if I dawdled and daydreamed just long enough after he gave an order, he took more time with me and showed me how to do stuff. Then when I did it, he said something approvingly like, "That's my girl." It was hard to reconcile the dad who gardened with me and the dad who spent time with me and my uncles with the dad who surprised me one day by uprooting my mom, sister, and me from Fort Lauderdale to Louisville, and in a very callous manner.

I awoke one morning to hear my parents arguing. My dad bellowed, "Cookie, we're moving. That's all there is to it." I padded into the living room, security blanket in hand. "Is Nonnie coming with us?" I asked. He callously replied, "No, Rach. You'll make a new best friend in Kentucky."

I remember my heart shattered; everything felt jagged. I couldn't get air in because I was crying too hard. My long, unbrushed hair was matted with rivulets of snotty tears. I hated my dad for the first time. I blamed him for threatening my safety and turning my world into a frightening, unpredictable place. I hurled all my fury at him, screaming, "I hate you for taking Nonnie away from me! I'll never find another best friend and it's all your fault!" I didn't want to be uprooted from my best friend, the Banyan trees, the playground that my dad helped to build for me and the other kids in our community, or my uncles.

I know that we were the ones moving away, but I vividly remember feeling a sense of abandonment. That feeling was another first for me and caused by someone I revered. He moved us to Louisville for a solid waste-related job. I was only six at the time of our first move, so I called him the Trash Man. I knew he wasn't the guy who rode on the back of a trash truck, but it took me growing up a bit to realize what his role as a middleman in the recycling and solid waste industry was.

A couple of years later, when I was eight, he moved us to Gaithersburg, Maryland, because he was offered a position with JCPenney related to recycling plastic hangers. When we moved that time, I told myself that there was no point in getting too close to anyone because we'd likely move again. I was too young to be making solemn vows such as swearing to be thicker-skinned "if only we didn't move."

CHAPTER 4 – INITIATIONS

I have one great adventure that my dad and I went on together before the move to the house I grew up in and the divorce and it involved Indian Princesses.

I wasn't a girly girl. I didn't like frills, ruffles, overtly flowery prints, or bows. Pink was as far as I went. I also wasn't a joiner. I was more of a lone wolf. I don't know how it came to be that I joined the alt-version of Brownies or Girl Scouts, an organization that fostered daddy-daughter cohesion in a group forum, whereby multiple daddies and daughters convened to howl at the moon and make drums. I don't know how an entity with that name could exist.

It was a blatant appropriation of Native culture. I found learning about Native heritage and customs enthralling. I didn't know that the episodes of *The Lone Ranger* I watched were reruns or that Tonto wasn't representative of all Native tribes. It was 1979 and I was a girl who loved horses and dirt, ritual, and song. I identified with Native culture, which embraced animism and nature. The only reason I stayed in Hebrew school so long was because I loved the traditions and songs of my Jewish ethnicity and culture. The music was the only thing that made being cooped up indoors in school on Tuesday nights and Sunday mornings bearable.

In Indian Princesses, my dad was Chief Run Amok and I, Princess Sunflower. Later, I renamed myself Princess Thunder Cloud because it sounded more powerful. Our self-given "Indian" names were indicative of our respective personalities. My dad thought that Chief Run Amok was hilarious. I didn't know what it meant, but it sounded cool. Evidently, he was a lost soul and I alternated between being a sunny flower and a big, moody cloud.

One weekend my dad, the rest of our tribe, and I went to Camp Letts on Maryland's Eastern Shore to become "initiated" in a ritual for new recruits like my dad and me. It was our first or second night at camp and we were at the sacred ceremony. Three hundred dads and daughters were gathered around the biggest bonfire I ever saw. My dad told me that there'd be an amazing display of fireworks. He wasn't wrong because the sky exploded. In fact, fireworks were headed right for us!

My dad and I ducked our heads and closed our eyes out of primal fear and instinct. My dad wasn't hurt, but I was. Three hundred dads and daughters were gathered around a raging bonfire, and I was the only one who got injured? This is the type of Murphy's Law or anti-luck I've always had. I reflexively moved my right hand to my left thigh. It felt warm and wet, and my chest hurt. I was dazed but my dad's hazel eyes surveyed the scene like a hawk. And like the raptor I often compare him to, he flew into action. My dad hoisted me in his arms and ran with me through the woods. I was hurt, but I felt protected as he held me against his chest.

I stopped my dad at some point and told him I was okay enough to walk the rest of the way to our cabin. He gently set me on the ground. Seeing me walk, my dad's friend, who accompanied us, told me he was confident that I was going to get a Purple Heart. Terrified, I wailed, "I don't want to die! I don't want to die!" As if on cue, they started laughing so hard that tears streamed down their cheeks. "Hello, I'm dying!" I repeated. I had no clue that a Purple Heart was a military badge of courage. As it turned out, I ended up with a second-degree burn on my chest, which thankfully healed quickly and without scarring. I also had a hole in my thigh that required stitches inside and out. Forty years later, I still bear the scar. Good riddance, Indian Princesses!

Indian Princesses was my first organized initiation and communal ritual, but it wasn't my first trial by fire (no pun intended). That occurred in kindergarten and set the stage for how I would interact with others, as well as see myself for many years.

At the age of three, my mom enrolled me in a ballet class but quickly plucked me out of it because she observed that I struggled more than the other toddlers in coordinating my movements. She noticed that I wasn't good. In kindergarten, my eye-hand coordination hadn't improved as evidenced by how I valiantly tried to form my printed letters but couldn't connect the straight line of my lowercase "a" to the circle part (mine looked like O I versus a).

To determine what was "wrong" with me, my mom had me tested by a child psychologist who conducted a battery of tests over the course of a few days. The tests were extremely frustrating and made me angry with myself. I thought, *I'm stupid! I can't print my letters and I can't run or skip or hop!* I understood how to do all the things the psychologist had me do, but I couldn't satisfactorily perform many of the tasks except for those that tested my verbal and comprehension capabilities.

I knew I wasn't stupid, but I told myself that I was. How else could I make sense of the fact that I could read books better than other kids in my class or that I had a bigger vocabulary than theirs? I already read the *Hardy Boys* books while the rest of them were stuck on their ABCs. It just made no sense to me that the other kids couldn't read but could legibly print their names.

The stress and anxiety I felt daily caused me to gnaw the insides of my cheeks, as if chewing cud. I constantly ruminated on what made me so different and my life so much harder. I would continue to wrestle feeling like a misfit or an outcast until I turned 27 and was given a diagnosis that made sense, but until then, I had no clue that I had a disorder that today is as common as Charmin or Kleenex and its name then was "minimal brain dysfunction." I only understood that my brain worked differently from everyone I knew, and, because of this, I often dealt with its sinister companions: anxiety and depression.

I learned that I had Attention Deficit Hyperactivity Disorder (ADHD. There is so much information out there on the Internet on ADHD today and a whole generation has been over-diagnosed and over-medicated, but in the mid-'70s, there was no Internet yet, so information on ADHD was hard to find and established support groups - even harder.

My family dealt with my "otherness" the way most families did: alone. My mom did the best she could with the information at her disposal — especially since I wasn't hyperactive in a visible way. I don't think my mom realized that it was my mind that was always moving and churning things over and obsessing. Outwardly, I was what's referred to as "inattentive."

My mom didn't want to hold me back in kindergarten although that was suggested. She knew I was already self-conscious of being "slower." When we moved to Kentucky, I was placed in a special education class-room because that was the only option for kids with special needs. My classroom was modular and wasn't even inside the main school building. By first grade, I already read at the fourth-grade level and I had the most extensive vocabulary in my mixed-grade classroom. I didn't understand why I was trapped inside a truck-like classroom and punished. I was the only one in there who wasn't on the autism spectrum or didn't have a behavioral issue.

We moved to Gaithersburg just before I entered the third grade and the Indian Princesses Incident. I went through another battery of tests with a child psychologist to determine whether my spatial relations and executive functioning had improved enough that I could be placed back into a "normal" classroom.

Like the last time, the tests occurred over a few days and lasted all day long each day. I completed Rorschach tests, aptitude tests, personality tests, verbal and written comprehension tests, spatial relations tests, eye movement and hand-eye coordination tests. I assembled confounding puzzles and tried to memorize and repeat the alphabet and numbers backwards. I only got as far as Z, Y, X and 10, 9, 8; it was traumatizing!

In one series, I was asked to choose which analogy made the most sense for each given example. None of them; none made sense. I had no clue how a flounder was like a vacuum. One swam in the ocean and the other made a lot of noise. They both sucked things up from the floors but in my mind a fish and a vacuum were totally unrelated. One was an inanimate object used to clean and the other was an animal that swam in the ocean. *These are retarded examples!* I exclaimed to myself. ("Retarded" was a term still largely in use in the mid-seventies and was even called this on occasion by my sister and other kids my age.)

I fumed internally. I wondered if this was how my dad felt when he got so mad that he exploded. I might've verbalized my thoughts because it was hard for me to not blurt the first thing that came to my mind: *When will anyone stop me and ask me the difference between a flounder and a vacuum? Why do I even need to know this? I'm going into the third grade. I'm supposed to focus on reading and social studies, not analogies and statistics.*

By some act of mercy, I was mainstreamed that year and attended classes inside the school building (there weren't any modular units at this school). I was so grateful to go to school with "normal" kids my own age that I didn't mind being pulled out of classes a few times a week to meet with special education resource teachers. They worked with me on my penmanship, math, and logical reasoning, and my difficulties with physical balance. I worked with resource teachers at least once a week from elementary school through the end of junior high school.

I could say that everything was better because of this but I continued to struggle. I was supposed to move on with the other students at GJHS into Gaithersburg High School (GHS), but I informed my parents that I was going to drop out of school if they didn't allow me to go to a smaller private school. I was so tired of feeling like a fish out of water. I felt parched and thirsted for a better education with teachers who would see me for who I was in my entirety versus the limited version of me they saw because of tracking.

In the 1980s in Montgomery County, students were academically tracked. We were lumped together based on where we fell along the below-average/average/above-average continuum. According to this system, no one cared if you were below average in math but excelled in English or other subjects. I was stunned that my English teacher didn't notice or care that I spent the entire class either staring out the window or at the back of my classmate Dan's dyed-red, spiked mohawk.

Sometimes, I was the only one who had read the homework or answered the teacher's questions. When this happened, everyone else had to complete assignments in class, leaving me bored beyond belief.

And in Mr. Prezbocky's remedial math class, my teacher viewed me as a nuisance, regarding my frequent interruptions to ask for clarification as impertinence. According to him, "Math wasn't to understand; it was to perform." Supposedly, math was logical, but it made no sense to me. Mr. Prezbocky made it his mission to ridicule me daily.

I had so much anxiety in junior high school, I was a frequent visitor to the health room, so, by association, so was my mom. She was often summoned to come and pick me up early from school. I called her from a pay phone in the hallways or from the health room if the nurse felt generous enough to let me use the push button office phone. If I called from the pay phone, I cried, "I need a mental health day," our shorthand for "rescue me!" To her credit, she usually did.

CHAPTER 5 – YOU'VE GOT A FRIEND

Despite the emotional upheaval caused by my mom and dad's divorce, growing up in Gaithersburg in the '80s wasn't all doom and gloom. But it was boring. We weren't close enough to anything except the newly built Lake Forest Mall and the Shady Grove Metro station. Plus, I avoided Ride-On buses at all costs unless Leigh, the teenage daughter of a family friend, was with us. Ride-On buses were too dangerous for kids to ride on alone, and even teenagers like Leigh had to be careful. The only place Stacey and I walked or rode our bikes to without supervision was to the pool or Montgomery Village Mini Mall, the same strip mall where my dad and I used to walk to for donuts on the weekends.

There wasn't much development. Our subdivision bordered farmland, empty fields, and a creek. My childhood played out amongst the creek, the pool, a hill with a puny play structure, and a strip of pine trees and forsythia. The latter was close enough to the house that I could hear my mom if she hollered for me.

We didn't have the Internet or cell phones or cable television. I only got to see the latest and greatest - MTV and Betamax - at Leigh's house. What I wouldn't have given to have cable TV at home so I could watch MTV whenever I wanted to. It helped to catapult the careers of many of the musicians I loved, including Duran Duran, Billy Idol, The Culture Club, and The Police. Sadly, the coolest piece of technology we owned was an Atari video game console that Stacey got for Hanukkah.

I quickly grew bored of playing *Frogger, Donkey Kong*, and *Mario Brothers*. I was more into reading my teen magazines and playing at our nearby creek. And while Stacey and I could watch TV, we usually spent our playtime outdoors in the sunshine. Our mom encouraged us to be creative and to play outside before we resorted to spending time cooped up inside.

I relished the times I spent playing by myself or with Stacey and a few other neighborhood kids, but I always thrived on community. I love feeling that I belong to something meaningful and larger than my own small world. Having a sense of belonging allowed me to feel more worthy than I felt on my own. In school and at home, I always felt sorry for myself. In communion with others who shared my interests, I got to maximize my different abilities.

Stacey and I are just shy of being three years apart. We enjoyed the freedom we had to enjoy each other's company in an environment that was comparison-free. We loved one another and were close, but we were also compared to one another a lot by my mom and DP and neither of us cared for it. I was referred to as "the bright one" and Stacey "the graceful one." Our parents did the best they could but, in hindsight, they agree that they did us both a disservice by comparing our deficits to one another's.

While it was true that I lacked grace, I was strong and excelled at swimming like a fish underwater, holding my breath underwater, horseback riding, and archery. Stacey, while not interested in scholastics, wasn't dumb. She simply found dance, gymnastics, swimming, and sailing more interesting than school.

We enjoyed each other's company and the closeness of community at both our neighborhood pool and at summer camp from the time we were in elementary school until we graduated from high school. We swam until our fingers and toes were shriveled prunes. We went home for lunch and then returned to swim and play until the stars came out. We played Marco Polo and Shark in the Water with the big kids and we dove in the deep end. We thought we were so cool. We were strong swimmers and wanted to impress the male lifeguards we idolized; especially when they let us stay after they had kicked everyone else out at 9pm

The closest neighboring town to YMCA Camp Tockwogh, is Chestertown, Maryland. The camp sits atop eroding bluffs that buffer the Chesapeake Bay. Its waterfront is positioned directly across the channel from the Aberdeen Proving Grounds. Although Stacey and I sailed and swam in the Bay for seven years in a row, we never got used to the reverberating crescendos of the Proving Ground's sonic booms. They resonated within our lives on the water, where we sailed amidst large wakes and booms.

At camp, my talents shone through. I leveraged my passion for music and my gift for on-the-spot creativity at sing-downs and campfire singalongs. I helped our cabin win accolades and I helped others who were shy or frightened around horses to feel more comfortable around them. I loved the musty smell of horses and the way their noses wiggled at you when you pet them. I was an intuitive rider and wasn't afraid to canter or jump. The barn horses were so large yet responded to my smallest hand and leg commands. I craved the connection I formed with these gentle giants. My favorite horse, a white gelding named Gomez, stood at 15 hands.

Whenever I wasn't at the stables riding (something Stacey lost interest in after she was stepped on or kicked by a horse), we were together at the waterfront. Camp was segmented into waterfront, woods, and fields, and was also divided into boys' and girls' villages. I lived in various bunks over the summers in Ute Village.

Stacey and I were fishes in water since we could first swim, so we both passed our swim tests on the first try. The waterfront was ours. We made the long trek down to the waterfront together every day. We traipsed past the tennis court on the right and athletic field on the left, past the arts and crafts building, the canteen, the outdoors chapel, the drama cabin, and the mess hall. Lastly, we passed the flagpole where we lined up every morning for revelry. Then we delicately navigated our way down a steep, pebbly path that meandered through the boys' villages. Finally, we ended at the Bay's edge.

Although Stacey was younger, she was the better sailor. I was comforted whenever I got to sail Sunfish and Flying Scot boats with her. We had to carefully navigate jellyfish-infested brackish water to rig up our boats and set sail.

Stacey and I made a pact to look out for each other and enjoy spending time together at Camp. It was a secret that, away from our parents, we ceased to be frenemies and were friends. We weren't part of the same village or "tribe," but we still got to spend a lot of time together. We learned all about sailing from our hunky counselors, Mike and Bobby. We did everything we could think of to attract their attention without seeming like we needed any help. Every day, Stacey and I would "accidentally" make mistakes so that they needed to check in on us. If they were onto us, we never knew.

We were so young, but we were strong and brave. It felt awesome to know that we could sail all by ourselves — if we only applied our strength and knowledge. We were free! No parents. No teasing classmates. No homework. No one to supervise us except Mike and Bobby. Music had its own rhythm and lyrics to it. Ready about? Hard to the lee! Push the tiller, pull the jib sheet, shift the boom. If we underestimated the wind, we got stuck in irons and went nowhere. But if we overestimated the wind or were too hasty coming about, we capsized. It was the first time we were responsible for our own outcomes, and potentially our survival. Stacey and I realized that we depended upon one another and valued one another at Camp, in ways we didn't at home.

We took turns sailing and laying on the small Sunfish deck, while we worked on our tans. We twisted the words to The Clash's song, "Rock the Casbah" and bellowed, "Fuck the crab pot" instead. When Stacey and I didn't sail, we water skied or went tubing. We had so much fun doing these sports, but we had an ulterior motive.

Mike and Bobby supervised these waterfront sports, and we went wherever they were. They liked to mess with us. They waved one hand, and we waved back. Then they waved both hands and before we realized what we did — we dropped the tow line to wave both hands in response. Being towed and tossed around by the Boston Whaler was an experience that's hard to imagine was legal, let alone had been given parental consent.

I didn't even weigh 90 pounds at the time, and I know this only because 90 pounds was the minimal weight requirement for windsurfing. Stacey weighed even less so it's hard to imagine the way our light and little bodies were tossed about over the wakes as we took turns laying spread eagle atop a massive inner tube wending its maniacal way across the Chesapeake. We shrieked, laughed, and cursed because it was especially painful and embarrassing when the bottom part of our bathing suits hiked up into our crotches.

It was equally awkward when our tops began to ride down. Where Stacey had Skittles for breasts, I was much more developed than most girls my age. After so much physical exertion, we rested on the sand and scooped up handfuls of clay-like mud. We used our fingers as sieves and sorted out sea glass and sharks' teeth. Then we schlepped back to our respective villages delirious, starving, and reeking of brackish Bay scum.

Stacey and I spent most of our time on the water, but we also engaged in land activities that taught us to further hone our senses. We played Capture the Still, a hybrid of Color War and Capture the Flag. It was a camp-wide event that required cunning strategy to win.

I had no clue what liquor stills were, so the intended humor was lost on me. Capture the Still involved water jugs, water guns, and bandanas. We played on the tennis courts, which served as team prisons, and throughout the woods where each team was still hidden. I learned nature skills playing this childhood game that served me well as a nature-loving adult who spent a lot of time in the woods. I learned to walk on the sides of my feet, to not make noise while I helped to hunt opposing teammates, and to identify their stills by using my frontal and peripheral vision to scan territories. If I didn't want to flush out the "enemy" or get caught myself, I had to tread quietly and stop and listen for footfall.

Tulip Grove

I have been initiated many times throughout my lifetime. I am lumping some of the childhood ones together because they had a profound impact on my entry into adulthood. Some involve family members and others are specific events and, in one case, an entity. Because until we moved to the house on Tulip Grove Road, Stacey and I hadn't experienced stability. We moved into multiple apartments and homes within a few different states. I didn't know how to answer the question, "Where are you from?" I always answered with "everywhere." I had accepted that moving was just something we did — a lot.

We often changed states but sometimes, we simply moved into new houses. Maybe my dad got bored with work easily or maybe he was in what my mom called one of his "manic phases," whatever that meant. When I was older and friends asked me what my dad did for a living, I sometimes answered that he was in the solid waste industry. Other times, I said, "I really don't know what he does, but he's in business." Sometimes, I think my dad took his hero, Bob Seger, a little too seriously because he always said, "Here I am, on the road again." And as I got older, I would silently sing the next line, "Here I go, playin' star again ...."

In high school, I told friends that he was in the CIA and that I couldn't tell them exactly what he did because it was classified and even, *we* didn't know what he did. The latter wasn't a fib, and the former wasn't outlandish because my sister and I didn't understand all his "projects" and we lived within driving distance of CIA headquarters.

Our house was considered California-style. It looked like a rambler from the outside, but it had an upper and lower floor divided by a central landing or entryway. I recently saw a special on the Brady Bunch and our house looked a lot like theirs. All the houses around ours were meant to look alike, and they were separated by an open strip of common lawn. If you wanted your house to have more character than your neighbors', you had to have changes approved by the governing body of the Homeownership Committee, of which DP was president.

Our house was distinguishable because it was the one next to the corner house bordered by Harkness Lane. The front yard was draped in cherry trees. Papery-bark confetti carpeted our front yard. We had a covered walkway that led to both the garage (aka DP's office) and the front door. In wintertime, the entire wall of the walkway was lined with cords of firewood that we used in our wood-burning stove. The other side of the walkway was lined with azalea bushes that bloomed in vivid shades of red, pink, purple, and white.

We had a large living room window that stretched from the left corner of our walkway to the left corner of the house where the drainage spout let out onto a sloped hill. The window was framed with window boxes that DP made with tools from his "office." In springtime, they were filled with a riot of color: blooming marigolds, petunias, and impatiens. A row of colorful azaleas stood sentinel at the base of the window boxes. Just before you entered the house, you were greeted by our mezuzah and "Cale Yarborough," a sculpture of a purple bird made from reclaimed metal. (My parents said it was named after a famous racecar driver. I wasn't curious to learn more about said driver because, back then, that required a trip to the library!)

As you walked into our house, you stepped onto our front landing. Grandma Mary's (my mom's mom) brown, antique hutch sat there and housed her antique aqua glass bottles that survived her family's voyage from Russia. Directly above the wooden hutch hung a framed piece of silver that said "SHALOM" in both English and Hebrew. To the left of that was the long window that housed David's window boxes. From the landing, you could walk up the cornflower blue-carpeted steps to the upstairs den and bedrooms or downstairs to the formal dining and living rooms.

Stacey's and my bedrooms were really 10' by 10' shoeboxes with windows, while our parents' master bedroom was the most spacious room in the house apart from the living room. The upper level also housed the hallway bathroom that Stacey and I shared, as well as the upstairs open loft. If you walked down the stairs and turned left into the living room, you stood under the long window. If you sat on the living room couch, the windowsill was easily eight feet above your head. It stretched the entire length of the living room. Our cat Ho would often launch herself onto that sill from the stairs' guardrail.

Our living room had an incredibly high, vaulted ceiling with sky-lights, which made the house seem much larger than it was. The far-left wall housed my piano and keyboard, and an abstract painting of a home in New Orleans. The corner of my synthesizer bumped into The Pit. Only I truly used The Pit. It had a tacky, working, but never-used faux-rock fireplace in it. An iron grate at the bottom was supposed to hold firewood, but to us, it served as a perfect Barbie doll stable. The only other thing in The Pit was our stereo system, which included an eight-track player. I used to pull out my parents' music and shove my KISS and Queen into the wanting player.

When you turned right when coming down the same set of stairs, you walked past the hallway closet to your right and the kitchen to your left. Tucked into a narrow hallway to the right was a teeny half-bath and an unfinished laundry room that housed our hot water heater and fuse boxes. If you walked past the kitchen and made a quarter turn to your left, you stood between the L-shaped kitchen island and the kitchen table. Both abutted a long sliding glass back door.

If you made a quarter-turn to your right, you stood in our family room. This was the most used room in the house. It held the black, metal wood-burning stove and featured a tall, long brass etagere, as well as a ginormous chocolate-brown sectional sofa. The sofa was home to mul-tiple decorative pillows, as well as Pea Man and Potato Head. Pea Man was a pillow shaped like a pod of sugar-snap peas with a smiley face, while Potato Head was a plush potato pillow shoved inside a burlap sack. They adorned the couch well into my college days.

The brass etagere housed our TV, several porcelain LLadro figu-rines, and a slew of Tom Clark carved wooden gnomes. In the middle of the living room sat a brass coffee table with three circular tiers that could be moved independent of one another. No matter what other objects it held, there was always the Mikasa bowl full of gumdrops, homemade trail mix, or other candies in it.

The open floor plan meant that all the rooms downstairs flowed into one another without doors, except for the bathroom and laundry room. Upstairs, the bedrooms and bathrooms had doors, except for the upper loft, which overlooked the living room. The upstairs loft featured a large, clunky Compaq desktop computer. It also housed our copy of the *Merck Manual* (the 1980s equivalent of WebMD), DP's engineering periodicals, a collection of encyclopedias, and my robust record collection.

This was my favorite place in the house because of its openness. For years, it was where I played my music and pretended to be a rock star. I sang to my audience in the living room 10 feet below, singing into my hairbrush and dancing to my records without anyone judging me.

I have so many memories of times spent in this house with my family that it's paradoxical that what I recall most vividly are the many hours I spent at home by myself while my sister and parents were out with their friends. My friends often spent more time at my house than they did at theirs. But I remember feeling like my family didn't understand me, so it was easier to be alone at home than to explain myself to them. So, when all of us were home, I often stayed up in my room. I liked the solitude. The rest of my family is extroverted and often too loud for me. When I did hang out with everyone, it was usually in the open-style kitchen and family room.

The dominant fixtures in our kitchen were the butcher block and the island. The island was topped in a horrid shade of puke-green Formica. Why the house's previous owners chose that specific shade of green I'll never know. Maybe they'd been inspired by the Brady Bunch. The island was L-shaped and wrapped all the way around the kitchen, ending at the sink. It served as our home base and was the center of most household activity. Stacey and I climbed onto tall bar stools that had to be pushed back exactly the way we found them — tucked into the countertop — when not in use. This was one of DP's many rules and it was one of the hardest to remember because we were always in and out.

We ate breakfast at the island every morning and completed our homework there after school every afternoon. I don't know why Stacey and I did everything sitting perched atop the stools at the island because our legs dangled like we were Muppet Babies sitting in highchairs. The island was also where DP stood every morning just before dawn. He was always stationed sink-side with *The Washington Post* propped atop the counter of the island. He valued his peace and quiet above everything but, sadly, I intruded upon it every morning. It might be the only thing I was ever consistent about.

Ain't It A Shame

I only have a few memories of my dad in the house, but the one that stands out is the one that signified the beginning of the end of our family. It was from the "before we got DP" era. It occurred during either Thanksgiving or Christmas break from school. Most of my dad's family was in town. Stacey, my mom, and Aunt Carolyn were watching *The Sound of Music* in our cozy, brown family room. Stacey and I were already dressed for bed. I vividly recall that I wore a long, lemon-yellow nightgown with rucking and a sunflower on the bust. The other adults kibitzed around the kitchen table and the countertop.

Suddenly Rocky, our beloved Schnauzer, and Stacey were in a tug of war of the lips. He accidentally got his hallmark underbite caught on Stacey's lower lip. My dad, who was drunk, flew into a rage. Usually, he was like Rocky — all bark and no bite — but this time, he meant every bit of what he said. He tossed his chair aside and began to chase Rocky, who had, by then, managed to wrest himself free of Stacey with the help of my mom. He ranted, "If I catch you, I'm going to kill you, you fucking dog!" Stacey wailed and I screamed at the top of my lungs, "Daddy, don't kill him! It's not his fault! He's simply scared!" My dad was in soldier mode. He didn't listen. His sole mission was to protect Stacey. I screamed so loudly and for so long that I lost my voice. It took days for it to come back.

Rocky's saving grace that night was that he ran under one of our kitchen chairs that my dad knocked over in his pursuit. My dad's stumble bought Rocky just enough time to run up the stairs and under my parents' bed. It was bad enough that Stacey, my mom, and I witnessed this awful scene, but my entire family was there. They saw everything. I learned it's possible to feel more than one emotion at a time. I was relieved that my dad didn't kill Rocky and that Stacey was okay. The two small puncture wounds where Rocky accidentally bit her healed quickly. I, however, never fully recovered from this incident. I was conflicted about my feelings for my dad. His reactions were usually unpredictable but, until that night, I had never felt ashamed of him.

After that terrible night, my memory of time and sequencing gets fuzzy because so much happened in quick succession. It was such a painful time, I unintentionally blocked out entire memories. There were times my parents fought openly and times my dad went away on extended business trips. Many times, Stacey and I were left alone. It wasn't so unusual back then for parents to leave young kids home while they ran errands. We were always by ourselves after school. By that time, both my dad and mom worked full-time and, as a result, Stacey and I became, like many other others our age, "latchkey kids."

Corned Beef and Cabbage

There was no way, in writing this book, that I could separate my Judaism from my childhood even if only to avoid making the book front-loaded with my childhood.

I loved the joyous and melancholy music of my culture as young as nursery school. Some of my earliest memories involve schlepping to and from Sunday and Hebrew school. When I was three, I remember I'd sing "Shabbat Shalom Hey!" all the way home from Sunday school. It touched me to the core in ways that I didn't understand, like I was even Jewish in a past lifetime.

I connect my culture and my religion to love because I loved Grandma Mary intensely and I knew that she, her parents, and her siblings had fled Russia (now part of Belarus) to escape Christian Pogroms just before 1910. Grandma Mary spoke Yiddish with her family when she was growing up. Although she was fluent in English and only spoke to our family in it, she interjected a lot of Yiddish idioms: Stacey and I were called *boobeleh* ("dear"), *tatteleh* ("young one"), or *shayna punim* ("beautiful face") all the time.

Grandma Mary ate the same thing for breakfast every morning

and had ever since her family's arrival to New York's Lower East Side: beet borscht and toasted Rye bread topped with a slice of Swiss cheese. She loved when my mom made her corned beef with mustard or corned beef with cabbage or brought her home beef tongue from Katz's Deli on Rockville Pike.

We ate dinner together as a family every night and on Friday nights, assuming we remembered, my mom lit the brass shabbat candlesticks that Grandma Mary's family had managed to sneak out of Russia with them. As a girl, I loved to polish those candlesticks. I longed for the day when one of the two sets would be given to me (which they were not long before this book was published).

Aunt Sister (her real name was Lillian so everyone else called her "Sis" except for Stacey and me) was integral to our family dinners whenever she drove down from her shoebox apartment in the Bronx. She piled our kitchen table full of everything that was on sale at Simms. And she always brought us an L & M Bakery cheesecake. Schmearing cheesecake onto bagels was one of our family's rituals whenever she visited. We swore that she was preparing for the "end of days," which, being Jewish, we don't even believe in. We do, however, believe in miracles.

The first time I witnessed a miracle was on Erev Passover, the day before Passover begins. I witnessed Grandma Mary peel an entire apple without breaking its peel. It made a long, red, concentric-circle slinky. This became the measure of adeptness by which my mom and I measured our Jewish culinary talents. I was well into adulthood before I accomplished this.

Even my first memory of DP involves Judaism. He called the day after Passover for the charoset recipe I made (a sweet mixture of apples, walnuts, cinnamon, honey, and wine). At the time, he wore thick-rimmed glasses, a pinky ring, and multiple gold necklaces. One of his chains had a large Star of David that dangled down to the middle of his chest.

Passover was and remains my favorite Jewish holiday. For a week, Jews the world over recall our bittersweet history of enslavement to an Egyptian Pharaoh. We commemorate our exodus from Egypt to the Holy Land, Israel. In our haste to flee Egypt, we didn't have enough time to prepare leavened bread. We journeyed through the desert laden with cardboard-like, tasteless bread until we came to the land of milk and honey. We celebrate our sovereignty each year by recounting our travails through food over the course of two nights of ceremonial dinners or *seders*. In fact, in Hebrew, the word *seder* means "in order."

I was teased for having to prepare for my fall bat mitzvah in the middle of summer. My mom ended every letter she sent to me at Camp Tockwogh with "Don't forget to practice your bat mitzvah lessons *and* kiss your sister for me." I'll never forget my bat mitzvah. It was my initiation into Jewish womanhood as well as my introduction to a Jewish mother's guilt.

Everyone and their mother and their mother's mother were invited and all I wanted was for mine to relax. So, I decided to do something special for her. I figured since she and DP had poured their hearts, soul, time, and money into me having a bat mitzvah, the least I could do was make the front yard beautiful for their out-of-town guests.

I seriously have no clue how I came up with a hare-brained idea like this; oh right, I'm impulsive because I have ADHD. I loved gardening. I was good at it and having my hands in the dirt reminded me of the fun my dad and I used to have gardening together. I watched my dad trim plenty of shrubs with clippers, so I wielded mine in a similar fashion. *This is going to be a piece of cake*, I said to myself. I worked tirelessly and took great care leveling them. I thought, *Mom is going to be so happy and surprised*. And she was surprised alright—just not in the jubilant way I imagined. She was dismayed. In fact, it was one of the few times I've ever seen her cry. She and DP had just gotten back home from running last-minute errands and they had to get right back in the car to go buy a yard full of new azaleas.

Moody Blues

I wasn't graceful enough to be a cheerleader or Pom, but I had a natural ear for music. I made so many mixtapes that I knew exactly how and where to stop and start songs so that they blended into one another without any static. This trait is what got me elected as Pom Manager. I carried around a boombox larger than I was to all our basketball games. I liked the recognition that came with being the manager, but I cared more about watching boys.

This was my ticket on the court and that allowed me to watch my heartthrob run up and down it. I had visions of the two of us running away together from the game where he scored the winning three-point shot. I didn't know what his ethnicity was, but I loved his exotic black eyes and feathery brown hair. I pictured us hugging, kissing, and dancing to Howard Jones's "Like To Get To Know You Well."

I was introduced to HoJo's music the previous year (1983) by my summer camp counselor. When I found out that he was coming to the Patriot Center in Fairfax, Virginia, that October, I used nearly all my allowance to buy tickets for myself and my friend Dana (pronounced "Dan-ah"). I had just enough left over to buy a sweatshirt. In 1984, $16 for a concert ticket was a lot.

Dana and I spent nearly all our free time together mooning over HoJo, Thomas Dolby, and Duran Duran. My bedroom in the early- to mid-'80s was covered from floor to ceiling in Duran Duran posters, as well as magazine photos of Wham! and most of the other rock celebrities in between the pages of *Tiger* and *Teen Beat* magazines.

I wasn't much different from other teenagers in that I was significantly impacted by an onslaught of hormones. Most sweet girls stopped being so even keeled around the age of 13, but I was particularly moody. My initiation into adolescence was a rocky road. In fact, it wasn't until I went to college that my gynecologist determined I'd been suffering from premenstrual dysphoria. I was always in a lot of physical and emotional pain in the middle of my cycle and right before it. I became despondent, irritable, and intensely sexually aroused.

My mom loves to tease me about how angst-ridden I was back then. I never knew how much that period of my life impacted my entire family until I was well into adulthood. In my nearly daily journal entries from this era, I ranted about my relationship with my father and then quickly shifted gears and documented the most minute details on my latest boy crush:

I saw Dad. We got along great. A while after I saw him, he called me. But now he owes child support, which he hardly ever pays. And so, he doesn't call again. I knew he wouldn't. When I had oral surgery and was half knocked out with drugs and spitting up blood, he didn't even call to see how I was doing. I was sick for a week and it was good to get back to school and to Pom practice. Oh, I almost forgot, I saw the Thompson Twins in concert. They were excellent. I've had a huge crush on Mike V. ever since seventh grade basketball.

My mom told me she thought that I suffered from depression whenever I got uber-maudlin. I vehemently disagreed with her because I thought she was trying to tell me that there was yet *another* thing wrong with me. I insisted that I was just blah sometimes. I argued that everyone experienced blue moods now and then. In skimming through those old journals, I was startled to see that I truly was grappling with depression.

February 2, 1986

Help! I'm sooo depressed. I've never felt like this before. Stacey and I aren't getting along at all! We're trying to work it out, but it seems as if it's of no use. School's lousy. Mom says I have a while to go and a good chance of bringing up my grades for college. I have a little higher than a C+ average. It's so hard! I thought it was good enough that I do my homework every day. I'm even studying now. I thought that was great. But it's not enough. I'm so lost! My timing isn't right for my work schedule. I can't study right, or it seems that way. And it's so boring. I try real hard, but this is just too much. I wasn't meant to be a genius. I want to play in a band or do something fun and enjoy life. It seems dumb but I'm not that happy with myself or life right now. I'm not giving up though. There's just too much to live for. I just don't know what to do. Science is too hard. I love Poms but it seems like I don't get enough credit for it. I like a boy but I'm not getting anywhere with him yet. I need to lead more of a social life but if I do, my grades fall.

I love and hate my father at the same time. He never calls or pays money or writes…. Everyone else wonders why I feel like shit, like nothing, when I hear his name. So, he got me what I always wanted, a keyboard. I'm happy with it and I'm thankful to him. But like the Thompson Twins say, "All the gold won't heal your soul, if your world should tumble to the ground."

I might've been an exceptionally moody teenager, but I was resolute in my promise to drop out of high school if my parents didn't allow me to go to private school. I was tired of trying my hardest and getting nowhere. I was done with teachers who didn't pay any attention to me because I was neither a "bad" nor a "great" student. I can only think of two teachers I respected and whose classes I looked forward to: Mr. Smiley and Ms. Pepperman. (Apparently, I have always been partial to individuals with last names that didn't match their dispositions.)

The former was my science teacher and he rarely smiled. He made students stick chewed wads of gum on the end of their noses if he caught them chewing too loudly in class. This is my mom's number-one pet peeve and I'm surprised that she never tried this tactic with Stacey and me whenever we smacked our gum to spite her.

As for Ms. Pepperman, she taught Spanish, and she was anything but spicy chorizo. She was short, obese, and quirky. I especially adored her for being the latter. I regarded us as equals in a way. She was as madly in love with Tom Selleck of *Magnum P.I.* as I was with Simon Le Bon from Duran Duran.

CHAPTER 6 – PUNK-ISH GIRL

"Punk rock girl let's go slam dance …
You look so wild
Punk rock girl …"

My mom's dad, William, died of cancer shortly after my mom was born. He was a Russian immigrant who made a fortune in America as a butcher. My dad told me that he was a pioneer in his field. He invented a process for cutting, packaging, and selling chicken breasts and wings separately before this was common practice. He was also a womanizer who cheated on my grandma. I don't know anything more about his branch of my family tree.

Grandma Mary dropped out of school in the eighth grade to help support her family by being a candy striper in a hospital. She was also a hat model, a talented seamstress, and a single mother to three children in a time when divorce wasn't common or widely acceptable. My mom's older brother, Uncle Bobby, was the first person in my mom's immediate family to go to college. He was an Army doctor who raised three kids and gave to charitable organizations. Aunt Sister started her career as a school counselor, then went on to become a skilled elementary school principal. She worked in the Yonkers public school system her entire career.

My mom began her career as an office temp, who worked her way up through the ranks in her profession. She went to graduate school at 34 for a Master of Arts in Human Ecology and then went back again for a second advanced degree in Human Resources Management when she was 47. She retired 10 years ago from her position as the vice president of human resources for a large, global firm. My mom's side of the family were resourceful, bright, and successful in their professional arenas.

My dad's side of the family were actors, musicians, and artists who grew up as at least third-generation Jewish Americans. Grandma Harriett was a radio actress who did voiceovers until she married and became a stay-at-home mother to four children. She earned almost $2,000 a week 80 years ago (probably around $30,000 weekly now [!]). As a woman during the World War II era, this was no mean feat.

Her sister, Great Aunt Blanche, was a gifted painter who didn't discover her talent until she was in her sixties. Great Uncle Julian (Juni for short) was a Spanish professor at Yale but was better known for being an eccentric artist. He was raunchy and fearless, as well as openly homosexual in a time when most other men wouldn't dare to "come out."

He painted amazingly textured oil paintings. In fact, I remember watching him work on a piece when I was no more than five or six. He crafted a gigantic, beautiful naked woman made of thousands of tiny scraps of colored paper glued onto canvas. Uncle Juni even dabbled in acting and landed a bit part as a taxi driver in *The Godfather II*.

Great Uncle Milton was an accomplished pianist and violinist. He was part of the Society Dance Band at the St. Regis Hotel in New York City and was once a featured guest on *The Ed Sullivan Show*. Great Uncles Lee and Aaron both played in the Benny Goodman Band—Lee played the drums (just before the legendary Gene Krupa) and Aaron the saxophone.

I presented both sides of my family because it is evident that my mom's side was greatly influenced by the "American Dream" of working hard and sacrificing to have a decent living without the benefit of much idle time to pursue hobbies, whereas my dad's side of the family were established and could afford to spend money on things like lessons. They also viewed the pursuit of the performing arts to be a viable means of employment.

My mom and dad were already divorced when I began taking piano lessons. My dad bought me a piano, for which I was extremely grateful, but he wasn't consistent in his duty to provide child support for my sister and me. My mom and DP needed to use their hard-earned money to clothe and feed us and send us to Hebrew school and make sure Stacey had Jordache Jeans and I had parachute pants. (I was not a fashionista like Stacey, so the brand name was irrelevant. I was simply happy with clothes that fit me and didn't have an Oshkosh label on them.)

There is evidence to suggest that artistic talent is an inherited gene: "Being artistic or creative is associated with the personality trait of being open to experiences. "Research suggests that there are neurobiological foundations for creative individuals. Based on all available information, it is very likely that the capacity for creativity is shaped by genetic influences—it's a complicated way of saying that creativity and artistic interests can almost certainly be inherited." Recent research also suggests that "it has long been described that AP runs in families, and there are several groups (Ashkenazi Jews, for example) with much higher rates of AP than the general population. (*AP is short for Absolute Pitch*)

If artistry is, in fact, an inherited gene, I believe that the Marks/Voloshin talent was passed down to my father's generation as well as mine and Stacey's. Aunt Carolyn played the piano, banjo, and harmonica, and sang. I recall her teaching Stacey and me folk songs when we used to visit her and Uncle Steve in Doylestown, Pennsylvania. Aunt Carolyn played for us, and Uncle Steve made us the best milkshakes on an old-fashioned machine. And my niece, Shayna, and I both inherited Carolyn's musical genes.

I play the piano by ear and can plunk out anything I know or anything someone plays for me. It might be in its most basic form, but many people don't have this ability. I briefly took piano lessons, but I quit because I struggled to read music. At the time, it was also too difficult for me to play complicated pieces that required coordination of my left and right hands simultaneously and at different tempos. Complex eye-hand coordination skills require your brain to be able to synthesize information that mine couldn't no matter how diligently I practiced. Besides, I argued, what was the point in learning to master Mozart or Bach when I wanted to play popular music like Tears for Fears and Madonna? My parents argued that there wasn't any point in taking lessons then. And that was the end of my formal music instruction.

I never stopped playing for fun though. I sold my piano when I was in a nomadic, unstable period of my life, but music was and always will be my first love. I've bought inexpensive Casio, Yamaha, and Panasonic keyboards, but I wasn't happy with any of them. I hated their warped electric sounds. I didn't want to play different nuanced sounds; I just wanted "piano." Aunt Sister passed away three years ago, and I used some of the money I inherited from her to furnish a new apartment and the rest on a digital keyboard that I can use headphones with. I don't play it often because, until recently, I commuted for work and worked nights. However, the 2020–2021 global pandemic held a few silver linings for our family: I work from home, provide individual, remote tele-behavioral health, and have more time to focus on my husband, animals. and passions (including playing piano, cooking, and baking).

I loved playing piano, but I longed to be a rock star. I have a decent voice that could've been trained to be beautiful, but my parents didn't want to invest in singing lessons since I had already demonstrated that I was a "quitter" in their minds. It is true that I didn't practice piano as much as I should've, but I didn't play because I was frustrated with my inability to get myself where I wanted to be. Practicing scales and playing "baby" songs wasn't fun or cool. If we had only known then what we know now about the nature of ADD and the way the mind rebels against learning if there's no perceived pleasure or reward, things might've been different.

Piano and singing lessons were nixed, leaving me to fall back on my passion for writing. It became my greatest love, as it allowed me to express myself (on paper) in ways I struggled to communicate verbally. It's free to pursue and I can do it anywhere. I've written in journals since I was in the third grade. I stuck to poetry and prose, except for one time ...

I once co-authored a short story with a high school girlfriend of mine. We were infatuated with horses and boys. Not surprisingly, our story was about two female and two male camp counselors who rescued horses from a fire that broke out at their summer camp. The four campers had to fend for themselves in the wilderness. It was a solid story, but my learning disabilities interfered with its ultimate success. My not-yet-diagnosed ADD made it difficult for me to sequence events chronologically.

I made the twin boys in our story different ages. One was twelve and the other was thirteen. I assume they could've been born at 11:59 p.m. and 12 a.m., respectively, but I immediately dropped all pretense of trying my hand at fiction—especially as my mom laughed hysterically when I read her the story. She was the one who caught the boys' age mistake, and it was silly enough that, for once, I wasn't offended by her laughter. My story writing proved to me that, despite being young, I was old enough to understand that I had limitations others didn't have. I began to sense the magnitude of my otherness.

No Barbra Streisand

I was okay with giving up my dreams of being a novelist, but I still clung to my aspiration of being a marine biologist rock star. I spent hours belting out my favorite songs by Sheena Easton, Laura Branigan, The Go-Go's, and Cyndi Lauper in the upstairs loft and in my bedroom. One evening, I was singing in the kitchen while setting the table for dinner. I reached into the top cabinets which I could now reach if I stood on my tiptoes while standing on a step stool. I was grabbing cups, or as DP ever fondly reminded me, "drinking glasses." I turned to ask my mom what she thought of my singing.

I don't know what I expected her to say, but what young girl doesn't want praise and encouragement? My mom is loving, supportive, and generous, but not always in the ways I wish she were. She's never minced words and has blown the wind out of my sails several times. There've been plenty of times when deflating my hopes was exactly what was called for. They occurred most often when I would've made catastrophic decisions had she not leveled me. Yet on that day, when I asked for her opinion of my singing, I wasn't at all prepared for her response.

She looked at me and said frankly, "You're never going to be Barbra Streisand." I was shocked into hurt silence.

I dropped my dream then and there on the kitchen floor. I wish I had braved sassing back or swept away the shards of glass and kept on singing for all the world to hear, but I wasn't that girl. I was furious with my mom. It would take therapy and sobriety to heal that wound and forgive her. Who callously dashes a young girl's dreams like that? I'm sure my mom meant her sarcastic remark to be more of a quip than a jab, but I wasn't a boxer; I was a young girl.

Many individuals who have the type of deficits I do have a limited ability to detect and respond appropriately to sarcasm. I'm creative, but I'm also a very literal thinker. My disabilities affect the part of the brain that processes social cues such as innuendo and sarcasm. A lot of humor I just don't get. I didn't understand that my mom's jab wasn't meant to be so biting. More importantly, I didn't understand that it was okay for me to disagree with her or to zing her back with a wry comment.

I was so dependent upon my mom because there was much I either couldn't do for myself or couldn't process. I desperately wanted her approval, and I was terrified of disappointing her. I avoided going against her opinions and values at all costs. My fear of her potential rejection and abandonment prevented me from doing many things I would've otherwise done. My mom never said she'd disown me or stop loving me, but her verbal communication and body language suggested otherwise.

What I didn't know until a recent exchange with my mom was that she was just as afraid of rejection. Only she wasn't afraid that I'd reject her; she was fearful that other kids my age, as well as the world at large, would reject me. I looked "normal" but acted so differently from others my age. By protecting me from others and from myself, my mom inadvertently fed into my low sense of self and self-worth.

My mom didn't have the patience or energy to teach me the critical coping skills I needed. She had Stacey and (initially) my dad to look after and protect, and truthfully, I only wanted to stand up for myself whenever I really wanted something or wanted to do something that my mom didn't agree with.

My mom and I were fully entwined in a codependent relationship that neither one of us could see for what it was. I didn't know where she ended and I began, or how her needs differed from mine. And is it really called codependency when only one person's happiness is tied up with the others?

My mom's happiness and actions certainly weren't dependent upon my approval. I figured out at a young age that my survival depended upon my ability to make my mom happy. My dad wasn't available enough for me to care about seeking his approval, yet I wanted his validation above all others. But I also knew I would only get it when he chose to give it. My whole world then became about making sure that the one who saw to it that my needs were met was happy.

What would happen if I disappointed my mom? If my dad was too self-involved to pay attention to me, then I had no one; I'd be an orphan. I don't think it dawned on me that having a sister, but no parent's didn't make me an orphan.

From my perspective, I sacrificed a lot to stay in my mom's good graces. In hindsight, I grieve for both my reality as a young girl as well as for hers. She didn't have a mother who paid much attention to her, but she hardly got a break from tending to my needs. Then, this pattern was repeated for her by her first husband. He didn't pay her the attention she deserved, and she was yoked with someone she mothered more than married. My dad used to tell me how carefree my mom used to be in the "good old days." How sad that I didn't experience this version of her. I do remember fun times with her, but even those times usually involved mine or Stacey's homework projects.

Minor Threat

Back to younger me …

More than anything in the world, I longed to do something so radical that my mom would surely disown me. I wanted to be a punk rock girl. I wanted to dye my hair, pierce my nose, and wear ripped-up clothing with safety pins all over them. I listened to bands like The Clash, Siouxsie and the Banshees, and early U2, and saw Fugazi play in a church basement in high school.

But I wasn't that into punk music. I was more into the punks *themselves*. They seemed so self-confident! I liked that you could look at a punk rock girl and be nearly certain that she was anti-establishment or a skater chick merely from her appearance. They were different like I was, but they were proud of their difference; I was ashamed of my otherness. I longed to join the punks in their nonconformity, but I wasn't brave enough.

I could pierce my ears once, but multiple piercings were out of the question. My mom passionately believes in the biblical thought that your body is your temple and shouldn't be marred. She only recently informed me that all of Grandma Mary's extended family had been slaughtered during Babi Yar, when the Nazis exterminated 34,000 Jews, in what was then Kiev, Russia. The Nazis tattooed Jews, gypsies, and anyone who was an "other" in their eyes with identified numbers that stripped them of their humanity. This knowledge helps me to better understand why my mom was appalled by the thought of my getting tattooed.

I wasn't totally without liberties, however. I could dress how I wanted, provided I was dressed respectfully and covered everything that "good Jewish girls" were supposed to cover. My mom grew more lenient over the years because my sister began to wear her down with her style demands. (Stacey has engaged in fashion wars with my mom since she was three years old. She has always known who she was in that regard. For many years, I envied her for that and her hazel tiger eyes, which resemble our father's.)

By the time I was preparing for my bat mitzvah, my mom caved. She consented to let me wear jeans to Hebrew school instead of a dress or skirt. And at age 16, I finally mustered up the courage to go punk*ish*. I was friends with a girl named Maddie in my confirmation class. I loved her dyed black-blue, iridescent hair and her cool nose piercing. I wanted to emulate her.

It was a 30-minute drive from where we lived in Gaithersburg, into Washington, where the punk explosion was in your face. I practiced being a punk rock girl on the weekends when my family went into Georgetown. We parked one of our cars in Georgetown and then jumped into the other car and parked it at Fletcher's Boat House three miles away. We then walked from the Boat House back into Georgetown and inevitably ended up at Commander Salamanders. It was THE place for punk and goth accouterments. It sold studded belts; Gene-Simmons-like KISS boots and Doc Martens; tiny tees with snarky comments or quirky graphics emblazoned on them; buttons galore to pin on jackets and bags; fishnet stockings; and gag gifts and other random items.

Best of all, the cashiers would aerosol-spray streaks of funky colors in your hair for free. They washed out when you showered. Perfect for playing punk for a day. I eyed silver-spiked belts and dog collar necklaces. I pictured myself wearing one of these with a checkered mini skirt and intentionally ripped nylons not very well held together with enormous safety pins and the crowning glory… black, calf-high Doc Martens. What did I end up wearing, though? A leather bracelet with slightly bumpy metal rivets, my gold Star of David, a jeans jacket with Duran Duran buttons, and penny loafers. I wasn't exactly a force to be reckoned with. My fashion statement read "confused," which I was.

CHAPTER 7 – LEAN ON ME

Until I was an adult, I didn't know that Bill Withers originally sang the song referenced above. In 1987, a rendition by Club Nouveau came out and it incorporated the reggae vibes that my mom, Stacey and I loved. Sadly, my introduction to reggae was through UB4. (Not that there's anything wrong with them, but it was just another example of how I grew up with rampant cultural appropriation. This is musical deviation, so ….) The point is that I loved the lyrics about friendship and reliance on others.

I was introduced to the concept of community as a camper at Tockwogh and I had felt a sense of camaraderie when my family belonged to Temple Beth Ami which was originally not large enough to be a full-on congregation but a large *chavurah* ("family"). But I didn't feel the same sense of belonging as my parents because I was still a kid. I found true belonging again however at Barrie (now known as The Barrie School), a Montessori school that ran from infant-care through high school.

Today, the entire school is housed on Layhill Road, but in my day, that campus supported infant care through sixth grade. The middle and high schools were housed in the old home of Argyle Middle School, on busy Bel Pre Road. It was bordered by remnants of an old farm on one side and townhomes on the other.

I wouldn't go unnoticed at Barrie because there were only about 80 students in the whole high school. I thought it was so cool that the teachers went by their first names. I still had a locker, but it was literally a stone's throw away from the school's lower level, where most of my classes were held. The classrooms were open just like the lower level of my house. Best of all, there were no obnoxious bells. Classes began and ended on time and we were responsible enough to know when to show up.

There was no working cafeteria so students either brought their lunch or walked across the street to Plaza del Mercado. At lunchtime, my friends and I often sat and ate at restaurants on our lunch break. There was a McDonald's, Pizza Stop, Giant, and China King. Best of all, we could shop for records at Joe's Record Paradise. I couldn't believe that the school trusted its students to go out to lunch and come back for classes afterward. Even the classmates I considered to be the bad kids — the ones that smoked and drank alcohol— returned for our classes.

I went from being a shy, self-conscious, and underachieving teenager to a secure and successful student. Many days, my friend Patty and I ate lunch outside. We sat atop the grassy hill that abutted the upstairs side entrance to school. We ate and gossiped while Oreo-patterned cows noisily chomped grass behind us. Patty was one of the first students I met at Barrie and was one of my best friends. She had long black hair, crooked, pointy teeth, and was extremely pale. She had a catlike grace and mystery to her. And she was practical, whereas I was idealistic and flighty.

I still struggled with math, and it didn't help that our math teacher, Bob, was an awful instructor. He was a brilliant mind in his field but a poor educator. He mumbled so much that no one understood a word he said, and he failed to explain directions on how to solve equations. I often argued with him for not answering my questions and for speaking too quickly. In turn, he sent me to the principal's office for being impatient with him.

He didn't know that sending me to the principal was more a reward than a punishment. The administrative staff were all kind and understanding. I adored spending time talking to Muriel, the school's administrator. She was Jewish too and treated me like a second mother. Kathy, the school's principal, welcomed me into her office to speak my mind and calm down.

I adored all the rest of our teachers, but I especially revered Marty and Garrett. Marty taught math and science and Garrett taught English and Government. Marty understood that as a staunch vegetarian (who sometimes backslid on pepperoni because it didn't resemble meat), I couldn't bear to dissect a sentient being no matter how small it was. Instead of dissection, he allowed me to write papers on nematodes and frogs. I don't think Marty stood a chance to tell you the truth. I had a conniption the one time I was made to kill and mount beautiful moths, butterflies, and beetles for biology. The memory of trapping insects and sticking them in glass jars full of ether still haunts me. I couldn't fathom why biology, the study of living things, encouraged murder and evisceration in the name of science.

Garrett was the teacher everyone adored the most. We competed for his attention because he was funny and real to us. He challenged us to become better human beings and he helped us to develop our own opinions about current affairs, as well as with the arts.

His specialty was poetry. I always loved poetry, but Garrett encouraged me to become a better writer. He gently suggested that I try to rhyme less often and use fewer, but more descriptive, adjectives. He had us make lists of freely associated words and then had us choose a few of them to incorporate into our poems. I came to understand that there was poetry in everything, including subject matter of both beauty and revulsion.

Here's an example of a poem I wrote in Garrett's English class:

MEMORIES IN GOLD

A big basket full,
Happiness in gold.

An aging man remembering,
his wife and marigolds.

Marigolds fading,
I spy an old and dingy pot.

Hidden,
in an alley.

We had Extension Days every Wednesday, which were essentially more laid back as well as alternative learning days. Some Wednesdays, we remained on campus but engaged in activities other than our regularly scheduled classes, while others were off campus. We once watched the movie Colors, which reinforced a lesson we recently had on racism. Another time, teacher Cindy's boyfriend, who occasionally substituted for her, showed us the movie *Hollywood Shuffle*. We had worksheets or assignments that went along with the subject matter, so we weren't free from paying attention on those days.

The same held true on the alternate Wednesdays when we were off campus. We usually had to find our own ways to get to these events. My classmates and I met up with Garrett at historical DC area landmarks, such as the Folger Theater, the Kennedy Center, the National Zoo and other Smithsonian museums.

On one extension day, we had to meet and complete an assignment at the National Gallery of Art. I don't remember which wing we visited or at which piece of art Garrett stood beside me. I was bored and didn't understand what I was supposed to get out of the painting. Garrett noticed my befuddlement and commanded me to stay in front of the painting until I could name three unique features about it. I don't know how the shift happened, but it did. Maybe it transpired after Garrett pointed out a few of the things he found most intriguing about it, thereby demonstrating how to scrutinize a work of art. Or perhaps it was simply his presence that assured me he genuinely cared that I got as psyched as he was about individual artworks. I suddenly was able to see things about the painting that hadn't been obvious to me before. I found myself pointing out to Garrett, the shading, angles, dots, and perspective that the painting elicited. I admitted, albeit reluctantly, that I was previously closed minded. I saw that art was another medium of poetry. Perhaps this is what Garrett had wanted me to see all along. My love of art literally sprang from that one experience curated by Garrett.

And All That Jazz

Barrie's teachers allowed us and encouraged us to delve deeper into subjects that interested us as opposed to being told by adults what we should find interesting. For one class, Garrett's assignment for us was to research and present on a topic that was of great interest to us. Doing so spoke not only to our interests but to our preferred styles of learning. The only requirement was that the subject matter had to reflect something we were passionate about. The presentation largely contributed toward our overall grade for the class.

I was infatuated with the Roaring Twenties, so I turned our classroom into a speakeasy. I was so into that era that I didn't mind spending hours researching. I highlighted the jazz of the time by recording my own jazz-inspired radio show. I draped all the round tables in our classroom with tablecloths and set out small vases of flowers and wine jugs filled with apple juice. I played my radio show and was surprised by the enthusiastic applause I received. I even created my own commercials. They highlighted products in use back then such as Fleischmann's Yeast and Palmolive. It was the first time some of my friends had listened to great jazz greats like Eubie Blake, Louis Armstrong, Billie Holiday, Ella Fitzgerald, and DC's own Duke Ellington.

I loved that the school's lower campus housed a mini farm. There were sheep, chickens, pigs, and most importantly, horses. Apart from Duran Duran and boys, I was most wild about horses. I rode every summer at Camp Tockwogh and was stoked to be able to have riding lessons at school. However, my stint with horseback riding lessons lasted if my piano lessons did. I wasn't keen on lessons because they required doing exactly as I was told. That's difficult for me to do because I'm rebellious by nature.

I loved pleasure riding. I pleaded with my parents to let me lease a horse that I rode for riding lessons. Barrie's stables closed over winter vacation because the barn wasn't equipped with heating and staff to tend to all the horses. Barrie let students whose parents could afford it or were otherwise bullied into renting horses for the winter. My parents caved and allowed me to co-lease a horse, a 21-year-old mare named Jasmine. I leased and shared boarding and care responsibilities with my classmate and friend Drea. We boarded Jasmine and rode her at stables owned and operated by Stephanie Mills on Muncaster Mill Road in Gaithersburg.

I sometimes rode Jasmine bare-back, and I once tried jumping her free saddle too, but I flipped right over her head. I surprised myself by landing on my feet, but I didn't repeat that feat again. I had Jasmine jumping as high as 3.5 feet, that is, until Stephanie informed me that I had to keep jumps under 2.5 feet. She said that as a senior mare, jumping Jasmine any higher was too hard on her bones. I didn't want to hurt her, so I respectfully heeded Stephanie's advice. Stephanie also instructed me on the proper way to groom and turn a horse out to pasture. I listened to her more than I did to other adults because she didn't push me. She simply suggested alternate ways of doing things and then let me be.

She must've gently reminded me a thousand times to double check that the pasture gates were locked before I left the stables for the night. I was conscientious about this and always double checked that the pasture gate was secured. But one night I forgot to do this, and my mom was awakened at midnight. Stephanie informed my mom that all the horses — over 20 of them — escaped due to my carelessness. It was a blessing that none of them trotted off onto the steep, high-traffic road. I don't know what I'd have done had any of them been hit by a passing car.

I can't say enough about the quality of my education at Barrie and how much it encouraged me to channel my creativity, to see things in new ways, and to learn new skills. It also taught me to be more open-minded. The fact that the school had no cliques helped. Everyone hung out with their own "type" of friends; we all interacted with one another and truthfully respected each other. I turned 15 a few weeks into my first year of high school, whereas most of my classmates were almost a full year older than I was. Because of this, most of my peers were more mature than I was. Classmates like Brooke and Seth were nice, but I thought they were "bad" because they smoked outside of McDonald's at lunchtime and bragged about their drinking, weekend partying, and sexual exploits.

I grew up in a household where alcohol was always around, so I never thought sneaking and drinking sounded fun. Additionally, my dad drank almost nightly when he was living with us and I hated to see him drunk. DP only drank sporadically. Occasionally, he made pina coladas for himself and my mom, but he rarely used our fully stocked bar. Alcohol held little allure for me as I didn't know it was usual for teenagers to experiment with booze and drugs.

Regardless of what I thought about Brooke and Seth outside of school, I loved being in classes with them. They made it fun mostly because they weren't afraid of speaking up and challenging Garrett or Marty openly. I didn't hang out with Katie, Ian, or Joe, but I secretly thought they were the coolest kids in my class. They were punks. They dressed the way I longed to but was too afraid to and they didn't need external validation the way I did. They were bright but disinterested. Joe and Ian skateboarded, and Katie had her nose pierced and her hair bleached blonde. Winston, one of my best friends, was way ahead of the mod and goth trends. He wore things like black leggings with black pinstriping and safety pins paired with a black mesh tank top. I, on the other hand, still hadn't developed my fashion sense.

It might seem arbitrary to drop in a few names of the kids I went to school with, but we were all we had. There were only 80 students in the whole upper school. Most public schools in the area, by contrast, had upwards of 3,000 students. And I graduated with only 20 other students in my senior year.

In public schools, odd pairings of friends didn't usually occur. If I had attended a public high school, popular kids like Julie and female Brooke wouldn't have given me the time of day. I wouldn't have spent time with "nerdy" students like Cosma or Andrew because they intimidated me. I wasn't nearly as bright as they were, and I had no interest in mathematics or politics. In public school, I'd never have been placed in classes with them.

That was the beauty of Barrie. Students learned in mixed grade classrooms and were not grouped based solely on scholastic aptitude. I learned to appreciate and respect Cosma and Andrew's intellect and I know they were at least amused by my spaciness and ardor for helping others. When we read adult literature in Peter's English class (the year after I was in Garrett's class), no one laughed when Jerome mispronounced the word "delight" as "dey-light." We just kept it moving. In public school, Jerome, like me, would've been teased mercilessly but for different reasons.

I grew so much during my time at Barrie that if I were able to spy on my junior high school self, I wouldn't have recognized her. I was obviously still small, but I had a much more developed sense of connection, sense of self, and more of a purpose. looked back got involved in student government and Keyettes, a volunteer-oriented, high school sorority. I earned some extra spending money by running errands and grocery shopping for senior citizens at Homecrest House, where Grandma Mary used to live. I ran for student government president and misspelled "Student" as "Stuent" on my campaign poster, a careless mistake that Cosma, the editor of our student newspaper, never let me live down.

Who cared about the sign? All that mattered to me was winning over Liam, my arch nemesis. Win, I did and in an odd twist of fate, he became my boyfriend shortly afterward. There were other guys I flirted with precisely because they were "bad boys," but Liam was a nice Jewish boy, both brilliant and arrogant. I spent the last three years of high school alternating between despising him and pining for him depending upon my mood or his actions on any given day.

Moodier Blues

I was a boy-crazed teenager, but I was also moody in a way that most other girls my age weren't. I experienced "the blahs" with increasing frequency, but I argued with my mom that I wasn't depressed and didn't need to see a therapist or a psychiatrist.

When I was elated, I was really elated but when I was blue, I was more raven-hued than cobalt. I was also exceptionally dramatic. Maybe this is a hallmark of being a privileged teenager, but I think it's the telltale signs that those in 12-Step recovery describe as feeling "restless, irritable, and discontented." I sought to fill a cavernous void deep within the recesses of my soul with anything and everything outside myself that I thought would make me feel happier and less like a misfit.

I felt like I was destroying myself with my own thoughts. Sometimes, I couldn't stand to be stuck inside my own mind. The first journal entry below was written just days before my true entry into "womanhood" (spoiler alert: my first-time having sex [I'll fill you in on it in the next chapter])

December 25, 1988

Out here on the porch, feeling the night air breeze through me. It cools my flesh and eases my thought process. I can hear the wind whisper eerie voices, mocking the night. Teasing, taunting me. I am only slightly afraid. The waves slap the underside of motorboats and yachts; daring them to struggle above its wrath.

Lights sparkle on trees at Christmas, reflecting mysterious shadows. I can see all around me. Millions of city lights and buildings. I feel so at peace but also small. Who am I among many other predators of the night? The silence is so loud. I feel like flying - circling around - upside down. Who knows, maybe I will fly with someone one day. You can own the world. Maybe that's why Liam wants to be a Naval pilot so badly. I understand this dream or obsession.

December 28, 1988
It's late and I'm thinking of you. But you're far away. May-
be I'm not thinking of you at all, but I'm bored, moody, and
lonely. Hell, I don't even know who you are anyway. Never seen
your face or heard your voice. But I've thought of you every day
and somehow, it's not the same without you. Maybe I'm just a
little lost or out of swing. And so, what if I'm a silly girl! What
difference does it really make?

I scream so loud and only the wind feels pity. Maybe I'm the
wind flying everywhere, every direction all at once. Who cares?
I need to do something. Anything. I see people on the docks, and
I feel sad. I think of Billy. I've called his house too much. His
mom must think I'm desperate... I saw my ship but no one's on
it. Why I search, I don't know. I just do. I must be an animal who
seeks a mate, a hunting partner. For what, I don't know. I think
other people don't destroy and act weird this way ...

There were times I tried to express the way I felt internally but it
came out all backwards. My mom became infuriated with me. This also
happened with other members of my family and at school among my
friends. It was like I suddenly became tongue-tied or randomly started
speaking in Hebrew and no one understood what I was trying to say to
them.

I was dying to graduate and make my mark on this world. I entered
school at Barrie not knowing who I was or what I stood for. Jessica, who
was one of my best friends, always told me to speak up, as in both talk
more loudly and stand up for myself. I know she wanted me to be outspoken like she was, but that wasn't my thing.

I often tried to speak up at home amid the din of family conversation
and I could never get a word in. At times like these, I chose silence. I
believed that if someone cared to know what I thought, they'd ask me. I
figured that if they didn't ask then they didn't really care about me.

Jessica also had a sibling but hers was older and a boy. Jessica was
used to claiming the spotlight as her brother didn't want it. She was the

apple of her mom's eyes and was a pretty tomboy to boot. She had a head full of curls, creamy skin, and full pouty lips. She resembled Lisa Bonet, who was the "it girl" of the day. All the guys wanted Jessica on their team, figuratively and literally. She was a competitive athlete who excelled in softball, basketball and running track. She wasn't vain, but I thought it was easier for her to speak her mind and make herself heard because of her looks. I adored her precisely for her lack of vanity. She was snarkier than I but she loved boys and music as much as I did.

Our friend Frances was similarly self-possessed and poised. She had lofty aspirations and was involved in everything from cheerleading and running track to singing in two outside choral groups at a time. I often wondered why Liam didn't date her our senior year, but they were platonic. Frances and Liam had both attended Barrie from the time they were little tykes through their graduations a year apart from each other. Frances was a gifted storyteller and DC historian. She always pointed out DC fun facts to me.

Many times, Frances, Jessica, and I were a trio. We drove around and hit up Benetton or Esprit. Oftentimes, Liam, Patty, Russell, and Dome met up with us somewhere along the way. We went to Silver Diner and the original Lucky Diner more times than I can count.

We were a perpetually bored lot. We went out to eat, went to the movies and the mall and played mini golf a lot. We struggled to come up with more creative ways to fill our time. I climbed the walls to go out and do something more fun. We were neither resourceful enough nor brave enough to get fake IDs and we all looked too young, except for Russell. Some nights, we were so dejected that we stayed in and did nothing except get on one another's nerves. A few times, Dome, Patty, and I drove all the way to Ocean City, Maryland, on a whim, bummed around for a few hours, and then drove back home. It was ridiculous to drive six hours round trip, only to spend an hour or so at the beach, but we were young and had the stamina.

I wish that Dome were alive today and could read about our silly antics and that he, Patty, Jessica, and I could get together after this book has been published and we could all laugh together. Sadly, Dome, the most positive of all of us back at Barrie, took his own life over a decade ago.

Russell was the one who unified us all. He was the bridge between our smaller circle of friends and his larger one, the one we all enjoyed hanging out with — and this held true over the years. It's always been "six degrees of Russ" because I'm confident that I could go anywhere in the U.S. and bump into someone who knows him. Even though we live relatively close to each other these days, we don't talk a lot, but he's the friend that I call if I need to hear a voice from the past. Time hasn't changed our love for one another. We used to have this pact that if we were both still single at age 30, we'd get married.

As much as my mom and DP adored Russ, they joked that they didn't know how to feel about our pledge to one another. They were conflicted and didn't know what bothered them more: that he was 6'4" to my 4' 10 ½"; that his parents were more educated than they were; that he wasn't Jewish; or that he was black. At different points in our lives, we seriously considered our adolescent vow.

I think out of our friend group, Russ and I struggled the most internally. I still struggled with an unnamed disability I didn't understand, and I still hadn't met anyone remotely like me. I still felt like an outcast despite our shared circle of friends. Russ had all the friends in the world but also felt alone. He wrestled with whether he was an architect who painted on the side or if he was an artist whose day job involved project management on construction sites. And he also had to walk his way through the murky waters of claiming his sexual identity. It took him a long time, but I'm so happy that he decided to live openly as a gay man. It allowed him to find the peace and true love he sought. I believe it is divine retribution that he ended up marrying a man who is much more introverted than he is.

I credit my close friends from Barrie and the Barrie community at large, for teaching me to speak up for myself. They helped me to trust that others wanted to be around me for who I am instead of who I was not. They also encouraged me to take myself less seriously. Before I met them, I didn't understand that I was truly likable or even lovable to others outside my family. My friends teased me affectionately for being spacy; for consistently forgetting where and what time to meet them; for mixing metaphors and fucking up the punchlines to jokes. But they did so precisely because they knew there was so much more to me than my weaknesses.

Seeds of Love

In 1989, the year I graduated from Barrie, Tears for Fears came out with a song called, "Seeds of Love." It was about the songwriter's political views at the time. I wasn't much into politics, but I loved that song because it referred to planting seeds within the spirit. My Barrie days taught me how to plant the seeds of self-reliance and advocacy. I learned to cultivate and trust in myself.

Similarly, the school's small student body sowed the seeds of communion within my heart. I was safe within the community and could be idealistic, creative, daring, and largely clueless as to where I was headed after high school. I didn't know what I wanted to be when I grew up, as I wasn't yet sold on the idea of growing up. But I loved the community. I thrived on helping others and I thrived in communal settings. I knew that whatever I ended up doing it would involve helping others—whether that was helping other people or animals or possibly both. A consistent thread that wove its way back and forth through my life has been how proud and happy I've been by belonging to something greater than myself. Conversely, my worst memories stem from feeling different, lonely, and rejected.

It wasn't a hardship for me to fulfill Barrie's graduation requirement of serving the community at large through internships and volunteerism. When Jessica, Patty and I were active in Keyettes, I served as its President for a time. Our most successful project was a junior high and high school Valentine's Day flower sale that my mom invented, and I coordinated. It was a fundraiser that benefited seniors living in local assisted living centers. We raised a lot of money, which all went towards amenities for the senior residents.

My passion for helping others didn't go unnoticed or appreciated. I received the McDonald's (as in the restaurant) Ray A. Kroc Citizenship Award. I was given a huge, brass plated medal with Ray A. Kroc emblazoned on it, as well as a $500 scholarship to the college of my choosing. I didn't know it at the time, but my affinity for helping others would lead me to become a mental health therapist.

Before graduation, Patty, Jessica, and I did an internship together at Greenpeace International. We were placed in its literature fulfillment center; in other words, we were unpaid envelope stuffers. We stuffed lots and lots and lots of envelopes. We mailed out packets and fact sheets about the organization's environmental conservation and protection efforts. We replied to letters from students of all ages who wanted to know what actions they could take toward saving the whales and possibly planet Earth.

I'm not making fun of environmentalism particularly, as I ended up studying environmental science in both college and graduate school, but looking back, it's funny that we took our internship responsibilities so seriously. On some level, we believed that our efforts would rescue belugas from becoming caviar. It was 1989 and environmental activism was still relatively a new frontier. It was the Rainbow Warriors and Earth Firsters against corporate America, and I got to be a small part of the action. I've never been one for large crowds and I've never believed that there is only one side to a story. While I was excited to be involved in the larger environmentalist community, I knew I wasn't going to be a radical environmentalist.

If there's one thing I've learned, it's that knowing what you don't want in any capacity helps to inform what you desire. I visited my Dad and Ona (his now-wife of 30-plus years) in Miami a lot during my last two years at Barrie. On a couple visits, I was fortunate enough to have actual encounters with dolphins and manatees as opposed to stuffing envelopes about them. And when I was 16, my dad and I went down to Islamorada so that I could swim with dolphins. It was one of those experiences packaged and sold as "a once in a lifetime opportunity." Would I do it as an adult knowing what I now know about the emotional trauma of cerebral marine mammals kept in captivity? No. Did I question it then, with my budding consciousness of environmental activism? Yes. Did I do it because I couldn't imagine doing anything more thrilling? Yes.

That experience convinced me that my inclination toward pursuing a college that offered marine biology was spot on. I had wanted to work with marine life since fourth grade, when I read Madeleine L'Engle's book *Arm of the Starfish*. I didn't know whether I'd become the next Jacques Cousteau, but I knew for sure that I was going to college.

Going to college wasn't optional in my household. In hindsight, I'm able to see that this was due to my mom's pride in being first generation American. Her mom didn't have the luxury of going to college because she had to work to support her family at a young age. At the time, I thought it was halacha or Jewish Law. There were similar things my mom told me "we" either did or didn't do - like "we" didn't shop at K-Mart or eat at Cracker Barrel. I thought those were weird things not to do but I rarely questioned her.

I ended my last summer of freedom before going to college working as a barn hand at Camp Tockwogh—and I ended my idyllic summer camp days by quitting said job. It turned out that being a camper was much more fun than being a Counselor-in-Training—especially if you were the only staff member to show up to corral two dozen horses and get them into their respective pens after an epic thunderstorm. I strode, bedraggled, across campus after this ordeal, hair soaked and matted, clothes plastered to my body and caked with mud. I barged through the Counselor-in-Training office and bellowed, "I quit!" Newly liberated, I stormed back to my cabin, packed up my trunk, and called my mom to come and get me.

The end of my summer camp days marked a definitive transition from adolescence into young adulthood. I had thought I was a woman because I had sex. Not so. Not so. Grownup life was not panning out at all how I envisioned it. I spent the remaining month of my summer of freedom dipping my toes into the murky abyss of existentialist philosophy. Garrett introduced me to plays like *Waiting for Godot* and Romantic poets such as Thoreau, Wordsworth, Keats, and Thomas. I devoured Thoreau's *Walden* and felt a strong bond with these long-dead men.

They had yearned to be left alone to write and lay in fields of flowers and sit idly by babbling brooks. They cared not for being responsible, productive men and adults. I'll never forget the first time I read Dylan Thomas's "The force that through the green fuse drives the flower." It was both hauntingly beautiful and desperately sad:

The force that through the green fuse drives the flower
Drives my green age; that blasts the roots of trees
Is my destroyer.
And I am dumb to tell the crooked rose
My youth is bent by the same wintry fever.
The force that drives the water through the rocks

Drives my red blood; that dries the mouthing streams
Turns mine to wax ....

In comparison, here's a glimpse of my mindset at the time regarding life and my place in the cosmos:

July 1, 1989 (A voyage into existentialism)
Almost seventeen years of feelings and I've never quite felt this way. It's not sadness, it's not peace. It's just "being there." The sun comes and goes while the wind frolics in my hair. The grass is dry beneath me and time just goes on. The night will fall. The moon will rise, and I will be lost in dreams.

All the while, time trickles away. Day after day after day. The world will keep on turning, and now, I'm only "here". A little thing in an awesome universe. This must be how B Wordsworth felt as he gazed at the cloudy sky above. I can watch a bee on a flower too, I feel it, and I can. Unselfish, am I? I am simply "there or here," wondering. Still the sand vanishes from the hourglass. And when the sand sits on the other side, what time will it be?

Israel

I learned through my synagogue of a once in a lifetime opportunity to study in Israel for two months. It was pitched as a study abroad opportunity to learn about the history of Israel from the time of Moses up through present day. In retrospect, I can see that it was an opportunity to see Eretz Yisroel, the land of Israel from a singularly Jewish cultural perspective. I cajoled my parents into allowing me to go.

I went to Israel from the second week of September through the second week of November 1987. Patty similarly convinced her mom into letting her go with me. I thought it was brave of her because she isn't Jewish and was usually too afraid to try new things. She usually needed a pep talk on the few occasions she went on dates with male classmates or college boys who were initially drawn to her pale skin and gypsy style of dress. I was so proud of her for asking her mom to go on the trip without too much pleading on my end, and that she cared enough about our friendship to want to embark on an adventure with me. I didn't want to go without her.

On the flight, I paced up and down the aisles until I wore a grooved path into them. I ate all my snacks, read, and uncharacteristically sat and cuddled with a strange boy who professed his love to me a few hours into our flight. Twelve hours after we departed, we touched down onto holy ground. I was ready to be off that metal bird and away from the weird boy. Thank G—d he wasn't on the same campus as I was. Patty and I met up with a group of students who were equally as fatigued as we were.

Once all of us had collected our luggage and made it through customs on the Israeli side, we hopped on a bus and drove about 25 minutes outside of Tel Aviv to a suburb called Hod Hasharon. The High School in Israel (HIS) Mosenson campus was a rustic assemblage of dorms and a *moadon* (pronounced "moe-ah-dohne," like "dome" without the M), or "clubhouse." I spent a lot of my free time inside the *moadon* or seated at the scattered picnic tables just outside of it. It was made of cement and was little more than a large square room that held two couches, an end table, two cafeteria tables, and two chairs. The floor was covered in the thinnest layer of filthy carpeting.

The Americans' dorm on campus was a two-story building. There was one set of concrete stairs that connected the two levels. I lived on the ground floor in a suite with two other young women. I wasted no time in claiming the smaller room with the single bed. I was disappointed that it didn't have a door to allow for privacy but there was only room for me. I wanted it that way. I made my room as homey as possible, given its minimalist decor. It had a small window with a narrow mantle and four small shelves underneath it. I could almost touch the opposite wall—which held only a set of drawers—if I spread my arms out eagle-style.

The larger room was where my roommates bunked. Their room held a bunk bed, a closet, and a few shelves. That's how sparse our accommodations were. Our floors were cement. We were each given two pairs of scratchy sheets and an even scratchier woolen blanket apiece. Our bedrooms, and all the rooms, including our classrooms, smelled musty. Apart from linens, we were each given 63 shekels worth of Israeli currency. I briefly wondered if this was how Private Benjamin felt upon seeing her living quarters when she enlisted in the Army.

One of the first things our counselors, or *madrichim* (pronounced like "Madrich" but with an "eem" at the end), told us was to be wary of students who weren't American. There were local Israeli teens who attended a vocational boarding school at Mosenson. The restrictions were meant to prevent theft, relationships, and maybe unplanned pregnancies. I easily bonded with almost all my classmates. We learned together, worked cooperatively on assignments, and took intense field trips together. So much togetherness helped us to forge lifelong friendships with one another.

We learned all about the history of my people. We visited the Wailing Wall in Jerusalem, where Orthodox Jewish men *davened* (rocked their torsos back and forth) and prayed, while women were relegated to their own section of the rock wall. I wrote a prayer for Grandma Mary on a slip of paper and crammed it into a minuscule hole in the wall. The profundity of that day has stuck with me all these years later.

We visited Yad Vashem, the Israeli Holocaust memorial. I will never forget the haunting, seemingly skyscraper-tall assemblage of tiny shoes that belonged to lost babies and children. Nor would I forget the vision of a cave-full of flickering lights representative of all those children whose lives were extinguished too soon. As you walked through the cave, you heard a recording played that listed all their names. I'd learned all about the Holocaust in confirmation class, but nothing could've prepared me for my visit to Yad Vashem.

We read the works of Elie Wiesel, as well as poems written by children about their experience of being imprisoned in ghettos and concentration camps. One poem clutched at my heartstrings. It was written by a young boy who saw a beautiful butterfly outside the barbed wire fencing of the ghetto. Our teachers meant for our hearts to be torn asunder. We were 16 and impressionable. Part of the school's mission was to encourage some of us to return to Israel upon graduation to make Aliyah, to become permanent citizens.

The last, the very last,
So richly, brightly, dazzlingly yellow.

Soundtrack of a Misfit

Perhaps if the sun's tears would sing
against a white stone ...

—*The Butterfly,* Pavel Friedmann, 4.6.1942

We explored Tel El Fool, where Saul built his palace; Wadi Qelt, where Jews forged a path through the watery ravine to escape the Canaanites; Qumran, where a band of ascetic Jews lived and where the Dead Sea scrolls were hidden; and Masada, a hideout for King Herod and was also where my people went to escape Roman persecution.

I have a photo of me from our tiul to Wadi Qelt. It shows sixteen-year-old me dressed in quintessential '80s regalia. My sun blond hair was tucked up underneath a Duran Duran-style fedora. In this photo, I wore a bright red oversized t-shirt tucked into and pulled out just a tad over a pair of matching red boxer shorts emblazoned with aqua waves, green palm trees, and the suggestion of fish outlined with white thread. Completing the ensemble were red scrunched down socks.

I kept in touch with the American friends I made at HSI for many years. I still keep tabs on my friends Lenny and Billy through Facebook, and I sometimes wonder what Adam might be up to these days. I was gaga about these three boys for different reasons. Lenny was all sweetness and goofball. He followed me around like a puppy dog and was the most opinionated and self-educated guy I ever met. He went to school, of course, but he also learned more voluntarily than anyone I'd met before. Lenny and Billy were mismatched best-friends much like Patty and I were.

Adam was a Sephardic Jew whose family was from Morocco. I'd never met a Sephardic Jew until I met him. I hadn't known that Sephardic Jews like Adam celebrated the Jewish holidays with different foods and rituals. I'd also never met anyone as openly proud of being Jewish or as knowledgeable of the Jewish religion. We were opposites. I was proud of being Jewish, but I knew little about our heritage in comparison to Adam. In my eyes, he was the epitome of tall, dark, and handsome. I was obsessed with him because he was the most impassioned person I knew. He was exceptionally bright and prone to melancholia, a combination I knew well. My dad was exactly like him, except where my dad is a big personality, Adam was a wallflower. He wanted to return to Israel when he was eighteen to serve in the Israeli army.

Billy was a sexy teenage boy who was 16 going on 21. He wore cologne and gold chains. I thought he was exotic because he is part Cuban. I didn't even know there were Jews in Cuba. He had curly, sandy brown hair and a wry smile. I won him over by being the bravest one to jump into a freezing cold river in my cobalt blue French bikini. It was one of my few skinnier periods in my life. Having nausea from recently having my nose fixed had helped me in the weight loss department. We were hot for one another but were not as emotionally mature as our physical bodies led us to believe we were. I could talk to Billy about anything ranging from Zionism to farts.

I had three distinct friend groups during my time at HSI. There were the Americans I traveled with. Then there were the three affluent local boys: Ohad, Barak and Yishay (the latter two being brothers). They didn't attend school at Mosenson but loved to visit with the Americans and practice their English. And lastly, there were the local Israelis that I wasn't supposed to befriend.

All Israelis learn English as a second language in school, but like most Israelis, they usually spoke in their native Hebrew, so their English wasn't stellar. Ohad, Barak, and Yishay improved their English by listening to the Beatles and Pink Floyd. I mean they listened to them nonstop. Patty and I swore we'd kill them if they sang "Comfortably Numb" one more time. We bickered with these boys like they were family. Sometimes, Patty and I sat back and watched "the boys" play shesh-pesh or backgammon. We thought we were brilliant as Weird Al Yankovic because as we listened to Suzanne Vega, we changed the lyrics "My name is Luka | I live on the second floor" to "My name is Loogie | I spit from the second floor."

I was especially close to Yishay, who shared my corny humor and was as enthralled with science fiction as I was with fiction. He was an avid reader as I and introduced me to the *Lord of the Rings* trilogy and Isaac Asimov. Ohad was the kind of young man even other guys couldn't ignore. He was vivacious and had the most mesmerizing eyes. His eyes and his maverick affability were just like Mel Gibson's. He was notorious for playing practical jokes. (Another spoiler alert: it shouldn't surprise, given my description of him, that Ohad was one of the first boys I had sex with. It happened the following year when he, Barak, and Yishay visited me in the States. Another spoiler alert: Billy was my first).

My third group of friends was the local Israeli vocational students I was warned not to befriend. They were the most fun boys I ever met. They always walked arm in arm, shoulders draped over one another's. It's common in Israel for guys to physically carouse and link arms without people assuming they're homosexual. I thought that was awesome. I didn't have that kind of physical bond with Patty. I didn't have that kind of kinship with anyone except my sister and she and I certainly never held hands once we were past elementary school.

CHAPTER 8 – DON'T YOU (FORGET ABOUT ME)

When I was at HSI, I met a boy. One night, I checked out a dance the Israelis put on in their *moadon* with Patty and some of our other friends. About 30 minutes later, I turned around to find that everyone had left me. My friends had left me dancing by myself. One of the local Israeli guys I'd seen around Mosenson told me he'd seen me around too. He introduced himself as Bono.

He was six feet-something to my four-something. He had feathered sandy blond hair and eyes that shifted from amber to topaz yellow, depending upon how the light caught them. Bono resembled Judd Nelson's character from the movie *The Breakfast Club*. He even had that same, "come hither and let me tell you how" vibe. I don't know how to describe our connection. It was instantaneous and yet it felt like we'd always known each other. Bono said he'd seen me with my friends walking around Mosenson campus. He added that his friends called him "Bono" because he loved the lead singer of U2. So did I. It had to be kismet!

He grabbed my hand and began to walk away, and I followed. Under a warm, starry sky, we talked and laughed for hours. He found a beat up red, plastic school chair to sit on. I sat on his lap. Then he asked me to read him a letter. It was from an American girl he'd met when she was at Mosenson. He said that he'd read it himself but that his English wasn't great, and he would become too frustrated.

Bono had that vampiric magnetic pull to him. From that night on, we were inseparable. We spent parts of most nights together, doing our homework and talking. He was darkness and light fused together. Bono loved to draw. He always sketched on my homework. He even drew U2 and "Bono Forever" on my hot pink, Chuck Taylor high tops which I solemnly vowed to never get rid of. We sometimes hung out in his dorm room alone, which I usually tried to avoid. Other times, we hung out with his friends, the Israeli "Lost Boys" (named after the movie).

I compare these fun-loving dudes to the vampires because they were accustomed to charming young, American women. Sometimes, they pushed their luck with young women just to see how many freebies they could get—be they sexual gifts or material. For instance, in Bono's case, he was so suave that he convinced me to give him my beloved plastic Swatch watch with its interchangeable colored bands.

My friend Veronica and I spent more time watching movies and hanging out in the Israelis' moadon than we did in ours. She dated one of Bono's friends. Sometimes, the gang just sat on the wall that bordered the campus football field. We spent hours just shooting the shit outdoors. They loved to tease me because I was especially naive and gullible.

One of their favorite pastimes was to play practical jokes on me. The best was Bono's. He sought me out one night: bare chested, denim jeans snugly resting on his hips, holding out a blanket behind his back like a soccer player holding its country a flag. The sight of him like that gave me butterflies in my stomach. He unfurled the blanket and wrapped me up in it so that I nestled against his chest. I pressed my palm into the hollow of his bare, hairless chest so that I felt his heartbeat.

I closed my eyes to savor the moment, but he insisted quite urgently that he needed my help. He said that he got so jealous of birds because they could fly. He added that he always wanted to fly but didn't know how and he was sure I knew the secret. He implored me to help him in his quest.

I didn't know what to say or do. He wasn't right in the head. Maybe he was hallucinating or was drugged or both. Before I could think of a game plan, Bono ran down the football field, his blanket flowing behind him like a cape. I couldn't believe he was coordinated and graceful enough at his height to leap onto the metal goal post. And he did just that, precariously balancing himself on the top. I was winded by the time I caught up to him. Bono leapt down onto me and we tumbled to the ground. He howled with laughter while I tried to compose myself. Belushi, Ilan, and the rest of the Lost Boys had been in on the prank. They ran onto the field echoing Bono, "Rachel, let's fly. Help me fly like a turkey." I hated to break it to them, "Um, guys … I think you mean an Eagle. Turkeys don't fly." Bono affectionately called me "Turkey" from that day on although with his Israeli accent it sounded more like "Tookey."

One night, Bono, the Lost Boys, and I were hanging out and watching a movie when, suddenly, Russell, my counselor, came looking for me. I was so nervous I was going to be in trouble. We were warned countless times about not mixing with the Mosenson Campus Israelis. Russell called me outside but instead of reprimanding me, he asked me how well I knew my father. My heart sank. "Knew," as in past tense?

I worriedly asked Russell if my dad had died. He answered, "No, but he's on the phone and he's getting married. Run to the Wohl dorm phone because I'm sure it's expensive for him to hold on the line." I was confused and replied incredulously, "Married, Russell? Are you sure? He just got divorced."

He's getting married? To whom? I asked the last two questions more to myself as I heeded Russell's instructions and ran back to take the call. Sure enough, my dad was getting married for the third time and to a woman I'd never heard of. Evidently, Ona knew Grandma Harriett well and had heard stories about my dad all throughout her adolescence and early adulthood. I didn't get how a woman my dad's age would be friends with my grandma, nor did I understand how they hadn't been introduced to one another before. My dad wanted to wait until I met her before they got married, but Ona's father was gravely ill. It was surreal. I was relieved to know my dad was still alive, numb to the fact that he was getting married yet again, and relieved that I wasn't in trouble with Russell for breaking the rules.

I ran back to Bono to tell him all about my call. To soothe me, he pulled me gently to him and kissed me deeply. Just when I despaired that no one would want to kiss me because I had old-school metal braces, Bono wasn't fazed. After that night, he took every opportunity to kiss me, as well as press his luck. He liked seeing just how "far he could get with me" physically every time we hung out. Sometimes, this happened in front of his friends, and I hated that. I wasn't into PDA. I insisted that I was saving myself for marriage before I had sex or at least true love. I was naive and innocent then.

Bono said things that made no sense to me like, "Babe, I'll get blue balls or Yellow cheese if you don't give me a hand job." I knew nothing about sex, but I was sure he wouldn't turn blue or yellow from me not doing what he wanted me to do. The cheese reference stumped me, but I wasn't about to ask him for clarification. I was sure he was just saying dumb stuff, but I wanted to make him happy. I hated to see him pout, so I gave in to his begging. I knew boyfriends and girlfriends did stuff like that and I thought we were a couple—especially as he got upset if I couldn't see him or if he saw me spending time with either Adam or Billy. Little did I know that he was also seeing and sleeping with one of my good friends all along. I thought his protectiveness and possessiveness toward me indicated how deeply he felt for me. I wrote many pages in my journal about how confusing my relationship with Bono was:

> **October 20, 1987**
> *Bono and I are good friends. I wrote him a letter and then we talked. I mean really talked for the first time. He said he has a real girlfriend but that they don't want people saying things. He has slept with lots of girls because they were cheap and because of that, he dumped them. He says it's different with me and I honestly believe him. He said I am the first person to last the whole time (meaning remain his friend) because we joke around and talk. We don't just have sex all the time. We don't have sex at all. We don't even fool around anymore. He says he likes it better this way. He says that we'll stay good friends because of it.*

Bono said things like that but then had a hard time staying away from me. We still spent a lot of time together and our interactions were still what I considered to be intimate. One night, I went into town with Adam. On the way out of campus, we passed Bono. I stopped and kissed him and said I'd visit him later. My friend Debbie, who was hanging out with her Israeli boyfriend, told me that Bono spazzed out and threw a table once I was out of his sight. I felt guilty, but I didn't do anything wrong. He was the one who didn't want to be my boyfriend.

He was in such a foul mood when I saw him later that night, and because I felt partly responsible and didn't want to disappoint him, I let him take my shirt off. He asked if I wanted him to be my first. Again, with the pressuring me! But again, I assured him that it wasn't because I didn't trust him, but because I needed to be in love with someone. Even though we'd only known one another a short period of time, I truly did love him, but I wasn't ready to give up my virginity. He settled for more fooling around. Bono whispered in my ear that he was jealous of Adam and sang me the John Lennon song, "Jealous Guy." What was it with Israelis and iterations of The Beatles? It took me over an hour to assure Bono through using my hands, that he mattered deeply to me and that Adam and I were just friends.

I was back in the U.S. by mid-November 1987, but Bono might've well been across the quad from me still. It didn't seem like he was far away—especially as he called me collect all the time. I spent mine and my parents' hard-earned money by accepting international collect calls from him. I told him countless times that not everyone in the States was rich. Bono either didn't believe me or didn't care. Then, in typical mercurial fashion, he sent me heartfelt letters with SWAK (*Sealed With A Kiss*) and airmail stamps all over the envelopes. This made me feel special all over again, so I always forgave the international collect calls.

Did I make the right decision by not sleeping with him? Most other girls my age had already had sex. They acted like it was no big deal. Clinging to my virginity made me feel more immature than my peers as well as uncool.

Like A Virgin

There had been guys I flirted with before precisely because they were "bad boys." I didn't know why I was so drawn to the never-available boys. There was Andy at Barrie who called me "Little Virgin Ears." I tried so hard to get him to like me. He was cute, skinny, and loved fast cars like the IROCs and Maserati. I'm sure he also liked fast women if you considered teenagers "women."

I skipped out on playing volleyball in Gwen's P.E. class to hang out on the stage and listen to Andy's constant droning about horsepower and car RPM. Gwen encouraged me to join the rest of my class on the gym floor but changed her mind when I inadvertently lobbed a ball that narrowly missed her face. "Congratulations! You're now our scorekeeper. Go sit next to Andy on stage and watch," she commanded.

I had beaten my nemesis, Liam, in the campaign for student government president and, in an odd twist of fate, he became my first real boyfriend. I *thought* I was in love with him. I wanted him to be The One. He was a nice Jewish boy whom I spent the last three years alternating between despising and desiring. He was insouciant, engaging, and funny.

He had the kind of big "Jewish" nose that I used to get teased about. I found his humped protuberance insanely attractive and his chocolatey eyes magnetic.

He flirted with me and then baited and switched whenever I reciprocated. He also did dumb things because he thought he was above rejection such as applying only to the Naval Academy without applying to any "safety schools." I felt like I had X-ray vision and was the only one who saw underneath his tough veneer. Having this "insider" knowledge made me feel a bit superior to my classmates, I suppose.

I was a "rescuer"—an unhealthy role, but it was a relationship pattern of mine that was coming more and more to light. I think it stems from a hybridization of my penchant for trashy romance novels and my own desire to be rescued myself. It was also rooted my relationship with my father and stepdad and NOT in any Freudian way. My dad was my archetype for manhood. My brain formed an impression of masculinity that was patterned after his traits. Based upon my knowledge of my dad, men were a complicated mix of arrogance and warmth. They were demonstratively affectionate and walled off. Ideally, they weren't just nice and predictable like my stepdad. I idolized DP, but I also considered him to be nerdy and therefore less masculine in comparison to my dad.

I wasn't attracted to "nice" because arbitrary kindness felt foreign to me. It prevented me from feeling attracted to what I refer to as "bagel boys"—guys like Lenny, my dear friend from HSI. I liked him but had no interest in dating him. I considered him to be dorky, preppy, and kvetchy. Lenny didn't want to spend time outdoors and he didn't have a clue how to wire stereos or graft trees. My stepdad might've been a bagel man, but he too, knew how to build or fix just about everything and anything. My dad and DP were my yardsticks for measuring masculinity. It was what I knew.

Flipping back through my journal from December 1988 to May 1989 (the year I graduated high school), I was surprised to see how frequently I linked my feelings to Liam's. I scratched lyrics from *Les Misérables*, and other Broadway sagas scratched into one page and the words to angst-ridden alternative rock songs on the opposite. I copied song lyrics and penned original poems in all my journals. I define time periods and pivotal moments in my life by recalling music I listened to at the time. For instance, "The Promise" by When in Rome reminds me of Liam whereas "Don't You Forget About Me" by Simple Minds and "If You Leave" by OMD is indelibly linked to my memories of Bono.

Liam was the first guy I consciously tested my feminine wiles on. He wasn't opposed to heavy kissing and feeling one another up, but sex was a no-go. *Oh my G—d, is this how Bono had felt?* I feel rejected! His indifference hurt. I visited my dad and Ona for Christmas break and literally threw myself on my close friend Billy. We'd been back from HSI for a little over a year and I had seen him and Lenny only once. Besides Liam, Billy was the only other person who made me feel happy and alive.

There wasn't much for teenagers to do at The Jockey Club, where my dad and Ona lived, except swim or play tennis. I didn't do the latter and the pool was already closed for the night, so when Billy came over, we went down to the docks to hang out. It was romantic on the water. We talked for a bit, star-gazed, looked for fish in the marina, then pounced on one another. Billy had intentionally doused himself with Drakkar Noir, the ever-present cologne of the moment—and I was gaga for it. I knew the moment I buried my face in his chest that I wouldn't end that night as a virgin.

We kissed one another until our lips were raw. It felt so good to feel Billy hard against me. I had no way of knowing when my parents would be home from their date night, so bringing him up to my room wasn't a possibility. He lived with his parents so that was also a nonstarter. We drove around for a while before agreeing to rent the kind of sleazy motel room one paid for by the hour. I felt so grownup handing over my credit card to the front desk attendant, but I also felt horribly self- conscious and wondered, *isn't it obvious that we're not old enough to be married? What do they think of us?* However, once inside our room, we ripped one another's clothes off and laughed. We didn't know what we were supposed to do next. I mean we did but we didn't know how to. Billy climbed on top of me and moved around a bit. A few minutes later, I felt deflated. *That was it?* Billy wanted to try again but only had one condom. I laughed and didn't know whether to feel disappointed or relieved that we couldn't get in more practice.

I had much more fun kissing and having my first experience with foreplay. Still, I was proud of us for finally crossing the threshold from adolescence into adulthood and we did it together. We cared deeply for one another but knew it wasn't love. I didn't regret our hastiness although part of me felt cheapened by his comedic timing. Immediately after we did it, he tritely quipped, "I need a cigarette now."

It's funny how something so innocuous and unintentional as a joke made me feel alternately foolish and giddy. It didn't surprise me to see that I copied the lyrics to "World Full of Nothing" by Depeche Mode after describing my first sexual experience: "She's lonely and he says it's for her only that he lusts | She doesn't trust him | Nothing is true | But he will do in a world full of nothing | Though it's not love | It means something."

The year after I returned from HSI, my good friends Ohad, Barak and Yishay came to visit me in Maryland. It turned out that Ohad's hormones were as revved up as mine were. Having sex was the only thing he was interested in apart from Pink Floyd and The Beatles. Every minute we stood side by side at the museums we visited with my family, he pestered me. He didn't care that my mom and sister were just a few feet away from us and might hear what he said. He flirted with me all day long so that, by the time I was ready to go to sleep, he knew he had me.

I was his equal where horniness was concerned, but I lacked his prowess. I had plenty of experience kissing but I wasn't prepared for how good it felt when Ohad's tongue swirled around my insides and his fingers explored places I hadn't yet touched myself. Ohad moved inside me without me needing to think about what to do or how to do it, but he was generously endowed, so it hurt. And then ... before I knew it, it was over. I went upstairs to my room and went to bed feeling raw inside and out. I was disillusioned. (An aside: Years later, my sister Stacey and I discovered that Ohad had seduced us both during his visit.)

I'm proud that my younger self at least aspired to wait until true love. At 17, I wanted to be in love and to be loved more than anything. Having sex with Billy and Ohad had felt like love. I was friends with these young men, and I felt emotionally and physically safe with them. Sadly, I later swapped my scruples for alcohol and promiscuous sex with strangers who I momentarily convinced myself I *could* be in love with. I repeatedly mistook lust and sex for love and true intimacy. I was always desperately lonely no matter how many people I surrounded myself with.

The sad reality was that drunken and debauched sex never made me feel more connected no matter how desperately I hoped it would. I felt like I was consistently deflowered.

Shock, Chills & Redemption

As constructs, timing and time have always been wonky for me. I get confused by the sequential organization of months. For instance, in organizing journals by year, I don't know if something I wrote was a few months ago in March or it occurred in March of the previous year. Similarly, if something happens at midnight, I forget if that means it happened "today" (if I'm still awake and writing about something) or if it happened yesterday. If you're reading this and you don't have ADD, this might be surprising or confusing. However, I'm guessing those of you with ADD know exactly what I mean. In that vein, I don't know if I had sex for the first time and slept with my friend Ohad or if the two experiences happened a year apart. (Mom, if you're reading this, no comments.)

Anyhow, in this scenario, it was Christmas time, my freshman year of college. I was visiting my dad in Miami and on that night, I had a sleep over at my girlfriend Monica's house. She was one of my good friends from my HIS days. Most students who attended with me were from the Miami-Dade area because the home office of HIS is there.

Monica and I were having a blast catching up, but then she dealt me a low blow. She informed me that she had been and still was the girlfriend of my old Israeli flame, Bono. She then added that he was still alive (you never really knew what might happen given that everyone in the country is conscripted into the military) and that the two of them had kept in touch and were supposedly in love. I wrote Bono countless letters since college started and they all went unanswered.

I didn't know which revelation hurt me more. I was happy to hear that he was alive, but he had been the one who declared that we were "special friends who would always be connected" and still had severed communication. I was also hurt to learn that my girlfriend had kept a secret from me for two years. Monica tried to soften the blow by saying, "Rach, we didn't know how to tell you and we didn't want to hurt your feelings." It was strange to know that despite broken communication, Bono was honest with me years ago when he told me that he had a girlfriend during the time I thought we were a couple at HSI.

What hurt most was that Bono hadn't liked that I had a tummy, yet my girlfriend was obese. I wondered if he was using her to try to get her to marry him so that he could come to America and get a green card. *Was it possible that he genuinely loved her? And if so, what was wrong with me?* I didn't know what to believe.

Call me stupid but after Monica broke the news to me about being in a relationship with Bono, I determined that I was going "make" him fall in love with me. I built him up in my mind as the "one who got away." Three years later, in my junior year of college, I returned to Israel. It wasn't my first choice, but it was one of the only options available to me at the time. I saw it as my chance at redemption.

CHAPTER 9 – EUPHORIA MOURNING

I applied to and was accepted to all seven colleges I applied to. Take that, learning disability! I hoped that my introduction to college life would be a smoother transition than my inductions into womanhood were. I didn't apply to top-notch schools or the Ivies. I knew that college was going to be difficult for me. I would still need the accommodations for untimed tests and set aside quiet study carrels for taking my exams, but my disability was still an enigma to me. I didn't know I had ADD at this point. All I knew with certainty was that I was more evolved than most people my own age in verbal and written communication, but I performed severely below grade level in math. I was still sorely deficient with eye-hand coordination.

I toured the University of Rhode Island, Franklin Pierce College, the University of Maine at Orono, and Rider College. I adored Franklin Pierce because it seemed like an extension of Barrie, but I didn't want to be anywhere that was too cold or too far away. I also didn't want to go to a school that was either too large or too small. Rider College (now University) in Lawrenceville, New Jersey, won my heart. It was just a few hours' drive from home but was far enough away that my parents wouldn't know what I was up to. It had a student body of 3,000, which is small by most people's standards but large to me. My number-one reason for choosing Rider, however, was that it offered marine biology as a major.

It was sunny and warm the day I moved onto campus. Girls sunbathed on blanket-sized sheets of aluminum foil and bare-chested dudes played frisbee on the short, narrow strip of Fraternity Row. Styx's "Come Sail Away" blared from someone's speakers. The sound carried across the duck pond. There was a low bar as far as dress code went, so I don't know why I bothered to dress up my first few weeks of classes. College life wasn't as glamorous as I'd envisioned. In fact, Rider was less about being showy and more about being hardly seen. Not many seemed to want to draw attention to themselves the way my classmates at Barrie had.

I thought students would dress more fashionably than they did due to the school's proximity to New York City. I didn't expect college students to look exactly like the high schoolers I had just left behind. New Jersey in the late-'80s and early-'90s was all about Billy Joel, Bon Jovi, and The Boss. It was an entire state full of women with big spiral permed hair and acrylic nails and men with mullets and muscle shirts. I quickly learned it was best to dress inconspicuously as possible so that you could get away with as much as possible.

It was also soon apparent that my college was what my mom called a "suitcase school." The campus bustled with energy all throughout the week, but it emptied out Friday after daytime classes ended. Freshmen weren't allowed to have cars on campus and there was nothing to do within walking distance if you were one of the few there on the weekends. You either knew someone who was old enough to drive into Princeton or you entertained yourself on campus. You didn't want to go the other direction into Trenton.

Most of my friends were New Jersey locals from beach towns, so the only direction they headed on weekends was homeward. They were fortunate enough to eat home-cooked meals and have their laundry done for them by their mothers; no cafeteria "mystery meat" or quarter-stealing washing machines for them. I stayed at school most weekends and became popular because I was tinier than everybody else. Plus, I had an extensive hat collection. Unlike most students who wore backwards facing baseball caps, I wore feathered bowlers, wide-brimmed hippie/Rasta hats, felt fedoras, and cowboy sun hats.

I might've been widely acknowledged, but I wasn't wildly befriended. I didn't have many friends. I was lonely and bored a lot—especially during my freshman and sophomore years. In fact, I might not have begun drinking if I had had a cadre or even a small pod of friends who enjoyed doing anything better.

I began binge drinking because the few friends I had spent their weekends imbibing alcohol. My school didn't have a lot of clubs or extracurricular activities. Just about everyone who stayed behind at school on the weekends or vacations drank to pass the time. I joined the party, but I wasn't thrilled about it. I hated the taste of beer, but when in Rome ....

I went to parties, fraternity-hopping on the weekends, and it was "party on, dude!"

> ### *September 13, 1989*
> *This probably sounds stupid since I just got in from a fraternity night party, but I despise parties! What is the purpose of drinking? I drank one beer, and something called a "blow job" because my hands had to be behind my back, and I was only allowed to use my lips to suction around the shot glass and kick back the liquor. I see no point in it all so why do I even bother drinking? I guess I expect to feel great. On nights or mornings (1:01 AM) I do weird little things by myself like go to the lake and see what the geese are up to.*

(Side note: The geese were outlandishly large, white, and notoriously evil. They hung out at the pond in the middle of campus. They waddled over to innocent bench-sitters and bit knees and shins. I had many unpleasant run-ins with King, unsurprisingly the largest of them.)

While I didn't date, I lusted after various jocks who knew I existed but weren't into me. There was Luis, who epitomized the male gym rat of the early 1990s. He always wore baggy muscle pants and "wife beater" tanks. I never heard this term applied to sleeveless undershirts before going to college in Jersey. He was stocky and bowlegged and had swagger. He had long, flowing, curly golden locks, and honey-cream skin. He knew he was a badass. I never saw him crack a smile—a smirk at my expense, perhaps.

I was hyper aware of Luis and he taunted me by being in the same place as I was all the damn time. He wasn't great looking, but there was something about him that turned my insides into a quivering mound of Jell-O. He once stood close enough to me in the cafeteria line that I could smell his intoxicating muskiness. He even acknowledged my existence with a grunt. This epic event caught me so off-guard that I ran into the bathroom convinced I was about to toss my cookies. I waited two years for this moment, and I couldn't even croak out "hello."

The first year of college was drab apart from frat parties (which I grew to like) and my daily afternoon jogs. My goal was to run to Princeton, but it was too far away; I never made it but was passed by Rider's track team. I waved to them from the opposite side of the street as they were beginning their daily run and I was ending mine. By the time the Rider women's track team became a thing in my junior year, I was too busy smoking pot and stuffing my face with Roma's Pizza.

I was lethargic and ill on and off since college started and three months was a long time to feel ill when you were young and otherwise invincible. One night, I sat in the gross shared hallway tub in the all-female Centennial Hall. I was so cold that I shivered, and my teeth chattered uncontrollably. I could hardly drag myself to classes the following week, so I went to see my doctor back home in Gaithersburg. I was diagnosed with mononucleosis. It was cruel that I got mono from drinking out of the same glass as my sister, who'd contracted a severe case of it during our family's summer vacation in Cancun.

I fell asleep in class every day. I usually sat in the front rows because it was hard for me to pay attention otherwise and I was too short to see over my classmates' heads. It was humiliating to fall asleep with my face on my desk. Most of my instructors were understanding and supportive. Somehow, I managed to get better grades freshman year than I did the rest of college.

Being the only one at college who had Mono didn't help my self-esteem or my social life. If I wasn't in class, I would be sleeping. If I had a spurt of energy, I would go to a party, but if I went to a party and was out until late then I was left depleted, and the cycle of sleep started all over again. That meant it took me a full year to shake mono.

Ch- Ch-Ch-Ch-Changes

The nominal lyrics above reference a well-known David Bowie song. I'm a huge Bowie fan (fortunately, getting to see him live in Philadelphia during the summer of 1990) and still grieve his 2016 passing. I looked up to him as a rock idol but also as an individual who wasn't afraid to speak his truth. He was cool with being different. He was cool with being androgynous and cool with changing his musical styles to match the changing times and fashions. He could write, sing, and act. Bowie had it all!

In contrast, I had nothing to offer the world. I couldn't do anything.

I didn't know if I wanted to declare myself deflowered or reclaim my virginity. I didn't know if I wanted to be a prep or a punk. I didn't even know what major to declare. I still wanted to be a marine biologist, but I was too inept in math and science. My dream was shattered. I no longer knew what I wanted to be when I graduated or what to do with myself. I wanted to have a fun career full of adventure and exploration. I never set out to have just any old job, so I declared myself a sociology major.

It sounds funny to me now, but it wasn't a joke. Anthropology courses were housed under Rider's School of Sociology and from what I could tell, anthropologists traveled all the time. I took every anthropology course offered and, essentially, majored in cultural anthropology.

I also declared environmental science as a minor. I didn't have resources to travel the world and live among indigenous peoples, which is also what I thought all anthropologists did. I was confident, however, in my ability to be a tree hugger. I already completed that internship with Greenpeace and nature was all around me even in cities. Since I was the first one to declare this minor, the School of Physical Sciences didn't know what to do with me, so they made me claim it as a double major. Being the trendsetter that I was, I started Rider's first environmental club. We focused on picking up trash to beautify the campus and we started the school's first recycling initiative.

If I wasn't busy beautifying the campus, I would be trying to beautify myself. I still spent a lot of time at the gym. My nemesis heartthrob Luis was also still working out there. I was only slightly less obsessed with him. Dudes like him still wore baggy muscle pants, dropped dumbbells at their feet, and made unattractive guttural sounds. Meanwhile, young women like me now wore tighter fitting clothing and practiced a new cardio routine called step aerobics (so much for our bodies needing oxygen to allow our lady parts to breathe, eh?). I remember being excited to sport my new cobalt blue leotard and shiny, black leggings that Aunt Sister bought for me that winter. I embraced the leotard-and-bunchy socks look and why wouldn't I? It was all booty-shorts and high-top sneakers in the era of MC Hammer and Vanilla Ice.

Dirty Dancing

I learned that as a female, I had the power to turn men on by gyrating my hips *Dirty Dancing*-style. I visited my friend Meredith in Nyack after seeing my aunt and we went dancing, our favorite thing to do. I had an epiphany: if you don't dance raw, fewer guys notice you, but when you danced like your hips didn't lie (predating Shakira by a few years), men thought you were "easy." It was thrilling to suddenly acquire a superpower that garnered attention. It was less thrilling to realize that by unleashing this power, I drew the interest of men who were interested in doing more than just gyrating their pelvises.

I pleaded and convinced my girlfriends to go dancing with me all the time. We went to this little dive club near Trenton. I can't recall its name, but I remember having a blast there. I wasn't old enough to drink legally, but if I was dancing, I didn't care. I was just so tired of being the odd one or the different one and dancing was a means of conformity and escape for me. And I could do my own thing while being surrounded by everyone else who was doing theirs.

We frenetically gyrated to the industrial music of Helmet, Front 242-, and Nine-Inch Nails. I got as close as I could bear to be next to the club's subwoofers and felt the music thump inside my body. Dancing gave me a sense of freedom and abandonment that I never knew before. I always started out dancing feeling uneasy and self-conscious. As the night went on and others began to feel the effects of their drinks, I breathed easier. I knew no one was concerned with what I looked like on the dance floor. I engaged in ecstatic dancing before it became popular; I danced well so long as no specific steps or moves were required.

The year I turned 21 and was of legal drinking age, my relationship with dancing and with alcohol changed. My dancing became less about fun and more about seduction. Drinking alcohol gave me liquid courage. I called the feeling of music pulsing through my body, my fingertips pressed either against a speaker or a man or woman's body, "liquid sex." How I wish I had stuck to the dance floor and hadn't taken my dance partners home with me after feeling that sensation pulsing through me. I don't regret enticing others, nor do I regret many of the experiences I had but there's no going back to innocence once you've pried the lid off Pandora's Box.

I wasn't really a hot-ass mess until my mid-20s, but I'd already set the stage for my fall from grace. In the early '90s, I was uber-aware of the dangers of having unprotected sex. For as much as I craved it, being underage and my fear of contracting HIV/AIDS made me too terrified to seek out sex with strangers. There was also still a part of me that craved my Sugar Plum Fairy idea of true love. This made seeking out sex less appealing than it did when I hit my promiscuous mid-twenties. I saw *Pretty Woman* with Frances and cried when Julia Roberts's and Richard Gere's characters made love for the first time. In my journal entry from that night I wrote, "I know it's a movie but how can something so beautiful as two bodies intertwining cause so much joy, pain, guilt, disease, and death?"

***

The second semester at Rider, I roomed with my friend Christine. She was studious and funny with librarian-like glasses, mousy brown hair, creamy skin, and freckles. I thought her study habits would rub off on me and help me to be a better student. She also intrigued me because for all her shyness, she somehow managed to snag a hunky, older, Italian boyfriend. We ate all our meals together, studied together, and spent hours talking and listening to music. She was a good influence on me, and she was one of the first women at school I spent time with because I genuinely liked her. I hung out with other roommates not because I liked them but because I just didn't want to be lonely.

We moved my things out of Centennial and into Wright. This dorm was also women-only, but it was much livelier. Most women in Wright liked to break the rules and I was surprised by this on several occasions, including the time I walked into a shower stall as a dorm mate and her boyfriend were exiting it.

Meanwhile, Christine and I went to bed at a decent hour while most everyone else stayed up all night and partied or crammed for their next day's exams. My brain had difficulty retrieving information from my short-term memory, so I was never able to cram for exams and resented that I had to spend so much additional time studying while everyone else was having fun.

A few months after Christine and I moved in together, there came a week where she completely ignored me. Our friendship was at an impasse. She abruptly decided that she couldn't live with me anymore and that she was moving out. She said that our differences were too great and that she was on the verge of a nervous breakdown and had severe depression. The last thing she ever said to me was "You're driving me to drink."

I didn't understand that Christine's response to me had little to do with me, but I'd never been treated so callously; she simply handed me a sheet of paper to sign acknowledging her move out. I was left to find a new roommate. I bawled my eyes out for the second time that week.

I called my mom expecting empathy and was stung by her lack of it. I couldn't believe she accused me of being selfish and of not thinking of the effect that my actions had on others. I knew that, in this instance at least, she was wrong. To me, Christine's vitriol came out of nowhere and caught me totally off guard. I felt mortally wounded. I didn't know how I'd rebound.

The experience was so painful that it contributed to the disliking of my own sex for years. It also resulted in me becoming even more of a "guy's gal." I felt safer with men. I didn't identify as a man, but I certainly didn't want to be associated with cattiness, manipulation and other traits ascribed to the kind of woman who is quick to throw her own sex under the bus if it means she'll land in a man's good graces.

D-I-S-A-B-I-L-I-T-Y

I thought I'd find a sweet college frat boy to date. I thought I'd join a sorority like my mom did at my age and go to pep rallies, football games, and homecoming. I envisioned becoming popular for more than wearing quirky hats. I assumed that Christine and I would stay besties forever, and that my learning disabilities would evaporate into thin air.

Although I was no stranger to feeling "less than," I hadn't felt so much "less than" due to my disabilities since before my Barrie days. I was surprised by how low I felt when I experienced rejection or felt inferior to others. I usually kept it all together but by the second semester of my sophomore year, keeping up a facade was too hard to do. I barely eked out passing grades after hours of grueling study. I lacked support, but I also refrained from seeking it out because I didn't want to be a "special case" yet again. It brought back too many painful memories of all the years I spent in special education classes.

But it was obvious to both my math teacher and me that I couldn't pass the exam, not even with all the studying in the world. It took being beaten academically and emotionally before I sought help.

I was in full-on crisis mode by then. After weeks of tutoring for my Finite Math class, the Math Lab Director dispassionately informed me that I needed to retake the test. I was told that if I didn't pass it, I'd have to drop the class and enroll in a remedial math class. I retook the test and doubled my score, but I didn't pass.

I ran to the disability's advocacy center on campus in hysterics. The Learning Disabilities Specialist grilled me about my academic struggles. The sheer number of questions she asked me overwhelmed me. I was given the accommodation of being tutored specifically to retake the types of questions I answered incorrectly on the exam. I was given another week to prepare and take the test one last time. I just barely passed.

I needed to escape.

Luckily, I went on my ISP trip to Jamaica shortly afterward.

CHAPTER 10 – POETESS OF PROTEST

I got my first retail job and began saving up for the spending money I'd need for trips to Jamaica and Israel. My mom and DP still gave me some spending money, as did my dad and Ona for a while—that is until I accidentally let it slip that my mom and DP were supplementing my needs, too. Then poof—my dad and Ona stopped sending me any money.

My West Coast parents' retraction of "fun money" was a bone of contention. My mom and DP couldn't really afford to contribute to my penchant for pizza, mozzarella sticks, CDs, and clothing. Meanwhile, my dad and Ona were in decent financial shape at the time and could afford to help me out. My dad was still obligated to pay child support for Stacey, and he had agreed to split the cost of my tuition with my mom and David.

Unfortunately, my dad's reneging on financial promises, including child support, wasn't anything new. He bought us clothes sometimes when he saw Stacey and I for our visits, but he didn't care about paying for anything else. I don't think he realized that his designs to fuck with my mom and DP made Stacey and me suffer as well.

I was working, so his decision not to help me out wasn't financially as hurtful as it was emotionally taxing. Then, he skipped out on his portion of tuition the last semester of my senior year. I had to take out a loan, which put me in debt, and even that wasn't enough to cover tuition. If DP's elderly parents hadn't come to my rescue, I wouldn't have been able to finish college. My dad knew that Elsie and Sam paid my last semester's tuition but expressed no remorse for bailing on his financial obligation to me. In fact, he coldly told me over a pay phone conversation, "Rach, I gambled your tuition money on a business deal and lost. Sorry, kid. I don't have it. You might need to drop out."

At least I had a job to be able to clothe and feed myself so I could take a little bit of pressure off my parents. I thought working at a store made me more grown up. Plus, 5, 7, 9 (the store I worked at) was geared toward petite sizes, so I got employee discounts on clothes meant for "short stuff" like me. The mall was a fun environment to work in and

I learned new skills such as making small talk, something I'm still not fully comfortable with or understand. My bosses praised me for my work ethic, which helped me build self-esteem. Also, work kept my mind occupied and helped to make me feel connected to others. This, too, is something I've always struggled to feel.

Jamaica

I was more excited to spend time with people I thought were cool than I was about spending time on a tropical island. I had been waiting to have a true college experience that I could regale others with at frat parties and at family holiday dinners. The part of me that was enthralled by reggae music won out over the part of me that wanted to play it cool. I was excited to study. I couldn't wait to learn more about reggae. I already listened to Bob Marley, UB40 and Steel Pulse.

Studying Rastafarian culture sounded interesting too. I knew what dreadlocks looked like because Lenny Kravitz had them and he was hot. By association, dreadlocks were hot. But I had no clue what a Rasta really was. We were a white, white group studying and temporarily living amidst predominantly mahogany and onyx colored people. Suffice it to say that we stood out as tourists and Rasta wannabes. We were a band of perpetually horny young women and dudes with maybe the exception of our two senior teachers.

I think they were hot for one another, but I could've been reading into it because one of them was a white, female minister and the other was her best friend, a black, male professor. He was the only person of color in our group, but he wasn't Jamaican. We stayed at the agricultural center in Ocho Rios, which was a riot of tropical fruit trees and bodacious hibiscus. I'd never tasted fruit so sweet.

The agricultural center also housed free roaming chickens and goats. I hoped they were pets, but they were not. I discovered this one day while everyone else was off exploring, I'd stayed behind to get some "me time." I was peacefully reading for class when I was startled to hear a foreboding bleat. I refused to eat meat at dinner that night. I knew why the goat had been in distress. I barely made it through the meal because I was crying. Everyone else laughed it off and ate goat meat. It was a small affair given everything else I'd cried over in my lifetime, but it was yet another reminder that I was different, more sensitive than others. I felt sorry for myself and silly for crying over a meal.

We were ostensibly studying, but we spent our days hanging out at the beach and our nights dancing at rooftop dance clubs. I laughed more than I ever recall laughing before. There was laughter woven into the fabric of daily life in Jamaica. It was so different from our lives in the States, where everyone took themselves so seriously. It was liberating to laugh, dance, eat and sunbathe and just feel *irie*. I discovered a delicious tropical cocktail called a Dirty Banana, a concoction of rum, Kahlua, and banana-flavored liqueur. I had a few every day and every night; I mostly had them virgin during the day as I still didn't see the point in drinking alcohol when it was sunny and when I felt happy. I was at my happiest when it was warm and sunny out. On the flip side, I associated alcohol with nighttime, frat parties, and boredom.

The gang decided that Hedonism, a trendy renowned resort, wasn't as cool as everyone had told us it was. Ours were the only naked nubile and virile bodies on display. There's nothing cool about being on a nude beach and having old wrinkly willys dancing jigs in our faces.

We decided to stick to the local bars and dance clubs of Ocho Rios. I never experienced dancing outside under the stars at rooftop clubs before. For me, that was sheer hedonism. Elaine, Stacy, and I all met "men" as opposed to "college dudes." For the first time in a long time, I felt like perhaps I could fit in. We partnered up with local men. I met a soft-spoken guy named Miller.

He ran a Jet Ski kiosk on the beach. I caught his eye one day while I was walking along the beach. When I saw him the second time, he called out to me and asked me to go Jet Skiing with him. Always game for trying new things, I eagerly followed Miller into the shallows. What could be so bad about holding onto the back of a strange man while speeding along in potentially shark-infested waters? My hormones overpowered my fear of being chum.

I was drawn to Miller's dark skin and brilliant, straight white teeth. He was so soft-spoken that everything he said sounded sexy. We jumped waves and giggled and went for a swim to cool off in the ocean, but things became heated instead. I didn't know what was going on until "it" happened. I was caught up in the romanticism of being in Jamaica with a Jamaican and living daringly. I relished the feel of Miller's warm body as he embraced me in the tepid, azure ocean and I enjoyed seeing and feeling his muscled dark arms enclosed around my sun-kissed skin. I had only been in waters so crystal clear when my family and I were in Cancun. The clarity of the water contrasted with the murkiness of my thoughts.

I really didn't know what I was doing or what I was expected to do. I thought, "*Should I initiate more? Will he respect me if I do? Does he respect me now?* My brain was as busy as a beehive. I should've been more in the moment. My monkey-mind prevented me from recognizing that what I thought was a finger probing inside my bathing suit wasn't. Once again, sex just sort of happened to me and I just went with it because I didn't know what else to do. There was no protest.

I was upset with myself because without my willing it, my confusion and anger morphed into excitement. We weren't that far from shore and there were onlookers that could easily have seen us from their hotel balconies. They wouldn't have needed binoculars to see what we were up to. I'd never done anything so risky. The prospect of being discovered was exhilarating. It was more exciting than the sex itself.

First, it was sex in the water. Later, it was literally sex on the beach. The latter was rough and gritty—not all it's cracked up to be. It was also the first time someone put me on my knees with my back to them and it was such a vulnerable position to be in. I was pleased with myself for having pivotal explorations in womanhood. They made me feel more mature and less naive. Having had the experience knowing it didn't mean anything more than casual sex was something that didn't sit well with me. It took me to dark recesses within myself that made me feel unloved, all alone, and ashamed of my sexuality.

I'm almost embarrassed to admit that I dove into the rest of my Jamaican experience with much more gusto than the rest of my classmates. I was gently teased for my nerdiness. I've always loved to learn. I was enthralled with reggae culture, which I knew little about previously. I read *Catch a Fire: The Life of Bob Marley* and dug into our assignments about Marcus Garvey and his ideal of repatriation.

I found the concept fascinating because the resettling of the descendants of slaves and refugees back to their mother land of Africa didn't seem that different from my Jews who made Aliyah to Israel after the Holocaust. In fact, I was stunned to learn that a people other than the Jews, considered themselves to be G—d's Chosen People. Rastafarians even sort of kept Kosher by not eating pork or shellfish or milk. They grew their hair out and coiled it into dreadlocks to honor the part of the Bible that says, "They shall not make baldness upon their head."

The songs of Rastafarianism and Jamaican society at large were songs of war and redemption, much like many of the songs of my own people. The roots of reggae music ran deep, and I hadn't understood that for all my previous listening to Bob Marley and Peter Tosh. I felt a deep connection to the music.

Music speaks to my soul in the same way that the protest songs of the 1960s do. In an era where songs like *The Train* and *Ice, Ice Baby* were prevalent, reggae's lyricism was largely pure poetry. The downbeats of drums and bass guitar, the happy feelings it stirred in me, the combination of hoarse voices of Jimmy Cliff, Peter Tosh, and Steel Pulse. I loved how the mellow vibe was penetrated by staccato, soprano scatting and bursts of wild, raw emotion. But above all, I loved the lyrics and the political overtones of the songs—especially Bob Marley's.

I was into Bob Marley before going to Jamaica, but I didn't know much about reggae culture. I didn't know its roots were in ska. I listened to music influenced by ska like Save Ferris without knowing what it was. Studying about Bob Marley's songs in Jamaica took on new significance to me. When he sang about "Buffalo Soldiers," I understood he was referring to African Americans who fought in the Civil War.

I appreciated on a deeper level the social injustices and war that Marley and other reggae artists sang about. I identified with being part of a culture that has been misunderstood, stigmatized, and even misappropriated. I admired the chutzpah reggae artists possessed. I hadn't yet smoked marijuana but was behind the political sentiment of songs promoting its legalization and decriminalization. I even wrote a college paper on this contentious subject.

Babylon to Bible Land

Rider's study abroad program was odd. It allowed students with good grades to go to sophisticated places like Italy and Spain while the options for students with only average grades like mine were limited. The school's system of country allocation didn't make sense. My only choices for studying abroad were in Middle Eastern countries. I reasoned that the only safe choice for me was Israel, where a second intifada was happening. It was September 1991, the beginning of the first Gulf War. There might've been another safe option, but I also chose to return to Israel because I had an ulterior motive: to redeem myself with Bono – to make him fall in love with me.

I returned to Israel and lived there for five months studying and working in Nahariya and Haifa. I flew there without knowing anyone I would be traveling with this time. I resided for nearly three months at Kibbutz Beit HaEmek, close to the northernmost coastal town in Israel. It was about an hour's drive south of the Lebanese border.

Apart from reuniting with Bono, I was looking forward to learning conversational Hebrew as opposed to prayer-book Hebrew. The kibbutz I resided on was settled by Dutch and South African colonizers, so everyone there spoke English or Afrikaans as their primary language—even many of the Israelis. I was taught to speak Hebrew by Abner, a tall and rotund, pale Israeli. In addition to Hebrew and English, he also spoke Mandarin Chinese. I found it amusing as I hadn't given much thought to people from other countries learning foreign languages.

Abner was strict and rule-abiding. He told us that if we were more than three minutes late to class, he wouldn't let us in. I never intended to be late but couldn't always get myself together on time. I arrived at class a few times to find that the door was indeed locked.

Free from class, I'd walk out the kibbutz's main gates and hop a cab into Nahariya. I loved those solo escapades. It was nice to get away from the chatter and bustle of my fellow kibbutzniks and it was exhilarating to be on my own. I enjoyed the peace and solitude of the ocean and the freedom to meander to nearby cafes and restaurants, sip coffee and watch people.

One time coming back from the beach, I got in a cab with a taxi driver who was friendlier than I'd expected. I don't know how the swarthy driver conned me into sitting in his front seat. I was happy to make small talk but was caught off guard when he reached over and laid his hairy palm on my thigh then moved it to cover my left hand with his. I recoiled and told the driver in clearly articulated Hebrew that my boyfriend was in the Israeli Army and that he was big and strong. *Why did I think that would matter to him or help me to get out of the predicament I was in?* The balding, gap-toothed driver tried to pull my head close enough to his lips to kiss mine. I popped the lock on the door and jumped out. It wasn't moving quickly as we were already slowing down for my drop off, but I didn't wait for him to stop.

I roomed with two other Americans, Aubrey, and Janice. Our dorm was close to the pool and the abandoned play structure on the barren field. Aubrey was a petite, lovelorn brunette. She had a freckled face and always wore her hair in double braids, reminiscent of Pipi Long-stock-ings, albeit without her unique fashion sense. Aubrey couldn't have been more than 23, but she complained like an old yenta. "My nails will get chipped! I'll be too sweaty! My fiancé this, my fiancé that!" My inner commentary track turned on: *Get a grip; you're on a frigging kibbutz to work! Who needs nails?*

Aubrey listened to the *Robin Hood: Prince of Thieves* theme song by Bryan Adams at least 10 times a day. And she reminded Janice and me daily that it was her and her fiancé's special song. When Aubrey wasn't looking, I rolled my eyes at Janice or she hastily mimicked shoving her finger down her throat, fake gagging on sappiness.

Janice was the opposite of Aubrey. She was both a tomboy and a bombshell with unruly, brunette curls, equally wanton freckles, and big eyes that melted many male hearts with a wink. Plus, Janice had a laugh that was incongruously large, despite her model-like figure. Janice was a world full of contradictions. She was feminine and knew how to apply her wiles, yet she was also rugged, wiry, and incredibly strong. Plus, she spoke five different languages. She's the kind of woman every woman wants to hate but can't help falling a little in love with.

I adored her despite how envious I was of all the attention she got from both men and women. She didn't eat anything in the cafeteria or in front of others except for the lychees she picked during her work shifts. People assumed that she starved herself, but that wasn't the case. I took it as my sworn duty to protect her from anyone who pried into her eating habits. As a woman with a bit of cushion for the pushin', I knew what it was like to have body issues. I knew her secret. She was a changeling.

While the rest of us slept, Janice morphed into a hummingbird who flitted from one flower to the next looking for nectar. Her weakness was sugar and peanut butter and candy. Whenever she ate too much sugar (e.g., a whole jar of jelly), she couldn't rouse herself from her stupor the next morning. I didn't want to see her get into any trouble for being late to her work assignment; I know a bit about lateness too.

Janice was like a bear in torpor in the mornings. Whether she'd eaten too much the night before or not, I became her personal alarm clock. Each morning, I hollered at her to wake up. I shook her until she opened her eyes and sat on my bunk opposite hers until I saw she had not only awoken but also got dressed and left our room. We had an unspoken pact. I kept her secret and woke her up. In return, she ran interference between Aubrey and me as the two of us weren't fond of one another. Janice also introduced me to people who wouldn't look my way otherwise. It worked beautifully.

Mornings on the kibbutz began as early as they do on American farms. Despite knowing this, I wasn't prepared to rise and shine at 4 a.m. each day before the roosters even crowed. I headed off to the greenhouse as soon as I knew Janice was out the door. I was the one who wanted to be a farmer. I even wore a pair of farmer-style overalls. It was an overall jean shorts singlet, which I wore with one shoulder strap unhooked and a tank top sans bra underneath. But it was Janice, the one who looked more like she could be a Tom Ford model, that was chosen for lychee and banana field duty. She stayed in the fields for the duration of our stay, whereas I was shifted to kitchen duty.

I think the Russian mama and papa that ran the greenhouse realized I was of little use to them. I love plants and I inherited Grandma Mary's green thumb. This was nearly eight years after my pre-bat mitzvah hedge trimming adventure, but my job in the greenhouse wasn't to plant; it was to untangle strand upon strand of twisted irrigation tubing. I also had to delicately separate baby tulip plants and set them ever so carefully into plastic trays. I did this all day long—and it was boring!

It's also possible that I was kicked out of the greenhouse because I asked too many questions while the Russians worked. I asked a lot of questions because they hardly acknowledged my presence. It drove me bananas. "What are these wires for? Why do I need to be so careful? What are you doing? Am I doing this right?" Every question was met with a singular shouted word, "Nyet!" or "Da!" I also did a short stint in the *Gan* or kindergarten.

I'm not sure why I was pulled from that assignment. I'm going with it having to do with a staff shortage in the kitchen. Finally, I had arrived! I have always loved being in the kitchen. I thrived there or, at least, did better there. I learned how to cut near-black eggplants into even slices by using a bread cutter. Evidently, they liked me well enough to trust me with this dangerous object. I didn't trust myself half as much. I learned to clean floors with a squeegee and to set up for breakfast, second breakfast, and early dinner—each meal with cucumber and tomato *salat* and little else. I was mercilessly teased for my naivete and lack of work experience by Margaret from Wales and Tsipora, a *sabra*, or native Israeli. It was okay, however, as I knew they only teased me because they liked me.

There really wasn't much to do on the kibbutz apart from work. I walked Beit HaEmek's fields; swung on the creepy, abandoned playground equipment; and sang to myself to keep from going insane. My saving grace was befriending the *Garin*, a group of Israelis who would complete their military service and then build and reside on their own kibbutz. They were vibrant, funny, and kinder than most of the other kibbutz residents my age. I ended up spending a lot of time with them swimming and dancing in the Israeli *moadon*. The men were ripped with six-pack abs and the women were exotic with untamed curly manes.

Get the Party Started

Two weeks before we were supposed to shift residences from Beit HaEmek to Haifa University, Janice went AWOL. She was the daughter of a successful lawyer from California and, though rugged, she'd decided she had had enough roughing it and needed a proper holiday. She used her dad's credit card to book a room at the Hilton in Tel Aviv and I went to visit her for a couple nights.

We had so much fun being two carefree young women. So long Abner, so long Aubrey, and good riddance, boring kibbutz in the middle of nowhere! Janice and I jumped up and down on the beds like little girls. We were so happy to have some freedom. We were ecstatic to sleep on real, soft beds with springs and proper bedding versus hard bunk beds.

We ate and drank everything in the minibar twice over. We went to the beach and flirted with men and had expensive meals out. I had so much fun that I decided to book a hotel room of my own. Only I wasn't an heiress. Janice wasn't really one either, but I thought so at the time. Room booked, Janice and I repeated the bed jumping and minibar scene with a different view. I had no clue that the minibar and room service weren't complimentary with the cost of the room. I'd never stayed in a hotel by myself before. My parents threatened to disown me because they had to wire me money.

Once ensconced at Haifa University, Janice and I shared a suite with two Israeli women. Ostensibly, we studied. We spent most of our time exploring Haifa, Mt. Carmel, and Hadar. Many mornings we got up and jogged all the way down the windy main road that ended at Mercaz Horev, a local mall. We stuffed ourselves full of fruity crepes and then either browsed the shops or saw a movie. I remember thinking how cool it was that you bought movie tickets for assigned seats and watched commercials instead of previews before the showing.

I'll never forget the day Janice and I were browsing in the record store at Mercaz Horev when we first heard George Michael's song, "Mother's Pride," from his current album, *Listen Without Prejudice*. His voice was so mournful that it moved me to tears. It was surreal living in a country where there was compulsory military service.

I stood riveted as tears flowed down my cheeks. I listened to and thought of the soldiers I knew who were actively serving in the IDF. Soldiers like Bono, Ohad, Barak, Yishay and all those boys I knew at HSI, who were now young men in their early 20s and likely fighting during the second intifada.

I loved the time Janice and I spent at Haifa University. I can still picture the view from the top of the dorm all these years later. It overlooks the port below and with my unobstructed view, I could see water all the way to the horizon. The view at night was especially ethereal. The water was a calm, inky black blue. Above it, the city lights twinkled like fireflies far past Mt. Carmel.

Another favorite place that Janice and I used to explore was Switzeria Catana (Little Switzerland). It's a nature reserve located at the top of the university. It was just a short hike up the hill, then down into a lush, wooded area. We sang Harry Connick, Jr., lyrics and songs from the movie, *The Marrying Man*, including "Mr. Sandman" and "Let's Do It." We belted these tunes at the top of our lungs. We laughed without a care in the world.

One day, Janice and I decided to picnic in a verdant copse in the park that is known as Churshat HaArbaim, or "The Grove of the Forty." Our Druze friend, Zait, informed us it is a sacred site for his people. I could see why it was holy. It was awe inspiringly beautiful. We spread a large picnic blanket and took turns reading aloud from what was still my favorite book, *The Princess Bride*. We were sprawled out, lounging, and eating grapes, when suddenly, an Israeli soldier walked right through the middle of our blanket, M-16 in hand. He didn't stop or break a smile. His face was impenetrable and expressionless. He quickly left, disappearing as if he'd been a mirage.

The eeriness of our interrupted picnic made us question things. *What if the other pieces of information Zait told us were true. Was our favorite place really a hiding place for members of the PLO? What if men were lurking in the woods solely for the purpose of luring women away?* We weren't sure, but we didn't go back by ourselves again.

Although Janice and I were thick as thieves, we didn't spend all our time together. I also loved spending time with my best guy friend, Dave. He was built like Jean-Claude Van Damme from the waist down and had that same high-rise kind of tush. Dave was a sweetheart disguised in a bad boy facade. He was the kind of guy friend every gal wishes for.

I went on an epic adventure with him and our mutual friend, Mark, for Hanukkah break in 1991. The three of us took a bus trip to Eilat and Dahab, Egypt, just across the Israeli border. The three of us boarded a bus and traveled the length of Israel to Eilat. Eilat was beautiful, but we got there in the evening, and it was too late to swim. Dave wanted to "drink real beer like a real man," so we went to the oldest bar in town. While Dave and Mark had their beer, I went off to dance and have my own drink or two.

I cozied up to the bartender adjacent to the crowded dance floor. He made it clear that his name was Eagle, pronounced like the bird. Emboldened by alcohol, I asked, "What time do you finish your shift?" I had to wait two hours, so I danced alone while he looked on. I had never done anything so brazen before. I had sex on the beach with Miller in Jamaica, yes, but I didn't initiate it, nor had I known what I was doing. But I set this in motion. Who was I? Evidently, I was someone who had casual sex atop bales of dry, itchy hay used for stocking inventory in lieu of pallets.

The next morning, we boarded another bus bound for Dahab. It took two to three hours and then waited an interminably long time before we were cleared to cross the border into Egypt. I think Dahab is where Janis Joplin, Jimi Hendrix, Jim Morrison, and all beatniks go when they die. Dahab was alcohol-free because it's in an area largely populated by Muslims, but drugs were a different story. Hashish was everywhere, with little boys popping up hawking it around every corner.

We stayed in some tiny makeshift village huts. And by huts, I mean there were rattan-like doors which opened to rooms smaller than 10' x 10'. The only thing in these huts were adobe slabs that doubled as both benches and beds. There was a communal toilet outside that wasn't much more than a hole in the ground. For some reason, using it didn't bother me in the slightest.

Dahab was full of restaurants. They were open on all sides. We ate on slabs of adobe piled with pillows. The decor was like something out of Aladdin. Local men smoked out of shisha pipes, sipped Turkish coffee, and drank tea. Their camels (more tourist attractions than a mode of personal transportation) stood by outside enjoying some respite before returning to work.

On our first day in Dahab, one young guy yelled out to see if any tourists wanted to go to a place called the Blue Lagoon. It sounded intriguing, and he promised it was the best place to go swimming and snorkeling. I was game and mistakenly thought that Dave and Mark would be up for it too, but they wanted to find and smoke hash.

It turned out that no other tourists climbed into the unofficial tour guide's jeep. I was a young, blue-eyed, blond-ish haired Jewish woman alone with three strange men in a male-dominated part of the world. The other two men were the driver and navigator. They were dressed in full Muslim attire. Their heads were wrapped in white scarves, which obscured their faces. In hindsight, I realized that in addition to being religious garments, they are practical; they kept desert sand out of their eyes.

The young tour guide and I climbed into the back of the jeep and headed off. We drove and drove and then drove some more. We passed through undulating waves of desert bleached white as bone. There were miles of endless dunes stretched out in all directions. It was straight out of an Indiana Jones movie.

I was terrified. I was in the middle of nowhere in a jeep in the middle of a desert with strange men. Suddenly, the drivers motioned for the young man and me to get out of the jeep, which we did. They left us alone and drove off.

We walked for a bit and came to a narrow strip of the bluest water I ever saw. If this was a popular tourist spot, where was everyone? We spread out our towels, but a knot of doubt formed in the pit of my stomach. I realized that I had no way of knowing where we really were and there was nothing I could do but trust that I'd be okay.

We swam for a bit and then dried off in the hot desert sun. The young man, whose name I didn't know, massaged my back without asking me if it was okay. I didn't want him to, but he could do as he pleased because he was stronger than I was. I couldn't stop him and I was afraid to try. I calmly went with it. The only thing I remember him saying was "You're too trusting. I could kill you if I wanted to. No one would ever know or ever find you."

How I kept my cool, I have no idea. I think it had more to do with an innate survival instinct than it did with bravery. Thank G—d, I was stone-cold sober. I was grateful beyond belief that I didn't put myself in a position to make myself even more vulnerable than I already was. I don't know how much time passed, but suddenly, the Jeep driver and navigator reappeared and drove us back to Dahab exactly as the young man had promised they would.

I've done many dumb things in my life. That topped them all.

I later discovered that there are two similarly named but vastly different places: the Blue Lagoon and the Blue Hole. The latter is the deadliest dive site in the world. I was nearer to the latter.

The Blue Lagoon is where I went on another solo adventure. I had no fear about this excursion, as it was more populated. I was seduced by a local's promise that I could rent a horse on the beach and so I did. I galloped along the shore's compact wet sand just as I'd dreamed of doing since seeing *The Black Stallion* as a young girl. This was a dream come true. I had never felt more elated. I raced up and down the narrow strip of beach. It was just me and the *Black Stallion's* twin. It still stands out as one of my most cherished memories.

My next destination of note was St. Katrin, the oldest operating Christian monastery in the world. Dave, Mark, and I embarked on a pre-dawn hike, under a pitch-black sky. As we trudged up a never-ending hill where Moses supposedly had his burning bush moment, our eyes struggled to adjust to the darkness. Then, however, we saw shooting stars galore. I was so tired and still awestruck from our hike up the mountain that it was hard to take in the monastery. It was an ethereal experience. I still dream of returning to Dahab.

Owner of a Lonely Heart

What of Bono, the man I pined over all those long, lonely nights? I stayed with him on and off the few months I was on the kibbutz, but he visited me there only once and after much pleading. Margaret and Tsipora, my kitchen duty cronies, flirted with him shamelessly in front of me and he didn't mind at all. We walked around the banana and lychee fields on what I hoped would be a romantic stroll. However, he used our limited time together to encourage me to lose weight and to stand up straight. He told me that doing so made my chest look bigger and my stomach look flatter. He then begged me to give him a blowjob in the room I shared with Aubrey and Janice. I acquiesced. Afterward, he wanted little to do with me. He remained sullen and distant until his departure.

Bono lived in a tiny apartment that he shared with his mom, Yael. She had the bedroom and he slept in an adjacent room that had a sliding privacy screen but no real door to speak of. Their apartment was in one of Israel's most religious communities. Yael was in her fifties and cleaned houses for a living but wasn't in particularly good health. Whenever Bono left in the mornings to serve his military duties, she sighed deeply and sadly. We both keenly felt his absence during those interminably long days.

I was still groggy with sleep whenever Bono left the apartment early in the mornings. He gently awakened me by caressing my cheek. I quickly associated this endearment with abandonment, however, as he only ever touched me like this when he was about to leave. It was years before I let anyone touch my face in that way.

Yael tried to console me whenever Bono left by cooking chicken schnitzel. She knew it was one of my favorite foods. I accompanied her to cleaning gigs sometimes. It meant company for her and prevented me from going stir crazy in their tiny apartment.

One of the houses she cleaned belonged to the local Rebbe. I was taken by this adorable older man. He had a full, white beard and chubby cheeks that conjured up images of a Jewish Santa Claus. He was as jovial as Santa too. I hugged him and kissed him on his cheek upon leaving his home. Yael flipped out about this. I couldn't fathom why. How was I to know it was unlawful for a woman to touch another married Orthodox man, let alone a revered Rebbe? But the Rebbe just smiled and chuckled. He loved the genuine gesture of affection.

Bono and I had fun times, but they didn't matter. He broke my heart. He didn't know that by the time I was halfway through my Ulpan (Hebrew immersion course), I had learned enough Hebrew to understand him when he thought he was being covert. I overheard a whispered conversation one evening, which included *"Tevili nishikah. Gam ani ohev otach."* ("Give me a kiss. I love you too.") He sat on the edge of the narrow bed that I slept on and uttered those words to another woman, while I lay naked beside him. I couldn't believe it was possible to feel so hollow.

This was just a night after he uttered the ugliest words I ever heard, which left a permanent scar on my soul. I spent years fantasizing about how meaningful it would be to reconnect with Bono over evenings of tender lovemaking. I pictured the way it would be in my mind so many times. I thought he knew I wasn't over him and that I loved him or convinced myself that I did. I thought he cared enough about me not to hurt me.

I couldn't believe I was finally going to have sex with Bono. I still alternated between calling him this and his real name just as I did when we were in high school. My belly did somersaults on the night I was ready to give into what he always asked of me when we were teenagers. I straddled Bono, praying that our first time together would be special despite my misgivings. I'd never been on top before, so I didn't know how to move or set the pace. He curtly admonished me, "Go faster, go harder." He then rolled out from under me and clicked his tongue in a way that is so Israeli: "Tsk."

Instead of being kind and patient, he scolded me for being nervous and awkward. He callously told me that "all men want women to be good girls by day but whores in bed come nightfall." He laughed in derision at my ineptitude while I lay naked and vulnerable on top of him. I had never felt so belittled in my life. Although I wrote the poem below a year later, it evokes exactly how I felt at the time.

If I Were as Cruel as You

I always knew that you were as empty as all the masks you rejected.
I never was the ghost you believed me to be.
I just pretended because that's the only way you'd have me ...
As thin as the sheet you pulled over me at night.
I wanted to creep into your soul and rot.
You never would have gotten rid of me then.
You let my skeleton walk away.
You made your blood run through my veins eternally.
If I was as cruel as you,
I'd wish that you were dead.

From that day on, I vowed that I would be the best whore in bed I could be. I embraced becoming a Jezebel. I'd be the one with the power to inflict harm or induce lust in men—not vice versa. No man would ever laugh at me again.

Would I do it over again? Most likely. The lows were extremely low, but the highs were exhilarating. I know therefore many women stay in emotionally and physically abusive relationships, just like my mom stood by my father through 14 years of his infidelity and emotional abuse. I finally understood why it's hard to leave someone who makes you feel like you're going through the worst drug withdrawal. They wield the power to make you feel higher than you've ever felt. Feeling emotionally high was something I viscerally craved.

Lily Tomlin once said, "Reality is a crutch for people who can't deal with drugs." In my heavy drinking and pot smoking days later, I thought this statement was the epitome of hilarity. It was meant to be tongue in cheek, but for me, it was simply a matter of time before I learned to numb hurts like the one Bono caused by substituting reality for substance-induced stratospheres.

CHAPTER 11 – THE DEVIL & MARY JANE

I left my study abroad program three weeks before it ended near Christmas of 1991. I was heartbroken and homesick. It was hard to believe that only a couple of weeks before, I told my mom that I wanted to make Aliyah.

Time management has never been my strong suit, so I shouldn't have been surprised to learn that I checked in for my flight back home a day too late and literally a dollar short. I was miffed because I stayed up late just so I wouldn't miss my flight. I even told Janice and my friends exactly when my flight was: midnight. I should've shown them my ticket to verify I had my timing correct.

Nevertheless, belligerence is not a virtue. Somehow, I'd finagled a change in airlines from El Al to Delta and changed my arrival destination from Dulles to New York City. I was so desperate to get back home that I didn't even care that my parents were out of the country. I didn't pause to consider that Aunt Sister might not be at home in Yonkers. It was Christmas Eve. I did what I've done so many times before and since. Some would say I threw caution to the wind. I prefer to view it as taking a leap of faith like that saying, "Leap and the net will appear."

I got off the plane and wrangled my bags which were larger than I was. I couldn't afford a porter to transport my luggage and I certainly couldn't carry everything. I bummed a dollar from a fellow female traveler. I dragged and heaved my luggage onto the $1 schlep-your-own-shit cart to the nearest pay phone and placed a collect call to my aunt. Mercifully, she answered and here's how that conversation went:

Me: Hi Aunt Sister. It's me. I'm here.
Long pause
Aunt Sister: Rach? What do you mean you're here?
Me: I'm here—in New York.
More silence
Exasperated Aunt Sister: Rach, are you at LaGuardia or JFK?
My inner monologue: SHIT!

My external dialogue: I don't know. I'm at the big airport. The one you usually go to when you're closer to the city.
Aunt Sister: Rach. Don't go anywhere. Stay exactly where you are. I'll be there in 30 minutes.

Odd Couples

I returned to college after Christmas Break and pleaded with my parents to advocate for my getting a single room in yet another dorm. I had gone through a few roommates, and they were all odd. One blew her nose all the time and constantly moved it around in circles like a mouse to get her glasses to sit more securely on its bridge. And another roommate had a strange little boyfriend with bowed legs and a long mullet. My few other girlfriends and I cruelly dubbed him "Troll." He and my roommate were always on again, off again. I didn't much like "on again" because it meant Troll was around a lot more. But "off again" was worse because my roommate not only pined for him then, but also played sappy Phil Collins music all day and night long. She was a nice person who I considered a friend, but I was tired of roommates.

My parents were successful in their campaign, and I got a single-occupancy room. This time, I moved out of Wright and into Hill House. I was pleasantly surprised that this dorm was coed. On my floor, there were alternating male and female dorm rooms. My single room was located at the end of a hallway. The wall my bed rested against was the backside of a common sitting area, which was across the hall from the women's bathroom. Like Fonzie from *Happy Days*, I utilized the restroom as an unofficial therapy office. And sometimes, I was the one who received therapy from my girlfriends.

On the other side of me were John and Joe. Next to them were Amy and Alicia. They were the only ones who lived in a suite. It was like an apartment in comparison to everyone else's cinder block hobbit houses. Across the narrow hallway from all of us, were Linda and Stacey and Heather and Leia. We all became fast friends. Not only had I found heaven on earth in the guise of a coed dorm, but I also finally found my tribe. It seemed fated that we would forge friendships over our mutual love of music.

John, Joe, and I connected over our reverence of the original Van

Halen, Mother Love Bone, and all the metal-punk-grunge bands from the movies *Singles* and *Point Break*. Stacey and I bonded over our shared love of Nirvana and Pearl Jam. I thought Kurt Cobain was sexy but was drawn more to the looks of Michael Hutchins of INXS and was head over heels for Soundgarden frontman Chris Cornell. Stacey, on the other hand, was infatuated—I mean totally OBSESSED— with Eddie Vedder. She cried whenever she saw him in videos or magazines.

Leia and I shared a passion for Erasure and 10,000 Maniacs. It was she who redeemed R.E.M. for me. If I never heard "Stand" or "Shiny Happy People" again, it'd be too soon, but Leia turned me onto "Radio Free Europe" and "Don't Go Back to Rockville," which I was surprised to learn was about the town one over from my hometown.

Amy and I were gob-smacked with Nine Inch Nails and Ministry. We often hung out just the two of us in her room, headbanging and spinning around like long-haired, laughing, Kewpie dolls.

As for Alicia and Linda, they were "Jersey Girls' ' through and through, and we shared a love of, unsurprisingly, Bon Jovi and other Garden State favorites. Their only non-Jersey concessions were Meat-Loaf and ABBA.

I Kissed a Girl (or wanted to)

My junior year of college is when I began to inwardly acknowledge my attraction to women. When I was 13, I had a friend named Robin. We pilfered my stepdad's Penthouse magazines every chance we could. We riffled through the glossy pages together and tried to imitate the women's poses. We took turns sitting naked atop one another, but we didn't do anything else. And I didn't really think about women sexually again until I met Leia.

Leia embodied voluptuousness and earthiness. Her goddess vibe was endearing. I really wanted to experiment with her. She knew it and toyed with me. Her best friend was gay, and I couldn't figure out if she were heterosexual or not because she was an equal opportunity flirt. We showered together once but apart from that, nothing happened between us.

I also wondered what it would be like to date Amy. I was attracted to her in a different way than I was to Leia. I didn't know what it said about me that I found her attractive because what initially brought us together as friends wasn't music but a shared sworn devotion to Marcus Schenkenberg, a hot male model.

Amy was short and quirky like me, yet she embraced her ditziness. I was afraid of being type-cast. I worried about my ditziness all the time. My parents and friends adored me but always mislabeled my otherness as being ditziness. I was admittedly an airhead, but it was by design — not by choice. I didn't have any luck when it came to dating guys in college and I didn't have a clue as to how one looked for a woman to date. Plus, even if I had dated Amy, I wouldn't have known how to talk to my parents about liking her when I knew I was still very much attracted to men. I stuck to the safety of our friendship and left my musings about sex with women in the confines of my journals.

Alicia hailed from an Italian American Catholic family. She and Stacey were both devout. Stacey giggled and apologized whenever she let a swear word slip but not Alicia -- she cursed worse than a sailor. Alicia was uncouth yet a genius. She knew a little bit about everything and everyone. I was drawn to her dualities. Plus, she was friends with *all* the guys. She, Amy, and I spent a lot of time driving to Wildwood in Alicia's sweet little CRX.

Of all my college friends though, it was Heather who was the most like me. She was also Jewish and was similarly brought up in the Reformed traditions. She was also zaftig like I was, but even more so. We also both suffered from low self-esteem. However, Heather had less of a sense of self-worth. She apologized for everything, all the time. Our entire floor lovingly yelled at her because she mumbled, "Oops, I'm sorry" a million times a day. She apologized for not wearing a cool enough belt or for simply waking up in a happy mood in the mornings. Heather was a ray of sunshine—always positive and bubbly in the face of everyone else's cynicism.

The Devil's in the House of ...

I was yakking in the room Stacey shared with Linda. We were on her bunk schmoozing about who knows what when Linda walked in and joined us. The conversation turned to our upcoming spring break. Linda asked us what our plans for Easter were. We already knew that Stacey would spend time in church. Stacey was genuinely religious, but she spent most of her time praying the Rosary and going to church each Sunday because she hated this life and fervently hoped that her devotion would bring her better karma in the next life.

When Linda asked me what I was doing for Easter, I replied, "No clue. I don't celebrate it." Incredulous, she asked, "Why not?" and I blithely replied, "I'm Jewish. Jews don't celebrate Easter. We celebrate Passover." Linda looked at me, mouth agape, then asked, "Where's your tail and horns?"

Now, it was my turn to respond incredulously.

My what? You can't be serious! What I actually said was, "I tuck my tail into my pants and my horns are detachable. No, I'm joking! I don't have a tail and horns! Have you never met a Jewish person? You live one state away from New York. You know, where there's delis and bagels and knishes ….

Linda grew up in an Irish Catholic household and was evidently both very sheltered and lied to. I introduced her to Jewish holidays and ethnic foods. In turn, she introduced me to Mad Dog 20/20 and Killian's Irish Red.

Linda had an older boyfriend named John, who wasn't in school and didn't work. This befuddled me as my parents had raised me to believe that adults either studied or worked. When I admitted my confusion to Linda, she laughed and remarked, "He's a professional drinker." In response, I exclaimed, "Oh, that's cool! So he's like a sommelier?" Linda confessed she didn't know what that was, but before she added more, I noticed that her face had become ruddier than usual. "No. He's an alcoholic."

Linda explained that John lived in a halfway house and was trying to get sober. He wasn't succeeding at it. I thought alcoholics were all men who stood around on street corners and drank out of bottles wrapped in paper bags. My mom often referred to my dad as a "functional alcoholic" and I laughed in agreement because his fondness for alcohol wasn't something he ever hid, but I'd never considered that, like John, my dad might be a "professional drinker."

I thought back on my times visiting my dad and realized that I had only seen his hands hold something besides a drink when he was either gardening or smoking cigars. However, I never saw him throw up, nurse a hangover, or need to be sent away from home like John to try not to drink.

My conversation with Linda made me uncomfortably aware of alcohol. I thought about how often everyone in my friendship circle drank. I hadn't drunk socially until I went to college, but I had been drinking more since moving into my new dorm and hanging out with my new friends than I had during my first two years combined. I often worried that I drank too much, but everyone else drank much more often and much more amount-wise than I did. What usually happened was that I either got bored with a party and left, drank until I felt too sleepy to drink more, or didn't drink some nights that others did.

On a few occasions, I did too many sambuca or kamikaze shots and ended up crying that I didn't want to drink like my dad. Stacey or Alicia would rub my back and chuckle saying, "Rach, don't be silly. You drink the least of all of us. Sometimes, you just don't know when to stop doing shots." Their reassurance made me feel better. I would console myself with the knowledge that I wasn't a big drinker or an alcoholic. Alcoholics looked like John, maybe my dad, and certainly my friend Laura—or rather my ex-friend Laura.

Laura was brilliant but was what most people would call "rough around the edges." She wore a daily uniform of a stained tie dye shirt and frayed sweat shorts or jean shorts. Her long dirty blond hair was unkempt and always center-parted; pulled back in a tight ponytail at the nape of her neck. I'm forever grateful to her for introducing me to Crosby, Stills, Nash and (sometimes) Young, as well as The Grateful Dead. But that preceding the spring break from Hell (but still before Linda asked if I had horns and a tail).

We went on a road trip to Fort Lauderdale during my sophomore year's spring break. We drove in my Chevy Celebrity down to Pompano Beach because Grandma Harriett was out of town having her own adventure with her boyfriend Morrie. The two of them were hip and enjoyed traveling the world together well into their mid-seventies. Pompano wasn't Miami, but I was glad that Laura and I were anywhere but Rider.

She knew that I had no sense of direction and couldn't read a map to save my life, but she got trashed every night, rendering her unable to navigate. It was unfortunate because she had a photographic memory. One night I got completely turned around in a sketchy suburb of Fort Lauderdale. Laura had drunk so much that she passed out in the back seat, so I was essentially alone. I stopped and asked the only person I saw on the street for directions. The woman spoke no English, nor did she speak Spanish or Hebrew, the two languages I can speak enough in and understand well enough to get by. I'm not sure if she held out a plastic baggy containing a white powdery substance out of pity or if she was trying to sell it, but I didn't want it. I just wanted to get us back near the horse racing track because I knew my grandma's apartment was on a golf course almost directly across from it.

Then, toward the end of our break, we agreed to drive from Pompano to Daytona so that Laura could visit her uncle. She hadn't seen him in a long time and she was a bit nervous. She warned me that her uncle was nice, but also a rough guy. She surprised me by saying that she wasn't sure how her uncle would react to me. Maybe she was worried that her uncle would think we were a couple? I didn't think much of it nor could I as I was once again driving us to yet another bar.

I still couldn't fathom why anyone would want to be indoors drinking in the middle of the afternoon on a gorgeous, sunny day. I wanted to swim in the ocean and search for seashells like I always did when I lived in Florida. Call me Pollyanna, but I loved the ocean and back then, there were still plenty of beautiful, intact conchs and whelks to be discovered. Since Laura hadn't had a drink yet, we made it to Daytona without incident, but Laura wanted to go to a biker bar. I wasn't too bothered by all the Harleys outside the shack.

But inside, Confederate flags hung everywhere. I grew up in Maryland, one of the northernmost of the former slave states and still considered by some to be "the South," but I had never seen a Confederate flag before. They made me uncomfortable. But they didn't make me feel as skeeved out as seeing bras and panties strewn all about the rafters. I wondered why anyone would want their undergarments to be displayed publicly like that. Did the ladies with the missing underclothes even know they were hanging from rafters in Daytona? And why would anyone want to drink staring at bras and panties for decor? Surely if bikers spent all that money on beer, the establishment could afford nicer decorations.

I hadn't met a biker before, but I was confident they were just over-grown frat boys in leather. They beer-goggled just like the college guys I knew. Nevertheless, what kind of friend brings a naive, underage, Jewish woman to a biker bar? I positively crawled in my skin. I was too morti-fied to call my mom. Nope. I was with a tough chick, and I resolved to be open-minded like Laura. I'd survive—and besides, maybe Hell's Angels were like Three Musketeer bars: hard on the outside but soft and mushy on the inside.

Sufficiently liquored up, Laura was ready to visit her uncle, so we headed to his house. We'd been there for no more than an hour when Laura decided that we should look around her uncle's room. I thought it seemed weird to snoop around like that, but I followed her. I didn't want to be left alone with her uncle—especially if there was a chance, he didn't like me.

His bedroom was sparsely decorated with imposing and rich-ly stained wooden dressers. On top of one sat a porcelain figurine of a ghost. I exclaimed, "Look how cute! It's Casper!"

Laura was a stoner, hippie chick who usually sat immobile on her dorm room couch. I was caught completely off guard when she flew across the room as if the figurine had come to life. She pleaded, "Don't touch it! Rach, it's not Casper. It's KKK memorabilia."

Your uncle is in the Klan? I'm Jewish! Didn't you think I'd want to know this?

Only these words never left my mouth. I was too stunned and con-flict-avoidant. The possibility that her uncle wouldn't like me was evi-dently dependent upon whether I accidentally mentioned being Jewish. That was the litmus test? I was livid. I felt betrayed. Why didn't she just tell me to drop her off? I could've amused myself by going shopping at a mall or something. Anything made more sense than her knowingly bringing me to a house where my safety was compromised.

I mustered the courage to hiss through clenched jaws, "I'm driving us back home now. I'm stopping in Maryland and I'm going to spend a few days at home before going back to school. Sorry to cut our trip a few days short, but I'm done. I'll drop you off at Union Station in DC and you can take the train or bus back to school from there."

We drove back with nothing more than the music we loved in common. I don't remember if we talked during the two days' drive back. We never spoke again.

Hits from the Bong

I spent the rest of my college career with the friends I made in my coed dorm. We were misfits, stoners, and alt-rockers. Although I listened to Reggae and had spent time living in Jamaica, I had never tried marijuana before. In Hill House, everyone including the Resident Assistants smoked up. Ironically, I was the only one among my friends who knew what the fragrant plant looked like in leaf form.

I was already a social drinker. I figured there wasn't much more harm in becoming a social stoner (is that an oxymoron?). I didn't get high the first time I took hits from a joint. I coughed up a lung and it was embarrassing. I was frustrated because everyone else was in a happy headspace. I puffed some more and laughingly declared it a useless experiment. My friends pointed out that I had a shit-eating grin on my face and red, swollen eyes. Stacey snort-laughed, "Rach, you're higher than a kite." Much to my chagrin, I realized that I was.

Thereafter, I fell in love with Mary Jane and the ritualism of getting high. Nothing gave me the warm fuzzies like smoking pot did. The hard lines and borders of my world grew blurry. Everything felt soft and kind like a lullaby. There were no clearly defined margins to anything, and everything was punctuated with light and color. People seemed more interesting and even vapid subjects were profound. I despised the convention of making small talk and doing it stoned was so much easier.

I could never figure out how to inhale cigarettes and I didn't see why people would want to burn their lungs with harsh, chemical-laden smoke. I felt similarly about smoking joints. They were hard to roll, and I never got remarkably high off them. I couldn't get the hang of it and it made me feel stupid. Bong hits were my jam, though. I discovered I had quite the capacity for inhaling vapor through a tube.

Our RA didn't smoke pot with us, nor did she suspect that my friends and I were stoners. We were smart enough to alternate whose room we hung out in and we always lit incense which laid down over the smoke like DJ layers background sounds on tracks. To our delight, the RA assumed it was the swim team jocks who filled our hallway with thick, musky smoke.

I was bonded to my friends through our reverent communion with marijuana. We were part of a subculture and we relished that. Speaking in code—Mary Jane, M.J, weed, Purple Haze, kind bud, ganja, Sinsemilla, shrubbery—made us feel cool. We relished spending all our time together smoking and going on ethereal and literal trips together.

We were all tight, but Heather, Stacey, Leia, and I ended up spending most of our time together. Amy took some time off to attend to her mental health, and Alicia had grown distant after the unexpected death of her father.

Sometimes, we explored the woods and boulders just outside of Lambertville, New Jersey, before traipsing around New Hope, Pennsylvania. It amused us that our favorite nature spot was called High Rocks. I had climbed a few times and loved to watch the climbers on the rocks opposite our favorite perch.

One sunny day, we were sitting and sunning on the rocks when volunteer backcountry rescuers jogged towards us. They asked us if we saw two people fall off the rock face which, thankfully, we hadn't. They informed us that a mother and daughter were climbing when one of them slipped and fell over 100 feet. We were instructed to assist them by not moving or hiking back out downhill. The rescuers needed to ensure everyone's safety while they carried out an emergency rescue mission. We heard saws buzzing in the valley below us, followed by the crash of trees. The volunteers were joined by a professional search and rescue team. We watched in stunned silence as the crews rigged up a gurney attached to two lengths of climbing rope. Of course, we didn't see the gurney on ropes until it was a quarter of the way up the mountain.

We'd never witnessed anything like this, and we were shaken. We walked along the river and beside the railroad tracks so we could get high. We sorely needed to elevate our mood having just witnessed the aftermath of a climbing fall. We smoked up outdoors and then browsed the shops that lined New Hope's main strip as well as the town's more hidden side streets.

Before we drove back to campus, we paid homage to Now and Then (the local head shop) and Mystickal Tymes bookstore. Leia and I loved that shop especially as they sold tarot cards, sage bundles, and books on Wiccan and Shamanic practices. Leia was in a coven, and I longed to join her and be a good witch too. I was just a bit too skeptical to pursue it and too afraid that my parents would disown me if I did. I think a bisexual, Wiccan daughter would've been a bit too much for them.

While we were all good friends, I was primarily a loner. Marijuana and alcohol connected us at night, but daytime divided us. Underneath it all, I still felt different. Stacey and Linda both worked. Leia had her male friends who she was always on the phone with. Heather despised heat, dirt, and insects. I spent time alone outdoors. I spent a lot of time walking in the woods near campus, jogging, wandering through Quaker Bridge Mall, and taking solo road trips. During the daytime, it was easy enough to find things to do.

The Long and Winding Road...

I wasn't of legal drinking age until September of my senior year, but something changed upon my return from Israel. It wasn't biochemical in nature nor was it immediate. It might have been connected to trauma, but whatever its roots, the change was gradual.

I had a lot of stupid fun times with my friends. We drank and smoked pot and danced a lot. Even so, I felt different among even my closest friends. Most of them resigned to staying ensconced in New Jersey. They seemed content to graduate and return to the same jobs they had during high school. Only Alicia knew for sure what she was going to do post-graduation; she was bound for TV communications in New York City.

I had dreams that were so grand that I didn't know how to take my first steps toward making them a reality. I wanted to be a photojournalist for National Geographic or an environmental journalist. I wanted to see the world. I also wanted to move to San Francisco and live in the Haight and save the redwoods. I was hippie-esque, but I wasn't anti-establishment. I wanted to change the establishment without being remotely political. In other words, I didn't have a clue what my higher calling was, so everything sounded interesting. (This propensity toward becoming easily overwhelmed is a hallmark feature of ADD, by the way.)

Marijuana added color to these dreams, but it also kept me in the moment. It was my mind's unconscious attempt at mindfulness. I never liked being in my moments. I didn't know how to do it without marijuana. My mind raced because the world was too big, and time seemed too critical.

If I wasn't stoned, I would be stir-crazy. Einstein said, "Time is what prevents everything from happening all at once." My brain doesn't intuitively get time. I don't inherently know how to prioritize actionable items because everything seems equally important.

Marijuana slowed my mind down and prevented me from feeling an urgent need to create order out of entropy. If marijuana was my bosom companion who never let me down, alcohol was both a backstabbing friend and bad lover. Alcohol was wily and conniving. In fact, alcohol reminded me of my relationship with my father whenever promises made weren't kept. More than anything, I wanted to believe in alcohol's promise.

Everyone else on campus drank and seemed to have fun doing it. I thought drinking was stupid, but I did it anyway. In my experience, drinkers were too unpredictable. My dad's drinking both scared and scarred me. He was funny and raunchy enough without it. Depending upon what type of alcohol he imbibed, he could be mellow or lewd and lascivious. I could take Mellow Dad because he was calmer than usual. His degree of reserve bordered on vacancy. But Crass Dad said unretractable, misogynistic things to Ona or Stacey, such as "Fuck you, broad. Do what I say!" or "You women are all manipulative." When I visited him and Ona, he often embarrassed me in front of their dinner company: "Come on kid. Stick your chest out. Quit your moping. Go get me the carving knife."

I observed how drinking alcohol impacted my dad, as well as the male population on Rider's campus. They became reckless daredevils and clumsy dolts. They were too mouthy and handsy. To be honest, alcohol made Rider's females act stupid too. Apart from my friends and me who threw on jeans, boots, and low-cut, V-neck shirts to go to frat parties, most women were consumed solely with themselves when they consumed alcohol. They teetered in high heels, pulled at their skirts which were too short or too tight or both, and whined about the dumbest things. Gossip among women on campus was awful. I didn't see why most women had to put other women down to have fun or to stand out amongst the herd. I guess my thoughts on inebriated women weren't so different from my dad's views on my gender.

Rider had a few fraternities and sororities, as well as a handful of dorms. We had one pub, aptly named The Pub. The campus wasn't like the University of Maryland, which had restaurants and coffee shops. It was wedged in between tony Princeton and unsafe Trenton. As a result, my options for socializing without alcohol seemed limited. I started drinking more frequently during my sophomore year, but only drank intermittently and never in the daytime. I rarely drank during the week. If I needed to escape, there was always my go to gal Mary Jane. I could do that before bed and go to sleep peacefully.

Still, I began drinking in an uncouth way. It was Mad Dog 20/20, Bartle's & James, Ketel One vodka straight or mixed with Kool-Aid, and sambuca straight out of the bottle. I rarely drank beer. I thought Busch, Budweiser, Miller Lite and all other cheap beers available were vile. Beer was always my last resort.

I wasn't drunk that often and I never blacked out. I don't remember anyone holding my hair back over the toilet, but it must've happened at some point; it's a rite of passage for college coeds. I'm sure this only happened when I made myself throw up because I hated the feel of alcohol sloshing around inside my belly. One or two times, I recall crying, "I don't want to be like my dad or John."

I didn't get sick from drinking back then. In fact, the only time I recall being violently ill from drinking was the time Amy, Alicia, and I went to my third frat party. Alicia wandered off at some point, leaving Amy and me alone and clueless. The two of us decided we'd feel less self-conscious of being smaller than everyone else on campus if we grabbed drinks. There was a table manned by some frat dudes handing the ladies—and only ladies—Dixie cups full of red Kool-Aid spiked with Everclear. No one told us that that's what was in the punch beforehand. The dudes just assured us that the punch was good. It was, but only because it reminded me of the bug juice I used to drink as a camper at Camp Tockwogh. Not surprisingly, I drank mine in one gulp.

I instantly felt more tired than I was when I had mono. I went to the bathroom and decided that the floor was the perfect spot for a nap. I don't know how long I laid there. I don't think it was for too long before I was lifted by the strong arms of an unknown frat boy. I have a hazy recollection of him telling me I shouldn't be laying on the filthy floor. He whispered that he was going to bring me someplace nice. He brought me into his room and laid me down on a couch.

I was okay with him stroking my head over and over. It was comforting. He instructed everyone who came into the room to give me space and leave me alone, which was smart thinking as without any warning, projectile vomit shot out of my mouth in waves. I threw up so many times, I lost count. I'm surprised my intestines didn't come out through my mouth. Another frat guy informed me that someone had found my little friend (i.e., Amy) and we were escorted back to our dorm where we were told never to return to that frat house again, which I thought was harsh. They were the dumb boys who gave me Everclear and hadn't bothered to tell me what it was. I hadn't ever had anything that was 190 proof. I didn't even know what "proof" meant. Screw the couch I threw up on, it was shitty anyways. I wouldn't be reimbursing them for ruining their couch. I could've been raped had the guy who picked me up from the bathroom floor not been nice.

It only dawned on me recently that although I was positive, I only had that one drink at the frat party, I don't remember how much I drank before we got there. For years, I insisted that I only had that one drink. My drinking didn't make much sense to me even then. Nevertheless, it was easy to shift attention away from my drinking when everyone else around me drank so much more and more frequently.

***

By the winter of 1992, I was counting down the days until graduation. I was eager to leave my college days behind me. I debated whether I wanted to join the Peace Corps or find a job. I made it to the personal interview for the Peace Corps, the last hurdle before final applicants were selected. I was asked many hypothetical questions during my screening, including, "How would you respond if you taught English to children in a village and one of the elders smacked a child?" I gave the answer I knew they were looking for— "It's not my place as a Peace Corps volunteer to interfere with the customs of other peoples"—but in that moment, my decision was made.

I wanted to look for my first real job, but my parents forbade me from doing so. They decided that it was in my best interests to go to graduate school while I was still young. They added I'd be unlikely to further my education once I got a taste of what it was like to earn money. They insisted that I was too young and immature to work in "the real world."

Their overprotectiveness was exacerbated by the fact that our country was going through an economic recession. They feared I'd struggle to support myself. Their overprotectiveness conjured up images like those in Suicidal Tendencies' "Institutionalized."

In the end, however, I agreed to my parents' "suggested" detour. I still believed that my survival was dependent upon them. I was too afraid of the potential consequences of going against their wishes. What would happen if I knowingly disappointed them? Asserting my independence came at a price I wasn't yet emotionally prepared to pay.

CHAPTER 12 – HOP ON THE BUS

If I was going to go to more g—d damn school, it was going to be something more akin to Barrie. It had to be experiential and fun. There was no way I was going to spend more time trapped within cinder block walls.

My dad and I were in a close phase. We talked on the phone often and he and I still shared a love of the environment. He had been in the recycling industry for over 20 years by this point. The two of us enjoyed spending time together outdoors, whether it was walking through the city parks of Philadelphia, strolling along the beach in Miami, or down the quiet tree-lined streets of Palo Alto, where he and Ona relocated to a few years before.

My dad and I were both voracious readers, but our only shared genre was environmental periodicals. My dad's always supported causes he believes are intellectually fascinating. It was simply luck that fueled his support of my attending a graduate school program he had read about in E magazine. He thought it'd be cool if I attended "this hip graduate school on a bus" he'd seen an ad for. I was toying with the idea of pursuing environmental journalism and while what I'd later call "the Bus" didn't offer this as a degree, it would provide great source material to write about.

My father and I share genetic coding for novelty seeking. We get high off the new and the now of adventure. My dad doesn't do "new" in moderation and his enthusiasm is infectious. He instantly sold me on the promise of the adventure of earning a Master of Science in Environmental Education by exploring the country on a retrofitted school bus.

Audubon Expedition Institute was under the auspices of Lesley University in Cambridge, Massachusetts. The school welcomed undergraduate and graduate students alike to earn their bachelor's and master's degrees, while communing with nature and nature-loving folk. AEI's print tagline was "The environment is your campus." I applied and was elated when I received an envelope containing my invitation for an interview.

I had to drive to the school's administrative office in Belfast, Maine, for it. My dad was so excited for me/us that he flew out to New Jersey to meet me and drive up with me. It was like Steinbeck's *Travels with Charlie* minus the dog. Our road trip together was one of the few times I've gotten to spend quality time alone with him. I've often wondered if Ona limited the times I spent alone with my dad because she was jealous of how close we are. Ona and I have a rocky relationship. There's love between us, but hers is usually the tough love variety, which I've never responded well—no matter how well intentioned.

We took detours into Connecticut and Massachusetts so my dad could show me around both Mystic Seaport and Cambridge. It was important to him to impart his wisdom to me about places that were special to him in his youth. More importantly, he wanted to eat fresh, locally sourced seafood. I'm not a seafood fan, but it was a small price to pay for the scenery and the time spent with him.

Both of us were ushered into the interview with Colleen, the school's director. Like they had at Barrie, the staff at AEI went by first names only. I thought this made my introduction to the school more welcoming and less of an overwhelming prospect. We were stoked to learn about what traveling and living on a school bus would be like and were relieved to learn that the program was fully accredited. It would take me two years to complete graduate school. I would have multiple breaks over this period to complete requisite hands-on internships or field studies of my own design or choice. It was uncannily like Barrie in terms of placing value on students learning at their own pace in subjects they were interested in.

The bus drivers, or guides, were more like mentors than professors. Their role was to drive the bus and provide students with individual consultation and final grading. Additionally, they were instrumental in demonstrating how students could successfully learn and live in an egalitarian, consensus-based community; in other words, everyone had to agree to a decision when it affected the entire group.

Graduate students on the Bus would be free to set their own learning objectives, provided they met the overall academic goals of the curriculum. Students would travel by bus by day and sleep under the stars at night. Additionally, students were expected to plan and engage in at least two Bus-wide wilderness excursions per semester. Colleen explained that students were responsible for taking turns shopping for the community's provisions and cooking for everyone. They wanted to know if I was on board with these kinds of living and learning circumstances? Hell yes, I was! My classes would include:

- Philosophy of Education I
- Anthropology: Cultural Perspectives of Human Communities 1
- Overview: Natural History; and Ecological Theory 1
- Camping and Outdoor Education 1
- Applied Group Theory 1
- Systematic Investigation of Local Flora and Fauna

I spent the rest of the summer preparing for the Bus. I joined the REI cooperative and I shopped. I bought, I bought, and I bought. It was incomprehensible how unprepared I was for my upcoming graduate school adventure. Reading books for class was a no brainer for me since I've always loved to read, but the wilderness excursion part brought on a fresh wave of "camp stomach" (Stacey and I always got butterflies in our bellies the night before we left for summer camp or were about to engage in a great unknown) every time I thought about back-country camping. The items I needed to satisfy course requirements and wilderness excursions included:

- An internal frame backpack
- A small, lightweight tent
- Waterproof hiking boots
- Compression sacks
- A Thermarest pad
- Three Nalgene canteens
- Parachute cord (to hang bear bags, although I didn't know it at the time and I'm glad I didn't)
- A trowel (to bury or smear my poop; also, glad I didn't know its intended purpose ahead of time)
- Gators (What are they for? The only gators I was familiar with were the kind that live in Florida and I was sure I didn't need to purchase my own alligator. It turns out that they're waterproof chaps for your ankles intended to protect boots and feet from

getting wet while fording streams.)
• Two sets of Gore-Tex rain gear (I didn't even know what Go-re-Tex was.)
• A zero-degree sleeping bag (I was terrified of sleeping in the cold and prayed that this suggestion was just to make me cozier in my tent.)
• A tarp (I wish they had suggested three of these.)
• Camping utensils and a mug (I ended up using mine for everything from drinking hot chocolate, sipping soup, eating oatmeal out of, and washing my hair with.)
• Two headlamps (I referred to these as "dork lamps.")
• Moleskin (I hoped this had nothing to do with needing a mole's skin for anything. Turns out a thin but heavy cotton fabric that you can use to help with callouses and such.)

I'm sure I'm missing some things. My parents never forked out so much money for me in my life, but I was extremely grateful to them for funding yet another one of my misadventures. I was giddy with excitement and more than a bit nervous. The night before life as I'd known it ended, I got a bad case of camp stomach. With the Bus, I had no clue what to expect, so my stomach was in knots.

The next day, I departed for Portland, Oregon, to begin my first semester. I'd be exploring the ecosystems of the Pacific Northwest. I strapped on my extremely overloaded and top-heavy backpack. Then I trudged through the airport to meet my fellow campers/graduate school cohort. I was told I'd be traveling on a bus, but I didn't know the bus would be an old fashioned, yellow school bus with a white banner with "Audubon Expedition Institute" in big, bold lettering. I envisioned something more modern. The Bus had a set of black, metal steps attached to its rear which led to a roof rack on top. I wondered how I'd lug my stuff up all those steps. I thought, *what if I fell to my death?* I started to second-guess my decision.

There were some friendly women standing around the Bus, as well as a couple of older people who were maybe in their forties and fifties. I assumed they were our guides. There were also a few hot guys. *This isn't too shabby, Rach,* I thought. They were older than me but not too old. I mentally chastised myself, you're going to school, Rach —*not on a singles' adventure tour.*

A few people started up a game where they played soccer with what appeared to be a cat toy. I learned the teeny ball was called a hacky sack. I thought, *And* I'm a *hippie?* A few of the women had hairy legs and, oh my G—d, hairy underarms! *What am I doing here? I think I made a mistake.* I ignored my inner voice, which screamed *RUN!* Instead, I meekly introduced myself. We stood around for a couple of hours before we realized that school had begun.

Jeff, one of the hot guys, said, "I know of a co-op nearby." I didn't know what a co-op was, so I was already learning. Tracey, who was one of the pretty and cool-looking ladies said, "I know this area well and can tell you all about some campgrounds we could stay at."

At that, one of the guides motioned for everyone to hop on board the Bus, and in a mad dash, we all scrambled to find the best seat. I shoved my milk crate, which contained my journal, Walkman, hair dryer, and makeup under a seat toward the middle of the bus. I figured that the front would be uncool and the back too bouncy.

The Bus's interior resembled any other school bus, except for the last few rows of seating. Where rear seats usually are, the Bus had three large empty bins and three or four large, empty coolers. Above the bins and coolers on either side was a makeshift library full of books. There were novels, field guides, and reference books galore.

I was used to and could get on board with reading. We could read as many books as we liked, and I ended up reading nearly all of them by the end of my two years aboard the bus. I was introduced to Edward Abbey, Joseph Campbell, Barbara Kingsolver (my absolute favorite), Pattiann Rogers, Terry Tempest Williams, Mary Oliver, and other greats.

Having chosen our seats and checked out the decor, we hauled our duffle bags and backpacks onto the roof rack, tossed our hiking boots into an empty dry bin, and chucked our sleeping bags into another. A few students brought guitars with them, and we secured them with bungees next to the dry bins in the back of the Bus.

A few of the older people that I had thought were guides turned out to be fellow students. Our actual guides—Andy, Judy, Julie, and Susan—were older, just not as old as our two eldest students. Andy was nearly bald and had a red beard. He was wiry, funny, and temperamental. I didn't have much interaction with him, and he wasn't a part of my Bus community after the first semester and, unfortunately, neither was Susan, who I adored.

Susan, who cross-stitched beautifully, made a bag specially to house my Medicine Cards, a deck of cards displaying animals sacred in Native American culture that you pair with readings from a book describing the magical traits each animal possesses. You can choose a card at random or lay out a spread ala tarot card fashion. Susan was the one who turned me onto these cards. On black and white checkerboard cloth, she lovingly embroidered my favorite flowers, yellow dandelions. Knowing how much I loved poetry, she added the Walt Whitman quote, "Love the earth and sun and animals ... and your very flesh shall be a poem." I treasure it and still have it all these years later.

Julie was a kind spirit I connected with immediately. She looked like Joni Mitchell and wore her long blonde hair in a ponytail, which was often topped with a tam hat set jauntily off center. She was soft-spoken and warm yet there was a toughness and a sadness to her. She was compassionate to all and provided me with much needed emotional support. It pained me to see her stare out the window sometimes, lost somewhere deep in thought. I alternated between wanting to give her a bear hug and making her eat noodle kugel or challah or other soul-filling Jewish food. It never dawned on me to thank her for her ceaseless encouragement, but this was long before the era of Facebook. It wasn't easy to find someone when all you had to go on was their first name.

If Julie was the quiet, unwavering taproot of our community, then Judy was its spirit. She was older than the other guides but had more energy than all of them. She was like Tigger from the "Pooh" books, always bouncing around and laughing. She was sun-weathered in that Robert Redford good way and was physically and mentally strong. Judy was also fiery. She used her fire like a superpower to encourage us to live emotionally open and daringly. I loved to hear her stories of travel and fighting not just for environmentalism, but for social justice and women's rights.

I fell in love with so many things that were new to me, such as food cooperatives, hiking with a full pack on, and cooking without electricity.

Sleeping outside underneath a canopy of stars was also new to me. I'd only camped out twice ever: one night out of every summer during my Tockwogh years and once during my semester abroad in Israel. I vowed to stay awake all night at Tockwogh campouts to greet the sunrise, but I fell fast asleep just before dawn. In Golan Heights, my group had all taken turns sitting looking out for wild jackals. I stayed awake until daybreak then because I was too afraid to fall asleep.

Most of my classmates had chosen AEI after being in the workforce for a while. They had all figured out who they were or at least what direction they were headed. And they had all also spent significant time "roughing it." Missy did Outward Bound multiple times and Tracey rock-climbed, skied, and participated in other outdoor sports. The two of them looked like fashion models that stepped right out of the pages of a J. Crew or Eddie Bauer catalog. Jeff, Steve, and John looked like rugged adventurers or lumberjacks. You could tell just by looking at them that they had this camping thing figured out. And Karen, while I had also just met her, I knew she would be able to handle anything that came her way. I knew "tough" when I saw her.

Hey there! Remember me, old friend, your demonic inner critic? I'm back! I'm telling you that you're different from all the rest. You don't look at all like the others. You don't belong. I needed help and how! But that's what community is all about.

I bought a backpack that was too big for me. It continuously threw me off balance. The hiking boots I bought weren't waterproof, and they lacked ankle support. I fell headfirst into trees and other natural obstacles, and I was indeed the only one who needed pointers on how to shit in the woods. I had poor coordination on the best of days. *I'm too little and too weak! They're all going to know that I'm an impostor. Who am I and what am I doing here among these tree huggers?* My inner critic was relentless. Surprisingly though, while I couldn't carry a third of my body weight on my back and shoulders like I was supposed to on wilderness excursions, I learned to ask for help—and do so graciously rather than grudgingly and then humbly accept the help.

I was petrified of walking across felled trees or logs that were poor stand-ins for bridges. *Oh, my G—d, I'm gonna die! I'll fall in the river and my backpack will sink me!* Somehow, Missy convinced me that I could do it. She talked me through every log crossing— "Just pretend you're walking through your house and saying 'Hi, Mom,' 'Hi, Rocky' (our beloved schnauzer with a massive underbite), 'Hi, DP.'" I don't know how I would've survived without her.

Most female students on the Bus huddled together in a conglomerate dubbed The Slug Pile. I don't know if it was more about safety in numbers or sisterhood, but I didn't want to be part of an eternal slumber party. I loved listening to Annie and Lynn giggle long into the night, but it just wasn't my jam. I was "peopled out" as well as physically and emotionally drained by the end of the day. I still felt like a loner among The Bus community.

I wasn't mature enough socially to hang out with the women I looked up to like Tracey and Missy, nor was I about macrobiotic food, going makeup-free, or being otherwise "all natural" (i.e., hairy pits, legs, and nether regions). I wasn't down with the outright rejection of consumerism as many of my Bus mates were. I thought a lot of their talk was hypocritical and too "out there" to support.

What about the Gore-Tex gear we depended on to keep us dry or the Nalgene bottles we all used to stay hydrated? Everyone on the Bus purchased high-end outdoor gear from REI and Patagonia. Consequently, I didn't think it fair that I was chastened for wearing a bit of makeup and using a hairdryer. I knew L'Oréal tested their cosmetics on animals, but I'm sure there was at least one organic cosmetics company by the early 1990s. Why did my female travelers have to eschew the way I chose to enhance my self-esteem? It tickles me to recall that by the end of our two years on the bus, every woman borrowed my hair dryer at some point. It was often too cold to go to bed with wet hair.

I believed in the concepts of Gaia and cosmic forces, but I thought one of my female bus mates was crazy. She said, "I heard the voice of G—d talk to me through a rock. The voice said it was okay for me to displace it and carry it." Maybe she wasn't crazy at all, but I was uncomfortable with being that "woo-woo."

The hardest thing to get used to be the number of consensus decision-making meetings we had. We sometimes brought up the inanest issues, and for some reason, they usually coincided with bedtime. I was always too exhausted from hiking all day and was usually freezing.

Who cared to debate the merits of crunchy vs. smooth peanut butter or Charmin vs. more environmentally friendly toilet paper? I'm sorry, but toilet paper is not something to skimp on. Screw environmentalism when it comes to tush comfort! There were times I wanted to scream, "Just put your thumbs up for G—d's sake!"

There were times we did have to make big decisions, and it was important for everyone to be heard or, at least, speak up if they wanted to. It was also crucial to listen to multiple points of view before making decisions about who to learn from, where to go back-country camping and which critical tasks we each performed for the community. I think the guides prepared us as best they could to understand and practice group facilitation techniques, but not even the best of teachers can make sure everyone feels emotionally safe all the time. I didn't understand why, when I felt perfectly at ease speaking up, others were fearful. Where I was inexperienced in the ways of back-country living, I was an old hand at speaking my truth.

My years at Barrie, where I had been truly seen and heard, had given me confidence speaking up in a group. I realized that I was more adept in this area than my peers and this helped me see myself as more of an equal among the pack. The concept of emotional safety stuck with me. I lacked the insight to understand it then, but today, I embrace the notion of allowing us to be vulnerable among a group. In fact, it's something I often help others to understand and embrace in my work as a mental wellness and recovery-oriented therapist.

On the Bus, we learned that our emotional safety was in direct proportion to how closely we listened to and truly heard one another. Sometimes, our physical well-being depended upon how much trust we put in each other, as well as how much faith we put in ourselves as individuals. During our first semester, we thoroughly explored:

- the benefits of diversity regarding forest ecology and the environmental ramifications of deforestation.
- ways in which individuals build intentional communities.
- the ethicality of fish farming.
- human impacts on pristine wilderness; and
- varieties of learning styles and techniques.

We traversed the Hoh Rainforest—meaning, literally, "forest prime-val." Most of us read the book of the same title to better acquaint us with the amazing terrain. I never saw such verdant moss. I learned from Louie (short for Louisa) that Spanish moss is an epiphyte or air plant. It's a type of lichen, scientific name, *Usnea*. She was the one who also taught me another fun fact: banana slugs, while slow moving, are especially well endowed. (A gratifying note: All these years later, Louie was one friend who helped critique and edit this book during its writing.)

We traveled from Hoh to Sequim, Washington, where we set up camp. We also explored Dungeness Spit; a narrow finger of land surrounded by water. I have a photo of Harold (the Bus mate who told me how to pitch a tent on our very first day of school) and Tracey examining the largest starfish I'd ever seen. I read *Arm of the Starfish* by Madeleine L'Engle as a young girl. I learned from that book that a starfish's ability to regrow its arms was the coolest thing. But until our time at the Spit, I'd never seen a starfish that was alive.

The Bus community was usually regarded with curiosity. We received quizzical looks whenever we pulled up to gas stations to refuel or met with various instructors (e.g., naturalists, writers, Bureau of Land Management figureheads). Occasionally, we had to go incognito, however. These instances were rare, but if we thought we'd receive flack or the Bus might be damaged because of its environmental banner, we'd remove the banner. This didn't make us inconspicuous as a community, but it helped lessen any tension.

We encountered such resistance when we rolled into Forks, Washington. This was decades before Stephanie Meyers made the town famous for its association with the *Twilight* trilogy. Loggers didn't want to see a pro-environmental group shamelessly promote their agenda when they earned livelihoods by chopping down the primitive forest. While most on the bus were opposed to forest destruction, we sought to be respectful of others. We tried to discern different points of views surrounding environmental issues. It was important for us to appear as impartial as possible or at least to appear interested in learning views and practices that went against our own. Who were we to judge the local loggers, who depended upon the timber they cut to support their families? As I was curious at this time in becoming an environmental journalist, I loved listening to various viewpoints, to tease out the human interest vs. the environment-first angle.

I struggled to find my place in our community specifically because of my preference for people over places. I often felt like my classmates didn't understand that without placing value on people and economic security, the lands we held sacred didn't stand a chance. I wasn't an outcast. I belonged, but I struggled to maintain my footing sometimes.

Since I'd never seen wild and pristine parts of the country before my travels on the Bus, I think I benefited the most out of anyone on those travels. Everything was new and exciting. My Bus mates enjoyed seeing the country through the eyes of someone who was seeing it all for the first time. I existed in a constant state of awe and wonder. In Sequoia National Park, I saw live salmon swimming upstream (not smeared as lox on a bagel), but also my first clear-cut forest. The hillside was a bleached white graveyard of felled trees. It resembled the elephant graveyard in *The Lion King*. I'd truly never seen anything so spooky.

Our second and more adventurous back-country expedition was along an adjacent park's shoreline and grasslands. This area in Humboldt County, California, is known as the Lost Coast. It was refreshing to see a beach after being in the woods for weeks. We parked the Bus at the beach trailhead and camped on soft sand that first night. The sounds of the waves were deafening but hypnotic. I slept surprisingly soundly, given that I had a bad case of camp stomach.

I had never been on such a rugged adventure before. We'd be nowhere near the Bus if anything went wonky. We packed everything we could carry on our backs the next morning. Then we began a slow slog along the coastline. We trudged about a mile-and-a-half although on sand, it felt like a thousand miles. Putting one foot in front of the other was difficult. It reminded me of soldiers in Israel, who endured grueling basic training.

The ultimate challenge, however, wasn't sand but accurately timing and dodging waves, as high tide was quickly approaching. We buddied up like my sister and I had at summer camp years earlier. We read tide tables and relied on intuition to gauge our sprints from one rocky beach outcropping to the next. It was wild and scary, but once we passed the natural rock breakers, we were in the clear. We hiked miles along a worn path etched in dirt that meandered between low valley and beach bluffs. We walked over logs and scrambled down sandy, pebbly slopes. We took turns interpreting topographic maps, as California sea lions gregariously cavorted on rocky Pacific outcroppings. Below the sea lions, we spotted harbor seals surfing the waves searching for their next meal.

We passed a stranded seal pup whose mom was coated in oil from a recent spill. The pup was sure to die without the protection and nourishment of its mom. It was making cat-like mewls and stared up at us in dismay. No anthropomorphism here: it was aware that its mom was suffering. A little further down the beach, we passed by a beleaguered murre whose feathers were slicked to its sides with the black, tarry oil. We made our way back and forth along switchback trails that led down to the shoreline. I had never seen anything like it and was mesmerized. To this day, grasslands are one of my favorite ecosystems. Most of my classmates sauntered down the steep embankments of greenish yellow, undulating grass, but I fell repeatedly. They laughed from deep within their bellies while watching me roll repeatedly ass-over-tea kettle.

We made it to the beach overlook and set up camp. A handful of women, including myself, helped Karen stake out her new plus-sized tarp that a family member had lovingly made for her. Since there was still enough free time before dinner, Annie, Catherine, Ellen, and I decided to trudge back up the last bit of hillside to view the sunset from the highest peak. We set off unencumbered by our weighty backpacks. Before long, I found myself asking why I was doing this? Each time we reached the top of a grassy peak, we realized that we had another peak that was equally difficult to summit. But our trek was worth the effort.

Catherine was one of the women I looked up to. She was kind to me but was emotionally tough enough to hang with Karen and Missy and the men. When she bailed to go help with meal prep, our small remaining clan divested ourselves of our clothing. It was a mutually spontaneous decision. There was something about being among the safety of women and the way the wind was blowing. Call it hive mind or pack mentality. Why not celebrate our wildness in the wilderness? We danced circles in the breeze like a coven of witches engaging in an age-old ritual. We closed our impromptu ceremony by howling into the wind, then threw our clothes back on and sprinted down the grassy slopes to rejoin our community for a communal dinner.

In the middle of the night, the weather changed. Karen and the women who shared her shelter discovered that her tarp wasn't properly waterproofed. It was 2 a.m.—not an ideal time to vacate our sleeping quarters. Karen barked, "It's Vietnam, ladies! Each of you must fend for yourself!"

We all made mad dashes and dove into the nearest female's tent, but as with many musical chairs' games before, I was the last woman standing when the shrieks of frantic women came to a stop. I was left outside in the cold, driving rain to fend for myself. What else could I do but seek shelter inside a dude's tent?

I had a huge crush on Steve, but he had farted in my face often enough for it now to be payback time. I crawled into his tent where he lay curled up in a fetal ball of sickness. I truly felt bad that I was disturbing his sleep. I had no other choice. Soaked, cold and exhausted, I was dismayed when nature called only five minutes after I crawled into Steve's tent.

I didn't want to go back outside, but crawled back out, I did. No way was I going to pee myself or Steve's tent; that wasn't the type of payback I had in mind. I just wanted to be close to him and warm up, but not going out to pee in the rain would only make me colder and more miserable. I was terrified of wandering too far away from his tent. What if I fell off the bluff? What if a black bear or a mountain lion stalked chubby little me for a snack? I didn't have enough fat on my bones for a meal, but maybe an appetizer? I walked only as far away from Steve's tent as fear would allow me and took care of "business."

The next morning shortly after breaking camp, Judy made an announcement. "Steve is upset that someone took a 'steamer' outside his tent. Please, everyone, remember to eliminate as far away from our group as possible." I should've guffawed like everyone else. Instead, I owned up to my sordid deed and was thereafter called "Steamer" by Steve. So much for payback. (I told my dad this story and ever since, he's begged me to retell it every time we see each other. And every time, he laughs until tears stream down his cheeks.)

We ended our first semester in Half Moon Bay, California. My dad and Ona picked me up from the campsite. I spent a week with them relaxing and reconnecting to things that I previously had taken for granted, such as free showers with consistently hot water and strong water pressure. My showers had never felt so luxurious. And having a bed to sleep in, let alone a comfortable one, was divine. Best of all, I had an endless supply of coffee. On the bus, this is something we'd fight till our deaths for in *Lord of the Flies*-like fashion.

At the end of the week, my dad and I loaded up his car and drove to Fiddlers' Green Farm in Yolo County. The farm was a short drive from the University of California, Davis - known for the quality of its agriculture. Davis's town center attracted hipsters, artisans, students, and farmers alike. You were guaranteed fresh produce straight from farm to table every weekend from the farmers' market.

I stayed on Sue and Jim's organic farm, and helped Sue teach elementary school students about the principles and processes of organic farming. This was part of my first outreach project. I lived in their teeny pop-up trailer right next to the greenhouse. I always wanted to live and work on a farm, so I was grateful to Sue for the opportunity. I loved having my own tiny space. It was great to wake up early and jog down county roads. Hardly a car passed me by during my runs. It was freeing not to worry about cars honking at the sight of a woman's bouncing breasts.

I learned more than I taught. I learned that asparagus takes two years to grow; that the scientific name for mustards (including, surprisingly, broccoli) is *brassicas*; and that ladybugs are nature's alternative to pesticides since they eat crop-destroying aphids. It blew my mind to learn that some plants form symbiotic relationships with one another. In turn, I developed lesson plans based specifically on what went on at Fiddlers' Green and imparted this wisdom onto first-through-fourth grade students visiting the farm.

I discovered that I was a natural educator. I instinctively knew how to make teaching fun. They engaged in a circular lap-sit exercise. I informed some students that they were in the sunlight and had to wiggle their way out of the circle. This resulted in the "habitat's" collapse. This activity helped the students tangibly see that a successful farm habitat needs sunlight (among other things, of course) for vegetables to grow.

I also assisted the students in carrying out a plot study, which was something I learned on the Bus. Students roped off a square foot of garden each. Then, they took their time and carefully observed and identified everything their patch of soil contained. Students "oohed" and "aahed" over worms, ladybugs, and every living thing they discovered.

I accompanied Sue on her early morning commute to deliver fresh produce to customers participating in Fiddlers' Green Community Supported Agriculture (CSA) program. We made produce drop-offs along our route to the weekly Davis Farmers' Market. I learned to weigh fruits and vegetables and to price things out for sale. I never knew how critical these markets were to farmers. I also didn't know that only a small percentage of people in the U.S. could afford to buy quality, farm-fresh, organic products.

I felt grateful to my mom and DP who had stocked our refrigerator full of fruit and vegetables and encouraged us to try everything at least once. I have fond childhood memories of going to pluck strawberries from the ground at Butler's Orchard. I wondered how many kids never knew where their food came from.

On the road again ...

My second semester on the Bus began in Tucson. This semester, we traveled throughout the entire Southwest. A second group of graduate students was added to our learning community. I had been frustrated by the necessity of consensus decision-making among 18 grad students. I really didn't want to freeze my ass off debating the merits of tofu over texturized animal protein amongst 30 individuals. I didn't want to figure out our roles in relationship to one another all over again. Fortunately, it turned out to be easier than I imagined it would be. We swapped some students from each vehicle to form two new Bus communities. We also exchanged a couple of guides. In the end, then, instead of 30 students, we were still 18 but configured differently. Sometimes, the two Buses traveled together and at other times, we went our separate ways.

My Bus lost Andy but gained two new guides, Angel and Don. Julie bus-hopped and left at times to take care of personal business—seemingly at random. A few members of our community left the program altogether. I was placed in a new peer review group with Don at the helm. Sarah, who was previously part of the other Bus community, joined this academic group, as did Ellen, Jon, and Heidi. We called ourselves the

Javelinas named after the large and elusive desert pig.

I fell hard for the Southwest. I missed all the greenery but was tired of feeling like a captive within dense growth forests. It was refreshing to see the horizon again. I never grew tired of seeing the rise and set of the sun in all its pastel glory. My courses second semester included:

- Water Systems: Effects, Interrelationships, and problems.
- Life Systems and Their Communication I.
- Practicum in Educational Philosophies I.
- Science and Technology and Their Effects on Nature I; and
- Independent Study: Experience, Environmentalism, Writing and Literature.

Everything in the desert was dramatic, including the multitudes of cacti, wildlife, and rock formations. Even inconspicuous life forms had more to their stories than met the eye. In fact, you could only bear witness to many of the desert's stories after a hard rain had fallen. Then it was "game on" to see which form of flora would be crowned "Most Riotous." All the different shapes and angles that gave the landscape its dramatic flair during its driest periods added allure. There was the popular sentinel saguaro, arms akimbo; and the lesser-known cacti that dominated the desert floor, like the aptly named barrel cactus, prickly pear, beaver tail, organ pipe, and teddy bear cholla. (Pro tip: I learned early on that you don't want to mess with cholla. Jumping cholla is notorious for its ability to leap and impale. Its prickly tines were painful to extract from my tender flesh.)

Desert mountains and rocky outcroppings embraced trickery even more than the rascally cartoon character, Wile E. Coyote. Some boulders resembled lions or bears. There's Ship Rock, which needs no description. It's a behemoth formation on the Navajo Nation. I was in a constant state of awe traveling through the Southwest. I couldn't get enough of varnished rock forms coated in dark, thick, marbled slabs.

Most remarkable was how resilient desert life forms are—and everything came back to water. Survival depended upon how efficiently plants retained water and detracted predators. Animals were master survivalists. In this biome, bees weren't the only pollinators. Wasps and hummingbirds also pollinated desert cacti. Saguaros munched on by woodpeckers during the day became perfect hideouts for burrowing owls come nightfall. Miraculously, the desert's canvass could be repainted with the first torrent of rainfall. Prim pastels morphed into verdant greens, neon yellow, and raucous reds, transforming barren arroyos into tempestuous rivers with the season's first flash flood.

We visited the Hoover Dam on the Colorado River and met with an engineer who gave us a tour of the inner workings of its operations. I'd never seen anything so complex. The Black Canyon Dam prevents the Colorado River from flooding the valley. It supplies hydroelectric power and irrigation water to residents in Arizona, Nevada, and California. Its turbines take up the space of an entire submarine. We studied its antigravity technology and environmental impact since damming the Colorado changed the river's flow, as well as its ecosystem.

Our Bus group met with renowned environmentalist David Brower, a former director of the Sierra Club. We learned of his epic fight to protect mountains, rivers, and all wild places. I admired him because his passion reminded me of that of my cohort member Jeff's.

Jeff was a three-semester Bus colleague and ally who always came to my defense. He was patient with me and could get through to me where others couldn't. I trusted him. Plus, he was as passionate about writing as I was. I fell as hard for him as I had the Southwest's landscape. Like his heroes David Brower, John Muir, and Gary Snyder, Jeff longed to un-dam the Hoover and Hetch Hetchy. And like the unpredictable natures of rivers, Jeff too, had his own moods. I like to think I protected and defended his character as much as he did mine.

After seeing a river harnessed, we allowed ourselves to unleash our wildness by embarking on a weeklong canoe trip down the Green River. I felt like a fish out of water during our back-country adventure along the Lost Coast, but I was at home on the water. I was a confident and competent canoe rower and prided myself on being a strong swimmer.

This trip was as spiritual for me as my first back-country adventure was but for different reasons. The undulating grasslands of the Lost Coast captivated me, but the Green River's quiet waters lulled me into a meditative state. We occasionally talked as we paddled, but for the most part, the only sounds to be heard were oars dipping into water. The rhythm was punctuated with bursts of chattering swallows darting in and out of cliffside dwellings. Steve, our resident raptor expert, pointed out his sightings of peregrine falcons and kestrels.

I loved paddling on the Green, whose waters were liver colored. I reveled in the river's striated and multi-hued mud. I repeatedly got stuck in thigh-deep mud along the riverbanks. The mud sucked you in, making it nearly impossible to extricate yourself from. Once I overcame my initial fear of sinking up to my neck in muck, I embraced the experience and viewed it as a metaphor for living. *Embrace the Suck* was what came to mind. Just when I felt I would surely be pulled under, I learned to just relax and focus on my breathing. I found that I could slowly inch my leg up and out of the mire.

The mud was fun for all. Steve and Jon dove into it headfirst. And later, when all the men went for a hike, us women were left to freely enjoy a bit of nude mud bathing. I also reveled in the river's pink-, gray- and taupe-colored mineral deposits. That night, we slept under a blanket of stars on rock cliffs. This was years before *The Lion King*, but it felt like I was sleeping atop Pride Rock.

Two of my favorite places we visited during my second semester were Paria Canyon-Vermilion Cliffs National Wilderness Area and Mesa Verde. The former was managed by the Bureau of Land Management. Some among us referred to it as the Bureau of Land Mismanagement because it often designated wilderness areas for mixed-use, such as setting aside land for both preservation and recreation, which seemed to be at cross purposes.

Nevertheless, the rocks at Paria Canyon were water-gouged to the extent that I could comfortably sit in large hollowed out rock depressions. The desert rock in this ecosystem was smooth and curvaceous. There were large swaths of burnt sienna and dusty rose. Being a tactile learner, I touched rock face to memorize all its contours. It was as if I could learn the history of the landscape through osmosis.

The latter site, Mesa Verde, is in Colorado and is an ancient Anasazi homeland managed by the National Park Service. According to the NPS website, indigenous people shifted from living on the mesa and instead resided in rock face. On the day we visited the cliff dwellings, we walked through its valley below. The trek alternated between being dry and dusty and being a desert wash filled in some places with rainwater. Walking in the arroyo and looking up at the Anasazi's ancestral dwellings was otherworldly.

This sensation was amplified by the frenzied courtship calls of the mare and stallion we came upon in the arroyo. Their whinnies ricocheted off the canyon's walls and took me back to being on an HSI trip to Masada, which, in turn, inspired me to write the following poem. At Masada, my people screamed *Misada Lo Tipol*! (Masada will not fall!) In the arroyo, the echoes of the Anasazi people could almost still be heard, their voices gone but not forgotten.

Canyon de Chelly

April 12th, the 18 of us hiked.
I remember the slick rock walls stretching to the Blue sky.
How smooth and powerful, they screamed.
The mare and stallion courting each other.
Frenzied neighs and excited snorts ricocheting off canyon walls.
Kokopelli, the flute player, etched in the burnt-brown, crispy walls.
Anasazi eternal.
Toes pink, exposed to water, brown and cold.
Elation.
Wanting to soar like the seven raptor species Steve counted.

At the semester's close, I went back home to Gaithersburg and taught students at Watkins Mill, where I'd once attended elementary school, about recycling as part of my second Independent Study Project. I created a game like basketball in which students had the chance to toss waste objects into different bins, based on whether they held trash, plastic, cardboard, mixed paper, glass bottles, or aluminum cans. This was when everyone engaged in single-stream recycling versus how we do it now, by commingling all recyclables together.

I also wrote poetry and journaled nearly daily during both this time at home. I also went out dancing and bar hopping with Russ, my closest friend from high school. We often smoked pot before going out if either of us had a stash. As we headed out one night, a stoned Russ exclaimed, "Shalom!" I responded with awe. "Russ! I didn't know you understood Hebrew!" It wasn't just that we were, as Jim Morrison would say, "stoned immaculate," but I had forgotten the silver framed "SHALOM" sign that hung above Grandma Mary's hutch in the entryway.

Free to be (You And) Me

Our third and final semester on the bus was spent traveling throughout New England. Our final classes consisted of:

- Approaches to Research in Environmental Education.
- Environmental Education and its Applications.
- Practicum in Communication I.
- Independent Study: Sustaining the Planet; and
- Internship in Environmental Education.

I shifted my focus from environmental journalism to environmental education. I was excited to learn about different styles of communication and approaches to teaching. I was more excited, however, to stop traveling on a nearly daily basis. Instead of being nomads our last semester on the Bus, we had two primary base camps in Maine, not too far from Belfast and AEI's headquarters. We made camp at the YMCA on Hog's Island and at Hershey Retreat near French's Point. We also crossed the border and completed a backpacking trip to Grand Manan Island in New Brunswick, Canada.

After two years of constantly setting up and breaking down camp, it felt heavenly to semi-rooted. It wasn't glamorous, though. We didn't have heat during fall in New England, but I knew I wouldn't be as cold as I was when we camped outside of Tucson. It got so cold there that I shivered all night even in my zero-degree, mummy-style sleeping bag and ended up "sleeping" in a campground shower stall.

We had a home of sorts, but if home is the place where you go to feel connected, I wasn't feeling it. Being predominantly stationary meant that we could accommodate more students. As a result, we combined our two nomadic Bus communities into a larger, consensus-based community of roughly 30 students. This transition resulted in the shifting of individual alliances. Some friendships evolved and others diverged. The students I was the closest to suddenly became enmeshed with grad students who were part of the other Bus community. I felt abandoned and lonely.

During the second semester, I was closest with Jeff and Sarah. Sarah was petite like me but thinner. She was quirky, fun to be with, and was a talented artist. Where I expressed myself in writing, she expressed herself in drawing. As drawing is a more public form of expression, Sarah garnered much attention from her abilities. I wasn't jealous of that because I adored her, and she looked out for me just as Jeff had.

I had been close to Jeff since our first semester. We shared an array of experiences that spanned all three semesters of travel, whereas Sarah infiltrated our community second semester when we switched up the dynamics of the two buses. I remained friends with both Jeff and Sarah during this, our third semester, but they grew closer to one another through their mutual friendship with me. I inadvertently played the role of *yenta*. I knew Jeff was too mature for me to date, but I counted on his friendship. Likewise, I didn't begrudge Sarah her happiness, but it felt like I was dealt a one-two combo to the solar plexus. I was stuck against the ropes with no clue how to get off them.

There were a few highlights during my last semester: Rowing off Hog Island to the mainland every other day to run and our time exploring parts of Canada. We backpacked on Grand Manan Island and spent time on Money Cove. We were back in forest terrain. It felt good to be back in the woods again after our semester in the rugged openness of the Southwest. I was placed at the front of the line when we hiked for once. It was great not to lag for once, as I had on all other excursions. I finally had a chance to take in the scenery, catch my breath, and take rest breaks. We hiked through lush forests and into vibrant meadows. Flowers bloomed in a parade of colors. We had a day to ourselves during this adventure. We had only been granted this luxury once before.

Lynn and I shared a birthday and enjoyed hanging out together when she wasn't spending time with Carolyn. During our time in Money Cove, we hiked down to the ocean on one of our rare days off. We situated ourselves behind different "installations" randomly strewn about driftwood.

It was an unseasonably warm early fall day. Being as we were alone, we pulled down our bathing suit tops and enjoyed the sun's warmth on our bare skin. The only thing that could've made sunbathing away from the rest of the community better would've been spotting dolphins or whales. I was almost lulled into somnolence when I heard a loud whooshing sound followed by another odd noise, which was followed by a distinctly loud *pffft*. Lynn obviously heard the noises too because we both sat up at the same time exposing our bare chests. The unfamiliar sounds were whales! The noise was created by their blowholes opening and closing upon breaching. I've never heard anything as relaxing or as awesome as that sound.

The arrival of two men in a fishing boat offering us freshly caught salmon brought the day to a nice close. They were happy to spy two sun-bathing women. Lynn and I were happy because we made the community's night. We never had such a fresh meal while on the Bus. Too bad I detest salmon. (I often joke that I'm a "bad Jew" because I don't eat lox, whitefish, or liver.)

We concluded our semester in Maine at YMCA's Hog Island. It was a mile-and-a-half of rockiness with no escape. We slept indoors due to it being extremely cold outdoors, yet we had no electricity. The inside was as cold as the outside, but we had more protection from the elements than we'd had since our travels began nearly two years earlier. The cabins we stayed in lacked hot water and working showers. We could go off the island every other day and only for the purpose of showering. We had to take a buddy with us in the one available rowboat, our lone ticket off the island. There wasn't anything to do on the mainland except shower anyways, save for walking or running throughout the residential coastal community.

I usually rowed across with Jon, who was much faster than me. We ran (independently) and then took turns showering before rowing back to the island. Running and writing poetry were the only activities that helped me maintain my cool during our last, interminable days. Jon stepped onto the mainland and was off, whereas I had a whole routine to complete before I began my jog. I tightened my shoes, adjusted my Walkman, undid my laces to fix my bunchy socks, then walked for five minutes to warm up. I then jogged with *The Best of the Doors* at full blast. I blissed out on dopamine and jogged until I was too exhausted to think or care about how miserable I was.

My last semester of school felt uncomfortably like my first in that I felt like I was an impostor who didn't belong. I didn't knit or play hacky sack like some others did. I didn't play guitar like Tracey and Karen and I wasn't in a relationship like Heidi and Matt or Jeff and Sarah. I wasn't part of a dynamic duo like Lynn and Carolyn or John and Steve.

I was tired of school and even more tired of Bus life. It was hard to consistently rearrange my milk crate of belongings and interrupt whoever sat in "my" seat when I found myself in need of a forgotten book, pen, or cassette tape. My frequent trips on and off the Bus to rummage through my "House" became a source of entertainment. I wouldn't be surprised if my classmates placed bets on the number of times I'd go on and off the Bus. (Bear in mind that I still didn't know I was experiencing a negative consequence of ADD: difficulty with tasks of executive functioning). I was also tired of feeling chilled to the bone and having limited access to creature comforts. I felt ashamed that I seemed to be the only one who was ready for our schooling to end.

I packed my bags and was on the verge of quitting more than once. It was my stepmom Ona who convinced me to stay and graduate. I usually balked at her strongly delivered suggestions, but I was stunned that out of everyone close to me, she was the one who knew what would get me through—writing—a poem a day for the remaining 13 days before we left Bus life and commenced either writing theses or completing internships.

CHAPTER 13 – EMANCIPATION & REVELATION

To gain experience, I chose to do an internship. I volunteered to make mine four months long in the hopes that it might lead to a job offer. I was brought on as a rookie naturalist at Meadowside Nature Center. It was only a 15-minute drive from home. The directors had been in the field for at least a decade, so I was sure they forgot what being a novice was like as their assignments were too hard for me to carry out independently. I didn't have the slightest idea how to build an interactive learning exhibit. My only previous experiences with building were relegated to school science fair projects, which DP all but built for me by himself.

I don't know what it was like for my supervisors, but I was all too aware of my lack of work experience. I also knew that I was immature in comparison to others at the age 25—at least that's what my parents routinely told me. But what I lacked in maturity, I made up for in fearlessness. I was assigned to animal-feeding detail. Raptor, crow, turtle, and snake feeding all fell to me. I didn't like feeding dead, frozen "pinkies" (baby mice) to live animals.

I discovered that turtles were omnivores and ate veggies and pinkies. The crows were macabre, leaving mice entrails for me to dispose of. The snakes were the worst, however. I'm not scared of them, but I hadn't handled them before, and no one taught me how either. I did my best to move around them while cleaning their heinously poop-ridden cages.

The one benefit of my unpaid internship was that I was taught how to identify local flora and fauna. I've always had a keen eye for observing nature. I was familiar with most of the animals, but I enjoyed learning how to differentiate maples—silver, striped, amur, big leaf. I enjoyed being able to pass this newfound knowledge off to others on the student and family nature hikes I led.

I was good at teaching others because I knew what it was like not to know things and how fun it was to discover new things. If paid work could include walking and using teaching props like snake molts, bits of animal fur, and feathers, then I would be all for working.

Anything was better than the paid jobs I worked in the evenings and weekends when I wasn't at the nature center. I was a salesperson at both Kinney Shoes and Natural Wonders at Lake Forest Mall. The latter wasn't so bad, except for growing tired of listening to Ottmar Liebert, Enya, and the entire Putumayo international music collection playing on constant rotation.

The overlap of my internship with minimal wage employment marked the beginning of a slow emotional unraveling. I was disillusioned with retail work. It was fun in college when all I was responsible for was some extra fun money. At this point, however, I still lived at home rent free, but I had amassed credit card debt in college and on the Bus. I felt hoodwinked by my parents, who painted graduate school as the gateway to a rosy future.

To me, the word "future" is synonymous with "patience," which I lacked. I was dismayed to discover that I wasn't, in fact, the hot commodity my parents led me to believe I'd be upon graduating. I wondered how they could be so far off the mark when they had never let me down before. I painfully recall spending hours at the big box bookstore where I later worked searching endlessly for environmental jobs in *The Washington Post*, *The Baltimore Sun*, *Environmental Career Opportunities*, *Mother Jones*, *Mother Earth News*, and other environmental periodicals.

I could now boast having an advanced degree, but what did it matter when I was underqualified for most employment opportunities because I lacked the professional experience? The few positions I was qualified for didn't pay enough to live on and they were in the middle of nowhere. I was disheartened to discover that my fantasy of full-fledged adulthood didn't match my reality.

I quit my internship after the third month without any remorse. I needed to focus all my energy on finding professional paid work. I wasn't happy living at home, and I know my parents resented their short-lived stint of empty nesting. My parents and I constantly butted heads. They tolerated me smoking pot daily in my bedroom because they were concerned about my safety if I drove under the influence or otherwise put myself in a situation that was hazardous. I'm certain they didn't know I was going to my shoe selling gig stoned or that if I didn't arrive high, I was by the end of my shift.

My parents stayed up till all hours whenever I went out with friends because they feared me driving under the influence more than they feared me driving to begin with. I tried to be careful, but sometimes, I didn't know I was still drunk when I headed home. Usually, I was out dancing with Russ and I thought we had danced off all the alcohol. It wasn't until I crawled into bed at two in the morning and my whole room spun around me that I knew I was still under the influence.

I met my first adult boyfriend through the classified section of the local *Gazette* in April of 1995. We had cordless phones by then and the Internet was just coming into its own. However, "love connections" were still made primarily through friends, family, religious institutions, and the classifieds. The personal ads required subscribers to record phone introductions to potential mates. One day I got a message from a guy named Rick. I loved the deep tone of his voice. I thought I *could listen to him for hours*. I believe it's possible to discern a lot about a person by one's tone of voice. And I once thought it possible to tell if someone was soul mate material by the timbre of their voice. Rick's suggested strength and kindness.

Soon after our first date, it was clear that Rick and I were enamored with one another. He was a straight-laced, enlisted military man and I was an underemployed free spirit. He listened to country music, had recently become "born again," and had grown up in an observant Christian household. I couldn't have been more opposite. I was a fan of alternative rock radio, had grown up in a Reform Jewish household and had pagan and animist leanings. In other words, to say we fell in love quickly and acted too hastily would be an understatement.

I took Rick on a road trip to visit my Rider friends Heather and Stacey who would soon be graduating. I was so happy and proud to bring my man to meet them and introduce him to New Hope, Pennsylvania. This memory stands out—not so much because of my newfound love for Rick, but because I was high on mushrooms.

Stacey ate a handful and Heather and I a smaller amount because they tasted vile. Still, it was wonderful: it was the longest and sweetest highs as I laid spread-eagle on the football field surrounded by so much love. We stared up at the clouds and called out the different formations we saw. Rick and I held hands and, even though he wasn't high, he "oohed" and "aahed" over them with us. The world felt safe like it had when

I was a kid laying across my dad's feet "flying."

Rick and I cuddled up on Stacey's top bunk as my high subsided. I felt the warmth of being loved and accepted. The combination of mushrooms and love made me feel the way I'd wanted to my entire life. I was amazed that Rick and I were still together two months later, let alone moving in together. I hadn't dated before, but I assumed this is what couples did.

We hauled my belongings from Gaithersburg and crammed them into his small apartment on the local military base where he was stationed. My mom called my new neighborhood The Slums. The housing was reserved for married enlisted soldiers. I wasn't sure how Rick finagled our residence until he dropped a bomb on me: he was technically married. I didn't understand how someone could be "sort of" married. He and his "sort of" ex had gotten an immediate annulment but were still legally married and in the middle of the separation process when Rick and I met. I guess that meant that I was a "kept woman."

I understood why my mom called our community The Slums. It was poorly kept both inside and out. I didn't love our apartment, but it was my ticket to emancipation. Living on base got me out from under her and DP's roof and allowed me to play "house."

It offended me that my mom, a first-generation American, made fun of the neighbor's lawn decorations. The enlisted husband had just returned home from serving in Operation Desert Storm and was sick from inhaling poisonous fumes. Plus, his wife had just given birth to their second child, and they couldn't afford their hospital bills. Who cared that they drove souped-up NASCAR like cars and Monster-like trucks? I don't resent my mom for being outspoken, but at the time, it truly hurt my feelings. She never envisioned that one of her (Jewish) daughters would shack up with a born-again Christian and live on a military base.

Rick and I were idealistic and desperate to find salvation in one another. Three months into our relationship, we adopted a puppy from the pound. She was a Belgian Shepherd mix with sad eyes and a sandy coat. We weren't inventive with our naming conventions, so we called her Sandy. I spent that summer working and playing as a camp counselor, "playing house," playing with our puppy, and playing surgeon. My left leg was in a hard cast that entire summer because I had an extra bone near my ankle removed. After five weeks of being in a cast, my leg was so itchy and stinky that I enlisted Rick's help in removing my cast. We used pliers, a metal file, and a large, serrated knife. It took over three hours to liberate my ankle. My surgeon was livid with me.

When Rick was reassigned to Fort Campbell, Kentucky at summer's end, I made it clear that I wasn't going to live on or next to base. The area was rundown, full of pawn shops, check-cashing kiosks, and adult video stores. If my mom thought our previous neighborhood was the slums, there was no way in Hell she'd visit us at Fort Campbell. We agreed to live in Madison, Tennessee, a 15-minute drive from Nashville.

We were thrilled with our apartment. It was a sweet two-bedroom, two-bath unit on the first floor of a garden-style community. There wasn't a garden, but it was cozy and was bordered by woods and a creek. I hung bird feeders and planted a container garden out back. Our rent was only $550 a month including utilities. That was unheard of in Maryland or even around the Virginia military installation. We had such a sweet deal, but it was bittersweet.

I was still so desperate to work and couldn't find employment anywhere. This had become my personal soundtrack which played in an infinite loop. Then Rick was told that he was going to be temporarily deployed to war-torn Bosnia. I was deeply saddened by the daily coverage of ethnic cleansings but knew there was nothing I could do to change things.

Sadly, I was more aggrieved by the imminent departure of my man. What if Rick was killed? He was a military engineer not a combat soldier. My head and heart weren't very spiritually aligned. To wrest control over an uncertain future, I asked him to marry me. I didn't propose, so much as emphasize that I'd feel better knowing I had a ring on my finger to remind me that he'd be coming back home. I knew he felt pressured to say, "I do." Maybe that was because he was technically still married?

We visited my dad and Ona in Napa just before our move to Tennessee. To celebrate our betrothal, they bought me my engagement ring while the four of us explored San Francisco. We drove from there to one of my favorite places, Bolinas Beach. I was elated to show Rick this funky coastal town where I already envisioned us married and moved into. I'd teach kids about the environment, Rick would sort his future out, and we'd live happily ever after.

We toasted to our future, which Rick hadn't even been given a chance to envision. We strolled through the shops and art galleries and beach and then drank some more. In fact, we drank wine and champagne everywhere we went with my dad and Ona that week. They treated Rick and me like royalty and we glowed in their rapture of "us." They also helped to outfit our new apartment with finds from the Sausalito Flea Market. We bought a green, orange, and white folk art stool; a rose and gold gilded mirror; a complete set of blue rimmed margarita glasses, as well as an entire set of black stemmed wine goblets shaped like roses and a matching set of champagne flutes. We also scored all new dishware and Bakelite cutlery.

Back in Nashville, we enjoyed our newly, fully stocked apartment but began to feel more like kids playing make-believe grownups. Rick didn't want to be deployed. He didn't even want to be in the military. I was aimless because I didn't have a job or anything to keep me tethered. We intended to be happy together and settled. I found a synagogue I adored, and we made friends with a couple that I had met through attending shabbat services. We also befriended a couple I'd met through a temp assignment at Prudential.

Both couples were further along in life than Rick and I were. They were the epitome of security. We envied them and strove to create an illusion of contentment. We all but adopted a troubled 10-year-old girl named Autumn. We gratefully watched her whenever her dad was too busy to look after her. We allowed her to have slumber parties at our place with her bestie, Brandy. They weren't so different from Rick and I, in that they hailed from different backgrounds and had vastly different personalities: Autumn was tough and guarded, as well as sweet and silly. Brandy was demure and bordered on snobbish.

Rick and I spoiled the girls with treats, movies, and adventures. One weekend, we took them both hiking at our favorite nature center. They were as enthralled as I was with nature, but hiking ... not so much. I wasn't sure whether I wanted babies, but watching Autumn and Brandy together made me excited by the prospect of having a young girl or girls that I could share my knowledge with—just like my dad shared his with me.

I also was keenly aware of what it was like to grow up in a home divided by divorce. Fortunately, I'd grown up with a loving mom and stepdad to care for me and spoil me. Autumn wasn't as lucky. She divided her time between her parents and mostly looked after herself. Both of her parents worked full-time and even worked some weekends. Sadly, her mom was addicted to crystal meth. I desperately wanted to spoil Autumn to show her that she was loveable and loved. I thought that I could introduce her to the wonders of nature as a healthy means of escape.

In hindsight, I realize it was hypocritical of me as I began to seek escape through the effects of alcohol. I began to drink to feel numb versus effervescent. For a few months, my future with Rick looked bright. We had fun fixing up our apartment and exploring Nashville. We went to antique shops, hiked in state parks and nature centers with Sandy, and enjoyed scenic drives. Sandy and I roamed the woods behind our apartment daily—often accompanied by Autumn. I taught her everything I knew about the local flora and fauna that could all be viewed from our sliding glass back door.

Our seeming happiness made it easy to temporarily blow off Rick's parents, who badgered us to tithe at a church as they did. We didn't even belong to a church. Rick assured me that we'd raise our unconceived children in a household that embraced both Judaism and Christianity. Ultimately, his parents' relentlessness wore on him. Rick, who was once open-minded about our shared future, soon ended conversations about religion with recriminations. He said, "Babe, I have no problem with you being Jewish but at some point, if you don't accept Jesus as your Lord and Savior; you're going to Hell and we won't be together in the afterlife."

We began to argue more frequently and with greater intensity. Our fights were senseless and were fueled by Rick's insecurity. One evening while shopping at the mall, I noticed that a man's cologne smelled good. In response, he blurted, "Why don't you marry him then?" And one time, he accused me of a preposterous imagined betrayal: leaving him for Antonio Banderas. I hadn't picked up on the seriousness of his tone and flippantly replied, "Of course, I would leave you for him!"

Rick was deployed, but thankfully not to Bosnia. He was shipped off to Honduras for a three-month tour of duty. Winter started before November in Nashville that year. I cried nightly and drowned my sorrows with wine. I still didn't have a steady job, was working here and there as an office temp, and still waiting to hear back about the nature center position I'd applied for a few months earlier. January brought freezing rain and ice storms. It never let up. I was convinced that the rain would keep vigil until Rick returned. I've always loved summer rains, but winter rains brought melancholy.

The days I didn't have work took on a predictable pattern. I ran a few errands and did random activities. I painted a wagon I found at a local antique store in royal blue. The next day, I filled it full of potted plants and stuck it near the sliding glass back door. I needed something, anything, to remind me that neither winter nor Rick's absence would last forever. I had never felt so alone. I stopped seeing the two couples I befriended because I wasn't presently coupled, and I didn't know anyone else in Tennessee.

Temp gigs thinned out. I managed not to lose it during the days, but nights were torturous. I justified that it was perfectly normal to drink alone and that anyone else in my position would do the same. I started the evenings sipping my wine out of our rose-stemmed goblets, but as the night wore on, I just swigged sips from the bottle. It wasn't like Rick was there to witness my debauchery. No one was watching me; no one paid any attention because I was fucking alone!

The only thing apart from alcohol that comforted me was talking to my dad on the phone. I loved it when he was humble. Times like these were usually his dry periods. If he was drinking heavily in general, he must've called me when he wasn't drunk. I didn't know what to make of the fact that my dad seemed to have more time for me with Rick being away. I hoped it was because he intuitively knew that I needed him more. I found that he was softening with age. He no longer drank hard liquor, which is what always made him mean and nasty. He was still uncouth, but I found it to be oddly endearing.

He interjected a lot of "fuck yeahs," "home run," and "feeling like a million dollars" into his running commentary. He tended to talk like that when he was feeling depressed and drinking more heavily. I love my dad even when he drinks, but I especially love him when he's humble and speaks from the heart. He drops the clichés and bullshit. He was in a more genuine phase like this while Rick was overseas. I was overjoyed to have my dad's sincerity and emotional support at a time when it was so needed.

I counted each day Rick was gone and crossed off my calendar with big hash marks. He was due back home January 18, 1996. I made reservations for us to spend the second through the fourth of February in Gatlinburg. The place I rented for us was a log home with an indoor hot tub, a heart-shaped bed adorned with rose shaped candies. I used the promise of our romantic getaway as a means of dragging myself through my days until his return, but as the day grew closer, I felt his absence more keenly. I needed to hear his voice on the phone more often as if it would somehow expedite his arrival. I loved whenever he called close to my bedtime because he whispered goodnight to me and sometimes added sweet talk. I often fell asleep wondering how he would be when we had a baby. I thought he'd be an excited and proud dad. I knew that he found pregnant women to be adorable.

No matter how much I fantasized about our future, mornings always jolted me back into the starkness of reality. I was miserable and not just because Rick was away. I hated going to meaningless temp gigs when I was lucky enough to get them. I usually liked the people I worked for but found stuffing envelopes, assembling packets, affixing mailing labels, making endless copies, sorting mail, and filing all too tedious to endure. All these separate tasks reminded me how difficult it was for me to shift tasks, and how compartmentalized offices were.

No work was fulfilling or fun, and there wasn't anything inviting or warm about the worksites I was sent to. The confines of the office and the miserable rainy weather that winter made me feel like I was slowly dying. Some days, I stared forlornly at the white, splotchy sycamores with their nubby and leafless limbs. I imagined myself as a Member Services Representative at Prudential. I'd have my own desk where I'd hang my wilderness calendar by a thumb tack on my corkboard above my phone. My calendar would be a humble reminder of what I genuinely wanted to be: an outdoor adventurer. The wilderness panoramas would be a daily memo reminding me of my unattainable, unfulfilled dream. My desk calendar would define who I really was. It would serve as the official line between my office persona and the real me.

Sweet Little Lies

Rick returned from Honduras but wasn't emotionally present. Sex was never great between us, but it was unbearable upon his return. He criticized the size of my breasts, not because they were big (which they were even post-reduction surgery), but because he disliked the scars that were still mildly visible. He lamented that they weren't bigger. Rick liked watermelons on sticks. Did he think that my having larger boobs would make up for his inability to get a hard-on?

The beginning of our demise began within a week of his return from Honduras. I detected that something had changed for him while he was away. Shortly before returning home, he sounded disinterested when we spoke. He didn't seem like someone who couldn't wait to be back in the arms of the one he loved.

Our religious differences weren't a deal breaker for us before he left either. He said that he thought I was Hell-bound if I didn't accept Jesus as my savior before I died, but I didn't think that he thought I wouldn't be "saved." I didn't believe that my soul needed salvation, but as the days passed, Rick's comments about our having gods of opposing viewpoints grew more mean-spirited. He claimed that we believed in the same G—d but that "He" wouldn't be redeeming me or "my kind" come the End of Days.

I felt as if an imperceivable handheld serrated knife to our beliefs and every day, it cleaved a wider chasm between us. He had G—d and Jesus while I only had G—d. I didn't understand why G—d would intervene in true love? Maybe those who said "sometimes, love isn't enough" were right. I wanted to believe that we could make it, have children, and be content with our individual G—d(s). Part of me wanted to find a middle ground, a religion we could both get behind, but a bigger part didn't want to let go of what was mine. Rick's faith didn't come with deep roots that originated in eastern Europe like mine did nor did his religion have an ethnicity associated with it as mine did. I loved my culture and didn't want to exist in a world that was solely Gentile. It became clear that I wasn't accepted for who I was: a Jew.

I resented Rick's mother for being domineering and meddling with our relationship. She freely asserted her opinions on tithing and getting married in a church yet wasn't aware that her precious son hadn't stepped foot in a church since we started dating. It was as if she'd forgotten that she was the one who had kicked him out of her home just a few years before. Rick went into the Army as a result because he needed room and board, as well as a source of college tuition after his service.

I was drowning and could barely keep my head above water. I couldn't compete with Jesus and fight my own battles in the job arena. Rick was home for two weeks when my long-term temp assignment at Prudential abruptly ended. It coincided with my telling my former boss that I had a job interview in the middle of the week. I indicated my interest in working at Prudential numerous times during my long-term assignment and they hadn't taken the bait. I was hurt that I was terminated. I worked hard and it was shitty work that no one else wanted to do anyway. My naivete was coupled with an inability to perceive work-world norms.

I thought my honesty about having an interview elsewhere demonstrated that my financial circumstances were tenuous, and that they could offer me a job if they didn't want me to leave. I didn't understand that there are things that shouldn't be said in certain situations. I valued honesty but didn't comprehend that I could maintain integrity without verbalizing everything. I didn't understand what self-preservation meant. I was angry that my boss wasn't woman enough to tell me that my assignment was over. I didn't get that this is just how it works between temp agencies and their clients. I took and still take way too many things personally.

In February 1996, I applied to be a substitute teacher with the Madison County public school system. I was surprised by how easy substitute teaching was. I had an intuitive sense of how to approach different classes, but I didn't want to be a classroom teacher. I couldn't believe how little schools had changed since I was in the public-school system:

> I walked into the building and immediately felt small, help-less, and annoyed. So many schools are ugly and impersonal. Open bathrooms, metallic lockers, loud bells, and loud inter-coms. I think that school bells don't teach students to be re-sponsible for their own time. They're like a means of control. You wait for the bell to ring, then move in a frenzy like a herd of

*cattle ambling through the hallways. Is it the school system that
makes teenagers so apathetic or is it simply hormones?*

I felt let down by my lover and society. I couldn't afford to work my
tush off for poverty wages or a gross salary of $15,000 a year, the aver-
age salary paid by most of the environmental educator positions advertised. I hadn't realized until then just how much my parents had spoiled
my sister and me or how much they had sheltered us growing up. I wasn't
prepared for the harshness of adult life. I was grateful for the love and
protection, but I was growing resentful. I thought life was supposed to
get proportionally easier with age. I thought what we now call "adulting"
was easy because Mom and DP made it seem effortless. As a result, my
worldview, especially where work was concerned, was skewed.

My mom sometimes put on her human resources hat at home and
explained how to apply for jobs, educated me about what employers
valued most in prospective candidates, and cautioned me that finding a
"professional" job took time. I didn't know much more about working,
but finding work was lackluster and soul crushing. There was no novelty
or sense of adventure to it. Why had I been so eager to be an adult and
work? Rick was supportive of my efforts to secure employment, but then
why wouldn't he be? He let me pay for our electricity and groceries, as
he claimed that I used more of each.

I was fearful I'd never find work and fearful of Rick's mounting insecurity. I wanted him to be a little jealous of me if I flirted with strangers
to demonstrate that I was desirable to others. But Rick wasn't jealous of
who I was then but of my past. He came across Bono's number in my
address book while he was looking for the address of the couple from my
synagogue. I sensed his anger when he left for work that morning and
I found confirmation of it later that afternoon. He "accidentally" left a
handwritten list out for me to find. I couldn't believe that it was just like
one of the characters on *Friends* had written.

Rick didn't list many bad things about me. In fact, the two bad traits
about me were true. What hurt me was that my boobs had made it onto
his "bad" column. He believed I defied G—d by reducing the size of
them. I wondered why he never complained about my nose job. I explained to him that my breasts used to be too heavy for me and even af-

terward, I was a full-figured, 36C at the time of "The List." In any case, I would never fault him for something he had no control over. This debacle happened on the same day that I found out that I wasn't selected for the naturalist job at the nature center I loved.

One thing I've always done when I'm down is to dream myself into a brighter future through journaling and retreating into my mind. It's been a method of self-protection and survival. I used to think that I fantasized like this when life was good, and I felt happy. In retrospect, I dreamed of relocating or having babies whenever I had sunk to an emotional low. Fantasy then became my ticket out of the pit of emotional despair. In one of these episodes, I dragged Rick to go look at houses for sale. We weren't even on solid footing as a couple yet as Rick drove through Clarksville, I reinvented our lives in my mind. We had a home. Sandy had a fenced-in yard. I even had space for a garden. I was so persuasive with my make-believe, that I even had Rick waxing poetically about fireplaces and country cottages.

Then reality smacked me in the face. What was I thinking? We didn't save any money for a down payment. Buying a home would put us in even more debt. Armed with this knowledge, Rick and I solemnly returned to ourselves and our apartment. Unsatisfied desires and wants ran rampant through my core. I wanted to have babies. I wanted them to be cherished by our families of different faiths. I wanted a house. I wanted a yard. I wanted Rick to be out of the Army. My wanting made it impossible for me to sit still. I was never content with what I had or where I was in the moment. If I had waited just a few more days, I would've seen that elation morphed into discontentment as quickly as the wind shifted directions. I was high on my love for Rick that day but less than a month later, I wrote:

> All those people who say that learning to be humble is good for the soul, don't know shit. Even if humiliation makes room for compassion, there are no sweet words to pacify the pain. I can't find work as a tree hugger and so I sit here answering phones at Bridgestone, Firestone.
>
> They mine Native lands in the deserts of the Southwest.

They aide the enemy. The big off-road tires they sell are accomplices to rape—clearing our forests.

When it rains, it pours. I fear I'm going to lose Rick and my heart is quivering, on the verge of cracking. I don't know how I'm doing it—holding on, smiling. I know now what it is to be discriminated against. I am Jewish and his parents and family are not happy with his intentions to marry me. Our wedding date is set for September first. Rick's mom is ignoring me and accusing me of not doing my part financially. I'm a good person and I love Rick and take good care of him. It's all so hypocritical anyways—salvation. Rick says that he doesn't want to lose me but I'm not so sure. I know he won't stand up to his mother. I want to leave now if we cannot be.

No point in continuing. I will always love him but when Rick goes for BNOK training next month, I'll go back home. I need TLC and I don't want to be alone without a job. Maybe if things aren't resolved tonight, I will just up and leave. He might need time and space to think things through. It feels like my head is going to burst open through the back. And I sit here and wait for Rick to come home and either banish me or plead for me to stay. I'm impatient as they come. Lately all I've been doing is waiting for my real life to start.

CHAPTER 14 – METAMORPHOSIS

A month and a half after Rick returned from his three-month tour of duty in Honduras, I was back at my parents' home in Maryland. Our relationship lasted roughly 10 months and it was rocky for us half of that time. How could I possibly have thought we would live happily ever after? It was obvious that he was just as miserable as I was so before I left, I asked Rick what he wanted. "I truly don't know anymore," he replied. I snapped back, "If you don't know what you want, then I know for sure that you don't want me."

My only solace in leaving was that it allowed him to look within himself. He admitted that he had issues to deal with. I planned to stay in Maryland for at least the month Rick was away at BNOK. I decided to narrow my job search to Maryland and California so I could be near either my mom and DP or my dad and Ona. Rick and I had plans to reunite in May and see where things stood and whether we'd decide to remain together albeit long-distance. The only thing I knew with certainty was that there wasn't any point in my returning to Tennessee when there were no employment options for me.

Back at home, I was lost. I couldn't sleep or eat. Strangely, I drank water like a lioness who stumbled upon an oasis in the parched savannahs of Tanzania. I was dehydrated from crying all throughout the day every day for the first week since leaving Nashville. I missed Rick's kisses, him spooning me in bed at nights, and touching him.

I felt stoned. Time stood still. I couldn't move, but my room, my head, and my heart spun at warp speed. I realized how quickly we moved and how persistent I was with my neediness. I unintentionally pushed Rick to act on my agenda. I decided to take an honest look at what I valued and disliked about Rick. Ironically, I made my own "List."

Upon reviewing the pros and cons, I discovered that I had essentially been dating myself. This was a monumental revelation. Perhaps it was our similarities rather than our differences that led to our undoing.

Rick

Pro
Sensitive
Gentle
Bright
Giving, little touches
Compassionate
Likes movies, antique stuff, food

Con
Fear of confrontation
Tries to please others/hurts self
Easily overwhelmed
Lets/expects others to "do" for him
Doesn't enjoy "city stuff"
Gets angry w/ me keeping a journal

What solidified my desire to end our relationship versus trying to make a go of it long-distance was my discovery that Rick had thrown away a box of my journals. I knew with certainty that he'd toss out anything I'd written about him and our relationship. I'd like to believe that Rick didn't deliberately throw out a boxful of my past. Maybe he didn't toss them but didn't know he hadn't shipped them back to me. Nevertheless, I was missing the box of journals that spanned my years of college and graduate school. I lost proof of my adventures, my existence. Rick swore that he didn't toss them away and I did have all my other journals. He had shipped them back to me as promised.

But I still knew how insecure and jealous he was of my past. I wondered if he read them and if so, was he revolted by my admission of bisexuality. It would serve his Jesus-loving-self right for prying into my life before us. I felt betrayed. I labored and birthed my journals from the dark recesses of my anguished and creative soul. It sometimes still eats at me that I'll never know the truth.

I should've been grateful to be home, but I was resentful. Aunt Sister and my parents were protective of me and reminded me of all the reasons I wasn't with Rick anymore (lest I forget), but they knew that I was overly forgiving. Usually, it was my dad I was quick to forgive for each time he made an empty promise.

Aunt Sister in particular, said rude things about Rick because she lacked a filter. The only reason I have a filter is because I come from a line of women who don't. I never wanted to inflict a harsh tongue on others because I knew exactly what it felt like to be on the receiving end of a Tankleff (my mom's maiden name) tongue. I do take after the women in my family when it comes to being protective of those I love. It's taken me an exceedingly long time to see that I'm the defensive lioness I am today, precisely because I come from a pride of strong women who protect me at all costs. Until recently, I misinterpreted their harshly hurled words as being overly critical or dismissive of my emotional needs.

By the end of my first month back in Gaithersburg, I went on 10 interviews for various environmental nonprofits. By mid-May 1996, I was coming back to life. Sometimes, I hung out with Russ and other times, I went to events (including open-mic nights) by myself. On one such night, I bravely read my poetry to crowds of strangers. My bravery was a facade. On the inside, I wasn't confident:

The men's poems tonight were so eloquent and romantic. I felt like I was a puny fish in a sea of beautiful whales. Three high school girls read poems that were incredible, and one was about Hannah Semesh. I will read next month too. I need to practice. I was the only one there alone.

Here's what I read that night:

Slavery

As I was lying in bed
Thinking about you,
I realized that slavery is not a thing of the past.

Soundtrack of a Misfit

One could say you have no master.
That another human being does not own you – body, mind, and
soul.
That you were not forced to lead the life you do.
That you are not cruelly punished for disobedience.
That you have not been denied the beauty of knowledge.

But to me, you are a slave.
Your owner—the United States ARMY.

You signed a legally binding contract,
Giving ownership of all of you away.
You cannot leave now if you wanted to.

The ARMY does not encourage your freedom.
It tempts you with the promise of ever-lasting security.
It will never send you a rejection letter.
It will never make empty promises
.

It is helping you to "be all you can be."
Bullshit.
It is helping you to be all it wants you to be.

I find it ironic that the ARMY is based on the principles of freedom
and defense.
Overall, I buy it.
But where you are concerned ...

I am the voice of comfort when you are sent far away.
And I am the voice of encouragement when you struggle to make
decisions on your own.
And I am the one who finds it messed up,
That I am playing tug-of-war with the ARMY.
And I fear that I will not walk away a hero.
Because I can't make sugar coated promises.

Rachel Leigh Wills

I can assure you of nothing,
Except my love.

This described how I felt about Rick's desire to leave the Army and his inability to do so. I didn't see that he was playing the victim role in his life, just as I was doing in mine. I was no better than the Army. If I saw the writing on the wall and I left, then why did I leave it up to Rick to decide the outcome of our relationship? I either didn't see that I could call my own shots or I subconsciously didn't want to.

Upon reflection while writing this book, I saw that I didn't want the weight and power of making major decisions. I wanted a clean break but was too afraid of the consequence of being alone. I hadn't even been home for a month but was already thinking of moving to California. I knew it would be easier for me to temporarily live with my dad and Ona yet I didn't want to incur the ire of my mom should I make myself vulnerable and assert my mental health needs. My mom and I still had a toxic relationship. I was no better at separating my wants and needs from hers, or rather I did but was too afraid to assert myself.

My dad was happy to hear that I was thinking of moving out to be nearer to him. He pointed out the beauty of the timing. I had no job or friends to leave behind in Maryland and it turned out that Rick had already found my replacement. We had only been apart for three months. Twenty-six-year-old Rick twisted the dagger in my heart by letting me know that the "new girl" was 18—and his second cousin!

The only thing I knew how to do when life was hard, and I fell apart was to throw myself at something or someone else. I made new friends through the B'nai Israel Young Singles Club. I wasn't attracted to any of the guys. I was under stimulated by the caliber of conversation in general, but they were kind. Hanging out with them was more fun than I'd had in a long time.

In late May, fraternal twins Michelle and Lisa threw a cook-in (a cookout-gone-inside because of rain). Of course, I was drawn to the one non-Jewish guy. He had aquamarine eyes and brown hair that fell into his eyes. We played ping-pong and flirted. He told me that he was going to come to the twins' house for their next party that Saturday.

I knew he was only coming because I'd be there. I found my new fix, his name was Dan. We decided that we were going to do tequila body shots. I'd never done a body shot before and I was more than ready if it involved licking salt off his body.

I was hooked. I ignored everyone who said it was important to date someone with a good job. Most people I knew assumed you weren't worth much if you didn't have a professional job even if you graduated from college. This was and remains a very DC -rea mindset. Many people my age were employed in menial jobs or no jobs at all. What did it matter if Dan was 26 and still lived at home? I had an advanced degree and was back at home and without a job as well. Besides, he ended up getting a job sooner than I did that summer.

Two days after the party, I was still thinking about Dan. I no longer felt heartbroken, and I felt sexual again. I was back to "me" but was more confident. I was drawn in by Dan's eyes. I wanted to run my fingers through his brown hair. I fantasized about his nose, protruding and perfect. I wondered what his long, thin hands might be capable of making me feel. I wondered what his lips tasted like.

Two nights later, I went back over to Michelle and Lisa's for dinner for what I thought was a girls' night. I was surprised to find it was a coed gathering and that Dan was there. I didn't think I'd see him again until the weekend. My inner voice sighed in relief. *Thank G—d I decided to put some makeup on at the last minute.* I don't know if I was simply sexually deprived or if I was genuinely magnetized to Dan, but I knew that I hadn't felt so on fire in a long time. Maybe not even with Rick. Whatever it was, it was mutual.

We couldn't wait to sit close together and touch each other. We held hands and teased each other's palms with our fingers. He followed me downstairs to watch *Braveheart* because I got too scared during the first five minutes of *Copycat*, the movie everyone else was watching.

Dan whispered in my ear; "I really like the way you smell." I was wearing Safari, my signature perfume. It was so sexy having him lean in to inhale my neck and I was just about to kiss him when everyone else came downstairs. I didn't mind too much because I knew it would be more fun to drag things out, to give the sexual tension time to build up between us.

The following week: "I can't stop staring at you," he said. I boldly replied, "Me either. I'm drinking you in." We kissed for the first time and his tongue moved slowly but powerfully. Dan kissed my neck and ears in a way I'd never known. My heart was beating so hard that I needed to remind myself to breathe. I thought it would burst through my body. I was mesmerized by his happy trail. I traced the thin line of hair, stopping where it met his jeans. He huskily whispered, "Your skin is so soft. You're so cute. I love staring into your eyes."

Dan's words were short poems. I knew I wanted to sleep with him, but he wasn't very experienced. I didn't want to hurt him as I knew I was moving to California before summer's end. I found his innocence incredibly sexy. He was soft-hearted, fun, and easy to talk to. I was having a party at my parents' home that Friday. Stacey was coming home, and she was bringing Mary Jane. I couldn't wait to be stoned with Dan.

The next morning, I had a four-hour-long talk with my mom about dating. It went in one ear and out the other. "Rach, don't view every man you meet as marriage material. You shouldn't be a serial monogamist in terms of dating. Don't give of yourself so quickly. Spread yourself around so you can see what and who you want." My mom sounded scandalous. *Date multiple men at once?* I wondered.

I never did that before. It felt dishonest, but I knew she was right. I wasn't used to attracting attention from men, but I'd lost weight during my days of heartbreak. Men were drawn to me now; in a way they weren't before. I loved how it felt to be thin, sexy, and powerful, but I couldn't bring myself to date. Dan marked me and I only had eyes for him. By mid-June, he claimed what I freely offered.

We had sex for the first time in the morning, which I usually didn't enjoy. Yet for Dan, I'd do anything. It was inevitable after we went out dancing. We danced with our bodies touching all possible contact points. We also talked about sex all night long. I didn't regret it, but I felt a tinge of sadness. Once again, I knew it wasn't love. I rationalized that it was the '90s and that this is what modern women who knew what they liked and wanted did. And what I wanted was to spend time with Dan. I put seeing him above everyone else, even my longtime BFF, Russ. It was easy-breezy, and I desperately needed lightness.

I admired how attentive Dan was. He left no part of me overlooked or unattended to. Knowing how innocent he was, I egotistically thought that I would be a good thing for him; that I would give him an experience to remember by teaching him a thing or two. I wanted a chance to pay it forward because I didn't receive tenderness or instruction when I was initiated into the ways of sex. I was so wrong. He turned out to be good for me. I'd never been touched in the ways he touched me. He made me feel exactly how I always wanted to with a man: sexy and cherished. He excited me beyond my scope of experience and there was no rushing into sex; we savored one another. He even licked my legs and arms. I had never raked my fingers down anyone's back or begged for more before. No one told me that I made them hard just by kissing them or that they couldn't get to sleep because they were hot and bothered by me.

Dan was special in and of himself. However, he was also the best "fuck you" to the men I'd known who didn't appreciate me or treat me with respect. As a token of my appreciation, I wrote an ode to him and read it in front of him at an open mic night at Borders but neither he nor the "J Crew" (the other Jewish single ladies) knew it was about him. I didn't know how to express the way I felt about him face to face because it made me feel too vulnerable.

Existing in that quiet space,
Where security feels certain but is only an illusion,
Where words are coveted gifts,
That could be strung together and worn,
If they wouldn't wilt,
As garland of purple clover,
I would give myself completely.

I wanted to combine Dan, Rick, and Russ with someone I hadn't met. The mosh-up man would have Rick's body and mind; Dan's eyes, fun spirit, sexual generosity, and passion for movies; and Russ's education and love of art, issues, and life. If that person happened to be Jewish—even better. A tall order and evidence that I still had to work on myself to become a good partner for someone else.

My need to work on myself was the source of the most brutal row my mom and I ever had. We'd been at odds since I moved back home. Things came to a head just two nights after Dan and I slept together for the first time. I brought up my father, which somehow figured into our conversation regarding "what I needed to fix about myself." My dad was and always had been a point of contention between us.

I wish I could recall what I said to her that caused her to fly in fury at me. I'd never been afraid of my mom before, but at that moment, I was terrified of her. I almost wet my pants at the age of 25. My mom lunged at me and physically attacked me. DP had to pull her off me. She screamed, "Talk to me!" but there was no way I was sticking around to do that.

I took Sandy and fled to Dan's. I really wanted to go to Russ's, but I knew he probably wasn't home; he always went out at night. Dan insisted that I stay the night and I was grateful because I didn't want to go home. I was emotionally drained. He was so understanding and sweet. He even made pancakes for breakfast the next morning. No guy had made breakfast for me before. It was raining too hard to go anywhere, so we went back into his bedroom and crawled under the covers. We had sex twice in his bed and it was so good. We loved to talk about sex as much as we liked having it and we mutually discovered that it heightened our arousal even more.

Having fun with Dan wasn't reason enough to keep me in Maryland, though. I was miserable at home and had already mentally checked out. I needed to get away. My parents didn't see me for who I was or for who I wanted to be. My mom pigeonholed me by referring to me as her "urban tree-hugger." It incensed me because it seemed pejorative. I didn't know how to ride out the waves of emotional upheaval I felt inside. My mom essentially told me to "buck up and deal with reality like everyone else does." I didn't know how to do that because it required taking any menial job and doing any work, no matter how boring.

But most of all, it required waiting and I didn't have the wherewithal to wait for a professional job to come calling. I had waited it out the months I was in Nashville and all it got me was back home to my mom and DP. I wanted instant gratification. I needed it because I honestly didn't know that I could tolerate feeling lost, lonely, and jobless and survive it. I don't think my mom understood the degree of fear that came along with an indefinite period of waiting for things to be okay. I was doing the best I could, but I was in survival mode. I did the only thing that worked for me; I escaped.

My dad arranged for my car to be transported to Napa and for me to fly out there. I needed him to put me back together. I didn't know how to rescue myself. I set my infatuation with Dan aside and allowed my first knight in shining armor to save me.

Give It Away

Before I moved to California, I did the most difficult thing I'd ever done besides ending my relationship with Rick. I surrendered Sandy back to the shelter we'd rescued her from. She chewed up Grandma Mary's antique chair and my mom was livid. This sweet puppy brought so much love and stability to my otherwise tumultuous life. I didn't know how I could betray her by giving her away. It was more than I could bear.

I was about to start a new chapter of my life and I wanted her to be a part of it, but my dad and Ona didn't want me to bring her with me. Who knew how long I'd have to live with them before I found a job and a place of my own? I'd likely rent a room in an apartment or house and in northern California, the cost of living was higher than in Maryland. I wouldn't be able to afford to live on my own.

Plus, most apartment complexes didn't allow you to have dogs at the time. When Rick and I adopted Sandy from the shelter, they stipulated that she needed to be returned to them if she needed to be surrendered for any reason. It was one of the only times I did as I was told. My soul was cleaved in two. I solemnly vowed that I would never again surrender another pet, no matter what situation I might get myself into. (Apart from giving a dog to my dad, I've kept that promise. Digger, a beagle, was never really mine. He loved me but he worshiped my dad.)

I have a survival mechanism of distancing myself emotionally when I've decided to end one thing and begin another. In 1996, I distanced myself by drinking copious amounts of alcohol, getting stoned nearly daily, and relocating. The night after I gave Sandy away, I smoked my face off. My glass bowl was my favorite object du jour and I used it like a new lover.

June 29, 1996

All I can do is say, "it's going to get better." I've been saying that for a year and in some ways it has. I've had to give up a lot to gain myself ... Rick and Sandy. It hurt so much. I love Mom, DP, Stacey, and Russ, but I don't know what else to do. I'm so ashamed to be almost 25 and have nothing career-wise to show for myself. I don't want to live at home with my parents, whether it be in Maryland or California.

I'm smoking my face off to numb the pain. A little weed to heal the emotional garden. There's a brighter star out there and in me. Whenever I'm low, I play Simon and Garfunkel, Concert in Central Park. I'm stoned and everyone else is too. The New York air is beautiful. Everyone is peaceful and groovy, and your body moves to the music, its own music. I am that music!

On July 5, I saw the movie Phenomenon. From the opening scene, I could tell that it took place in northern California. I saw rolling hills, twisted oaks, and maize-colored grass. I knew that while I was leaving Maryland and the home I grew up in, I was returning, as Shawn Mullins might say, the home of my soul's core.

Cali-luscious

Even before I hiked the Lost Coast, I was drawn to the wild beauty and ruggedness of California. I was lured by Steinbeck and Kerouac. I was pulled by the promise of a Beatnik-like adventure. I was ready to explore the land and sip coffee in a San Francisco Cafe. In *East of Eden*, Steinbeck referenced plants with exotic names: lupine, Lily of the Nile, cypress, eucalyptus, madrone, manzanita, agapanthus. I yearned to see these plants and trees again.

From my father's home on the outskirts of the Mondavi vineyard in Oakville, I was surrounded by promising, knotty grapevines and lush jungle-looking forest. My fresh start was as invigorating as the morning breeze that blew scented strands of sage and dust. The massive eucalyptus trunks stretched skywards but extended their branches down, grazing my shoulders from time to time. Jackrabbits bounded from one row of grapevines to the next and added a touch of disorder to the homogeneity of the vineyards. Soft, rounded foothills rose in the distance.

After two weeks of living with my dad and Ona, I reflected upon my relationship with them and the one I had with my mom and DP. I had close individual relationships with my dad and Ona. Our bonds were so different from the ones that bound me to those who raised me. My dad and Ona treated me more like an equal.

We had fun cooking and eating together. My dad and I usually took walks together, which I loved doing with him ever since I was a little girl. He philosophized about how America used to be. He stressed the importance of bestowing his knowledge of the world upon me. "Rach, I never had the opportunity to know my dad as an adult. Your Grandpa Ralph died when I was only 28. Your mom and David might not talk to you like you're an adult, but you're twenty-five. You can do what you want but be smart about it."

I knew my mom and DP worked tirelessly to give Stacey and me good lives. I also knew that they were more responsible than my dad was. But they weren't emotionally open with me, and I longed to know who they were as Cookie and David versus my mom and stepdad. It upset me that I knew so much more about my dad than I did either of them.

My mom never volunteered information about herself. I couldn't picture her as a little girl or as a teenager, but I could visualize the pretty, skinny, vulnerable woman she was when she fell in love with my dad. I could say that my dad shattered her and made her soul hard, but if that was true, then wasn't he also responsible for making her strong, reliable, loving, and giving to her children? My dad's self-serving and self-centered ways necessitated my mom's ferocious independence and resilience. After my dad left, DP stepped right up, looking as comfortable and trustworthy to her as a pair of broken-in boots. This is when my mom's true self appeared. This is when she poked her head out of her hardened carapace and faced the world unreservedly.

So why was it that I felt as if it'd been years since my mom shared her spirit and creativity with my sister and me? Why didn't she give more of herself like she used to, like whenever Stacey and I needed her help completing projects and papers? It seemed an eternity ago that she sang to Neil Diamond on Sunday family cleaning days. I longed to know my mom's stories.

I knew that she was conceived in the hopes of salvaging her parents' marriage. Grandma Mary was 42 and my mom was only two when her dad died of cancer. Aunt Sister was twelve years older than my mom and

Uncle Bobby (who I barely knew) was 14 years older.

My mom always said that her brother abandoned both the family and his religion. Supposedly, he got his children hooked on prescription drugs. He was a pediatrician and had easy access to medications. I had no way to know whether this was true, as neither my aunt nor my mom had spoken to him in over a decade (likely more by then). I remember how hurt I felt for Grandma Mary, my mom, and my aunt that he didn't come to Maryland for my grandma's funeral. (I was furious with him because I couldn't imagine any scenario that would permanently sever my ties with Stacey. I loved her fiercely even though she often annoyed the shit out of me.)

I didn't understand why my mom wouldn't talk to her brother. I couldn't fathom why she wouldn't at least talk to me about him. I wanted to know more than surface details about my mom. Did my mom realize that she had a lot to offer and that she could reveal to me pieces of myself and my inner landscape by sharing herself with me, as my dad did? I might not live with her anymore, but I still needed her in my life. Part of my thirst for knowledge about her was due to the fact that my dad told his origin stories and his current life stories in greater detail and more frequently than my mom did. Where my dad is a textbook narcissist, my mom is guarded.

I was certain that if I knew more about my mom's roots, I'd have a better sense of who I was and where I was going. My familial and individual landscapes were disorderly and obscure. Tracing my family origins on both sides while simultaneously mapping out a future for myself was confounding and it used up emotional energy I should've been putting to better use.

I knew a job was just around the corner and that I couldn't use my binoculars to help me see down a nonlinear path. I decided that I wanted to be a teacher, but I was loath to go back to school to do so. I craved a new boyfriend and new friends. I was adrift.

July 15, 1996, was a significant day for me. It marked my decision to pursue certification as a Montessori elementary school teacher. Making this decision gave me more clarity. When I wasn't busy making cold calls to potential Montessori elementary schools to work at, I enjoyed the sweetness of burning off my anxiety by working the land.

My dad and Ona had a large garden in their rented house on Dwyer Road. Of all the places I've lived in, their tiny rambler felt the most like home. I wished the owner sold it to them so that I could've inherited it later. Six months before I moved to California, my dad asked me, "Rach, where would you choose to be if you could be anywhere in the world?" Without missing a beat, I answered, "At your house."

His house was both perfect and perfectly located. It blended in with its natural surroundings. It was a soft yellow that bordered on ecru. It had a rectangular profile that flowed with the way the land was parceled out and planted with grapes. From the sliding glass door in the dining/ living room area, you could see the gated garden. Beyond that, there was a dusty path bordered by large eucalyptus trees, their neighbor's fruit orchard and beyond that, a verdant hillside. If you looked to your right, you saw row after row of Mondavi grapes and the Franciscan monastery. If you turned around and walked out the front door, their narrow (and almost always cold) pool and blackberry trees were to the left. If you drove two blocks to the right, you passed a patch of bourbon and Meyer lemon-yellow fields. Those were opposite the restaurants Mustard's and Brix.

I have so many fond memories of spending time with my West Coast parents on Dwyer Road. Ona bought a million different vegetables and flowers from farmers' markets and other sundry vendors. She gave strict instructions on where to plant everything. She also barked orders like a drill sergeant and reprimanded us like my dad and I were bad dogs. "Danny, no, not there! I said to plant the Bells of Ireland next to the Birds of Paradise. Rachel, where are you going with my Early Girls? Who told you to plant them over there? They go next to the Zebra and Sun golds!"

That house was also where my dad and I baked freshly harvested peach pies and cobblers and drank copious amounts of local wine. There was always a bottle of buttery chardonnay or sparkling wine being chilled in the fridge. And the white wine was always followed by leggy Cab Sav or Bordeaux.

I spent what felt like an eternity searching for nonprofit work when I was in Maryland, but within a month of moving to California, I received not one, not two, but three teaching offers. I accepted one at a private Montessori school in Palo Alto. I was going to co-teach elementary school students in a mixed-grade (first through third) classroom.

Before I started work, however, I needed to find a place to live on the Peninsula. I thought interviewing for jobs was torturous but finding roommates was another hurdle altogether. I couldn't believe the types of questions I was routinely asked by potential housemates:

- Do you drink? *(Do I answer honestly? Yes—and often)*
- Are you a vegetarian? *(Does it matter? I'm not a cannibal, if that's what you're getting at.)*
  - Are you a professional? *(Professional what? Does "almost" suffice?)*
  - Do you smoke? *(If we're talking cigarettes - no. If we're talking ganja, then hell yeah!)*
- Do you watch TV? *(Are you for real?)*
- Do you volunteer all your free time to help the disadvantaged? *(What if I am disadvantaged?)*
- Do you like film noir? *(Do I like what?)*

I finally found a place to live, and I was so excited for my mom to see me being self-sufficient. We were stuck in old roles that no longer worked for us and were miserable with the way things were. I felt like I needed her for everything and that she needed me to need her. I now understand that there's a term for this: codependency. My move to California changed the dynamic of our relationship. Being away from my mom forced me to be more independent since my dad and Ona didn't coddle me the way my mom and DP did. I used to worry all the time about how I'd survive when my mom died. I still worried about this from time to time, but I had a growing sense that I'd be okay. I was learning that left to my own resources, I could maturely find my own solutions to problems. And when I couldn't, then I could confidently turn to others for help.

I wanted my mom to be proud of me and happy for me. She didn't call me at my dad's, which hurt, but I understood why. It saddened me that she refused to even say "hello" to my dad, but no amount of wishing things were different between my birth parents would make it so.

I was surprised to learn that the students I taught had similar issues with their parents—and they were only six to eight years old! In fact, many of the kids I taught were the resentful and oft- spoiled offspring of Apple, Oracle, and other Silicon Valley tech companies. They spent so many hours at school with me, including before- and after-care. They often unintentionally called me "Mom." This made me feel grateful for my mom having been a stay-at-home mom until I was in fifth grade.

I was assigned to teach geography, botany, and biology according to the Montessori method. I worked under the supervision of two lead teachers and worked alongside another teacher-in-training who taught P.E. I thought it was cool that our students held consensus-based meetings which they ran themselves; they had a facilitator; a reporter; a historian, and a weather reporter. It was like reliving my time on the Bus.

I commuted about 20 minutes from my new place in Foster City, which was an equidistant drive to both San Francisco and Palo Alto. Foster City is bordered on two sides by water. It reminded me of Miami's portion of the Intracoastal Canal. I loved riding my bike and roller skating along the paved path parallel to San Francisco Bay. The path was decorated with purple ice plants, yellow teasel, and wild fennel. The smell of fennel and intermittent petrichor was intoxicating.

My roommates Marie and Regina were both in their early thirties and were coworkers at Genentech. I was stunned that they wanted me to live with them—especially as I was so new in my career, young for my age, and unsettled, and they were both established and classy. Marie was in communications and Regina was a scientist. They weren't around much, and they both had boyfriends. This made me keenly aware that I didn't have anyone.

I was overjoyed that I finally achieved something resembling independence. It was great to have a large master bedroom after living in tiny ones. My private domain received full sunlight and there was usually a nice cross-breeze. I contributed most of our furniture and I paid more than they did for rent, but I was a shitty roommate. I was in and out all the time and until all hours. It took a lot of time and energy to be an active single woman. On the rare occasions I stayed home, I made impulsive redecorating decisions without giving them the courtesy of asking first. I had furnished the space, so I felt justified in arranging the furniture how I wanted to. Instead of owning my part, I blamed Marie for being anal-retentive. I didn't understand why it mattered that I moved her beloved indoor tulips an inch to the left or right of the TV. What did it matter if I forgot to put a glass or a bowl away? I wasn't a slob; I was just forgetful.

The worst was when I brought two total strangers back home with me from San Francisco. This happened after a drunken night of debauchery that had begun with dancing at Holy Cow in SoMa (South of Market) with my friend (and classmate in Montessori teacher training) Tuija. I didn't give Marie and Regina a heads-up or a note. Regina was scared shitless when she came across one of the guys (i.e., the guy I didn't take up to my bedroom) on the couch. I don't recall Couch Dude's name, but I remembered Travis, the basketball player upstairs in bed with me.

When I came to hours later, I was mortified by my actions. I woke the men up and drove them home in cruel, pre-sunrise hours. It was hard to drive that early with a vicious hangover. After dropping them off, I drove to meet my dad, Ona, and my girlfriend Cathy at Roche Winery in Carneros. Ona somehow conned Cathy and me into taking kids on short, circuitous nature walks on the marshlands. Meanwhile, she and my dad hobnobbed with high-earning sales reps of Sahara Jeep. It was obvious to them that I was in rough shape.

I didn't have true love, but I had work that was meaningful and enjoyable. I reveled in my newfound independence. It was hard to believe. I was no longer tied to my mom or anyone else—not even a man. I missed intimacy, but it was good for me to have time to evolve. I took on a second job, two nights a week in the Palo Alto office of my mom's company. I put labels on vials of oligos or synthesized DNA. It paid $13.50 per hour, which was $1.50 more than I earned from teaching. This work was tedious and required me to pay close attention to detail, which, of course, I struggled with. I needed to be incredibly careful not to mess up. Any error on my part would render the samples of synthesized DNA useless. The extra income helped me pay off the credit card debt I accrued in college and graduate school.

When I wasn't working, I didn't know what the hell to do with myself. I turned as I always did to my two besties: marijuana and alcohol. This is where and when my drinking escalated. I was either surrounded by kids or I was totally alone; there was no happy medium. I didn't have healthy habits or positive coping techniques to combat my feelings of isolation. It seemed always to be a party for one with me shuttered in my large bedroom.

Connections

It was heartbreaking that for as deeply connected as I was to my surroundings, I was so disconnected from myself. I made a few girlfriends through solo escapades: two at a Jewish singles event and one touring a wildlife rescue organization. It was stereotypical, but my Jewish girlfriends didn't want to get dirty hiking or camping. They wanted to go to dinners and services to meet professional and eligible Jewish bachelors. I had a professional career, but I didn't want to be domesticated just yet. I didn't share my friends' interest in settling down. I still craved excitement, be it hiking on the peninsula or bar hopping in San Francisco. My desire to attract men and drink the way I wanted to be outweighed my desire for sisterhood.

Not surprisingly, my Jewish gal pals didn't stick close to me for long. Cathy was the only friend I made a point of staying connected to, because she was the only person I knew who was as passionate about the outdoors as I was. I went to stay with her at the Marin Headlands; she received free housing in exchange for her service at the Marine Mammal Center. The Headlands was one of my favorite places as its peaceful inlet lagoon was a striking counterpoint to the tempestuous Pacific Ocean.

We strolled along Black Sand Beach, one of the city's dedicated nudist beaches. (Fortunately, there were others like us who remained clothed.) We were kibitzing about our mutual love of men and adventure and were so lost in our own bubble that we nearly stumbled into a crowd of people gathered around a dead, juvenile gray whale that had beached itself. Its tail was intact, but the rest was a morass of decay. I'd never smelled anything so foul. We joined the solemn crowd and paid our tribute to the gentle giant of the sea. The Marine Mammal Center wanted the whale's bones for educational purposes, but the hillside was too steep for the recon team to bring its equipment down.

We watched the sunset from Point Bonita Lighthouse, which offered a clear view of the Golden Gate Bridge and Point Reyes. The sea was uncommonly placid. The only observable eddies were near the rocks that bordered the lighthouse. The old lighthouse manager's wife planted cabbage on the hillside, and it was there, thriving in such rugged terrain. The lighthouse was nearly an ecosystem unto itself. Ice plants, coyote bush, fennel, sage, and yarrow grew in abundance. Harbor seals lolled on the rocks and birds of all kinds abounded, including pelicans, cormorants, and murres. Point Reyes was a sanctuary.

After sunset, I drove Cathy into the city. We wound our way up and over huge rollercoaster hills that my car barely made it up and over. My adrenaline was on overdrive. I had nightmares about driving up huge hills like these and worried I'd roll backwards too fast to control. We went to a club called Sol y Luna which played salsa music along with a mix of songs that were easier for me to dance to. Cathy danced with some guy and left me holding her water and my Corona. A guy sidled up next to me and made a comment about my holding onto two drinks at a time. We started talking and dancing and I couldn't stop smiling. It was the first time since meeting Dan that I had felt sexy. There were some pretty women who were all dressed up, whereas I wore baggy jeans and a T-shirt. I felt even better about myself when the guy asked me for my number.

Seasons of Love

California is beautiful no matter the season, but it's especially glorious just before and after January's rains. I went to stay with Cathy again and this time we explored Ano Nuevo, just south of Half Moon Bay (one of my favorite places). We saw huge elephant seals that ranged in weight from 200 to 500 pounds and moved with a speed that was incomprehensible given their mass. Cathy assured me that we were fine walking along their beach, so long as we steered clear of any seal pups. I cautiously followed her and even walked in her footprints. I was scared and riveted, but the sea mammoths were nonplussed by our presence. We saw four pups and the seagulls swooped in to provide their services cleaning up placentas. We also saw bobcat tracks and ancient trash piles, remnants of the Ohlone Indians.

In February, I went on a few arduous hikes with Cathy and one of her older sisters. It was one of those weekends that made you feel proud of yourself for moving your body, yet your muscles rebelled hours later and demanded a bath. Throngs of cute men passed us by on mountain bikes both days of hiking and I vowed to become a cyclist if it meant drawing the attention of men. On our second hike, we clambered up past trees clinging tightly to eroding soil. From a rocky vista, we saw clear from the ocean to the horizon's edge. On our gradual descent back to sea level, we saw banana slugs, madrone, poison oak, and horsetail.

In March, I went for a hike one weekend with a girlfriend who was also single and Jewish. We went to Peter's Creek and the Ridge Trail off Skyline Drive. It was the kind of day that made me never want to leave California.

I didn't do much in April and it was likely that I had a month-long sinus infection. I was exposed to many germs, and I had a sinus infection nearly every other month for my first year of teaching.

Come May, I went on a backpacking excursion with the local chapter of the Sierra Singles Club, which was more like the Sierra Divorced and Single Again Club. I was the youngest by at least 10 years. Many cute men and one or two attractive women passed our group by. They were young college kids but I was closer to them in age than I was to the group I was with.

Despite the disparity in age, I could easily relate to everyone. It felt like I was back on the Bus. It was refreshing to eat outside after setting up camp while it was still light out even at 7 p.m. I never had enough daylight or energy to hang a bear rope up by myself before. I finally managed it. If only my old Bus mates could've seen me.

I hiked eight miles with 40 pounds strapped to my back. I couldn't figure out how my pack weighed that much. I carried food, but apart from that, nothing else felt like it weighed that much. We hiked the still snow-covered peaks of Trinity Alps. It was only 45° out and there was a chance of rain. I was too cold to socialize much that day, so I opted for snuggling into my sleeping bag and enjoying the solitude of my tent. It was nice to listen to the camaraderie of others' conversations from afar. When I ventured out later that night, others were telling stories about the "good old '70s." One man asked me, "Where were you in 1970?" I sheepishly replied, "I wasn't fertilized yet."

That July and August were crammed with social activities. I saw the movie *Contact*, starring Jodi Foster and Matthew McConaughey. The intensity of the movie wiped me out. I don't know many others who leave movies feeling like they just scaled the peaks of Yosemite. I've always had a hard time shaking off the vibes post-viewing, no matter if they're good or bad. Sometimes, the emotions that movies elicited in me stayed with me for hours and even days.

One Friday night in August, I went to the H.O.R.D.E. Festival with friends from my teacher training program. I was high, drunk, and as peaceful as a hippie at Woodstock. I felt safe enough among my friends to lay down on our picnic blanket and rest my head on Bill's shoulder. I knew no harm would come to me on our patch of space with Bill protecting me. His girlfriend Paige knew I was infatuated with him, but she didn't mind our spending almost all our free time together. We hung out all the time by ourselves, drinking and smoking pot whenever she went away on business, and I even slept over. We were attracted to one another but had enough mutual respect to not cross the friendship boundary.

On another weekend night, I spent the afternoon at the beach in Alameda with Tuija. She was a tall, leggy blonde from Finland who was even more boy crazy than I was. She also smoked more marijuana than I did, which said a lot. Tuija was an Amazon version of Marilyn Monroe, and men went crazy for her. That night, I drove us to North Beach, so that she could get tattooed on Broadway and Montgomery near Columbus. We went dancing at Holy Cow afterward. It was our third time there and this time, I met a nice guy and his much hotter (but not as kind) brother. They were Nicaraguan Jews. I was dancing among strangers. Under the spell of alcohol, some part of me still believed that true intimacy could be found in a crowd.

November 1997 found Cathy and I on a camping trip along the Lost Coast. This is the place I literally fell head over heels for while on my second backpacking expedition nearly four years earlier on the Bus. It was great to return as an experienced backpacker. I helped Cathy with her pack and gave her advice on weight distribution just as others had helped me back then. My second experience in this wildness was equally mystical. We explored tide pools and hiked along the beach where we spied green sea anemones, an orange ochre sea star, a few hermit crabs, and limpets.

I was awestruck by our findings. It brought me back to innocent and happy memories of girlhood playing on the sands of Pompano Beach. I marveled at the ocean-smoothed stones and shells. I found broken bits of green and purple urchins and an intact chiton with a turquoise underside. Cathy and I also found an animal vertebra that possibly belonged to a porpoise.

As we approached the Punta Gorda Lighthouse, we came across a suffering beached baby sea lion. It was emaciated and it looked up at us with sorrowful eyes. I hadn't seen many animals like this, and I was overcome with grief. Despite knowing death is part of life, I cried for it.

And we saw still more suffering that night. A murre's breast and wings were coated in oil from a recent tanker spill along the shores. It tried to peck off the oil with its long, black beak but was unsuccessful. Cathy and I asked the father and son we met at a nearby camping hut if they had any soap so we could use it to try to save the murre. The dad informed us that we wouldn't be able to save it and that it would be better if we kept on moving. "McWorld" people, my term for individuals like oil refinery workers, were responsible for the 15,000 gallons of oil that spilled into Humboldt Bay. Cathy pontificated on birds, stating that fewer than 20 percent of all birds, seals, and other animals that were cleaned off survived the stress.

We discovered evidence of a mountain lion. There was a deer's chewed leg and cleaned ribs covered in dung and fur. I was frightened that the lion was lurking in wait for us. That night, I lay awake and wondered if a hellcat would tear my eyes out. I didn't get how Cathy was unperturbed. There were no nighttime visits by mountain lions, but we did hear the call of coyotes. The next morning, we saw irrefutable evidence of their presence in the form of scat.

I was exhausted after our hike the next day. It felt heavenly to lay inside my tent and listen to the crescendo of the ocean below us. I never slept well on backpacking excursions and existed in a state of walking somnolence during the day. It took us forever to get to an elevation of 1,000 feet with full packs on our backs, but the next morning, we scrambled down the mountainside with ease. It's funny how motivating the promise of a meal is. We set up camp again close to the shore and wolfed down our second breakfast: avocado smashed onto bagels (the first breakfast had been bananas smashed onto bagels).

We combed a stretch of beach and I again found myself in awe. I was excited by my finding of a whole chiton and sponge but was even more amazed by the basalt rocks we found in an array of colors and patterns. Some of the rocks were marbled, others were oblong, and many were smoothed and flattened from being tossed and polished by waves and sands over years untold. I collected so many shells that my backpack weighed just as much hiking out as it had when we hiked in.

Homecoming

When I wasn't off on adventures with Cathy or exploring Northern California on my own, I was consumed with the concept of "home." I was growing tired of not knowing where I belonged. I was restless again and questioned not so much my teaching career, as the lifestyle being a Montessori teacher would afford me. For the first time, I comprehended what my mom had been telling me for years.

She advised me to do something that made me happy, if it afforded me the lifestyle I craved. I had champagne tastes on a beer budget. I couldn't understand the logic in this when I had lived securely at home. I didn't understand the value of money because it had never mattered to me before. We weren't rich, but we were hardly poor. All our basic needs were met. Any time I got myself into financial trouble, my mom bailed me out. I never paid consequences. I couldn't comprehend the freedom that having money afforded or the misery it wrought by virtue of not having enough.

It was humbling to live in a well-to-do bubble of California yet feel like I was among the poor. I could pay my rent and afford groceries, but I truly needed my second job. It helped me to pay off debt and afforded me a bit of fun money. I didn't know if I wanted to remain in Silicon Valley and struggle or wanted to move to another part of the country and call it home.

One thing was certain: my classroom didn't feel like home. I questioned the beneficence of Jud, my head teacher. I observed him acting rashly and erratically on several occasions. He once pushed one of our students down and it was only partly accidental. He often lost his temper, and he was rude to parents. I couldn't believe the inappropriate comments he made, such as "Go away. You make me nervous." I understood that I was the apprentice teacher, but I often felt that my judgment was sounder than his. He frequently disregarded my input and lost his patience with me. He disrespected me yet passed off responsibility to me without hesitation. He designated me as the lead instructor of biology, but he didn't give me enough time to prepare my lessons.

I didn't fully know what I was doing yet. I was fed to the wolves and left to deal with poor classroom management. I wanted a raise since I did most of the work. My male coworker earned $10 per hour without a college degree, where I made only $1.50 more with a master's degree.

It didn't help that our classroom lacked essential supplies, atlases, and textbooks. Jud informed me that I had to pay for classroom necessities myself. I didn't see how I could provide supplies and pay my rent and bills. I didn't get to observe Montessori Key Experiences required for my teacher training, which would've made it easier for me to consider our classroom as my work home.

I went back home to visit during winter break just before New Year's 1997. I visited my favorite teachers from Barrie, who still worked there. I wanted to see if my experience at the school I worked at mirrored those at another Montessori school.

I observed three rooms of first through third grade combined classrooms. It moved me to tears. It was exactly the kind of homey environment that I wanted to work in. I wanted to feel a sense of belonging to a school's larger community. All the students at Barrie were engaged and actively learning. There was no running in the classroom, no talking back to teachers, no fighting, and no whining for help. The rooms were large and set up in a way that was more conducive to group learning. At my school, students sat in cubicles that blocked off access to other students, thus fostering dependence because it emphasized individual work. It placed the teachers in positions of power whereby we were the keepers of all knowledge. They had to come to us versus seek out one another for support.

Barrie's students were more engaged in everything. They recycled more, had more classroom animals, and even had a farm. More commercial and student artwork was displayed in classrooms and throughout Barrie's administrative buildings. Youth were honored, cherished, and treated with respect. All of this led me to give my resume to Barrie for consideration, as well as to other Montessori schools in the Bay Area.

Rachel Leigh Wills

But if I wanted my Palo Alto school to fund my American Montessori Society teacher training, I was obligated to stay in my classroom with Jud for another year post-certification.

Either way, I needed to prepare myself for transition. I was unhappy with my circumstances. Transition was a phenomenon I always struggled with. I didn't know how to be in the moment. I was either anxious about the future or I was stuck in the nostalgia of the past. I romanticized my past despite knowing that it wasn't ever as good as I remembered it.

In the winter of 1997, I was flummoxed by how dispersed my family was. What I really wanted was to have all my family reside in one geographical location. California felt more like home to me than Maryland did, but home was not necessarily a fixed place. It was where my loved ones were. It was where I felt I belonged. And it was intimately connected with the natural environment. I didn't know how to live or be present in my life and be content, while most of my family lived on the East Coast in Maryland, Pennsylvania, and New York. I longed to exist on both coasts with access to both halves of my family. Ideally, I wanted to have all my loved ones with me in California. My East and West Coast family was vastly different but equally as important. My visit home had made me feel more secure in the direction I was headed professionally. However, it triggered old feelings of being emotionally afloat:

There's a four-letter word I've been thinking about lately—H.O.M.E. Is home the place where one grows up? Can it be found in the man or woman you're in love with? Is it determined by the areas where we study and work? Can more than one place be considered home? Can home be defined by something other than place, such as inside you? Can home be an object?

I am a part of Generation X. As Alanis Morrissette sings, "I haven't got it all figured out just yet." I've succeeded in figuring out who I am, but I am still trying to figure out where I am. It's like that game my students love, "Where in the world is Carmen San Diego?" I'm approximately 10 hours north of Carmen, however, my internal compass has not yet located "true north." Where or what is home for me?

I know I should find some comfort in the fact that all my friends are asking themselves the same questions. Then again, how reassuring can a lost generation be? We'd like to reach the summit of all the obstacles we twenty-somethings face daily ... finishing college, grad school, getting our first job, finding our first apartment, mapping out our career path, keeping our first jobs, paying our rent, and buying groceries. Maybe some of us are closer to the peak but there are plenty of us breaking in our hiking boots.

I've concluded that both Forrest Gump and Morrissette are right. Life is like a box of chocolates, and it is also full of irony. There are plenty of opportunities to stick your hand back into the box or make many wrong turns, U-turns, and right turns. The more I mull it over, the more certain I am that home does not have to be a fixed place or be found in only one place. Home can be both physical and spiritual. This perception is appealing to me, as I have eclectic tastes and desires but strive to strike a balance in my life.

Two months later, I settled down enough to realistically assess what was in my best interest career-wise. I stayed put both in California and at my school. I did move but only from the Peninsula to East Bay, and Tuija and I became roomies. The adventure was a fiasco the likes of which I never experienced. We wanted a "city-living" adventure. Mind you, we didn't move to Berkeley or even Oakland, but to San Leandro. We found an apartment close to our teacher training center there. Oakland wasn't considered very safe in those days unless you lived in the tony hills, but I think even it was nicer than San Leandro, considered the armpit of the East Bay.

My dad offered to pay me not to move in with Tuija or to San Leandro. He saw the writing on the wall. There might as well have been actual writing on the wall. Graffiti would've looked nicer than our apartment did when I unexpectedly had to flee from it.

Within two months of moving into the apartment, Tuija got involved with a man who had just gotten out of prison. She moved him into our

Rachel Leigh Wills

bachelorette pad without even asking me if it was okay. I didn't love the idea, but I didn't ask her to kick him out either. It would've been nice if he contributed to our rent. They spent weekends getting drunk and stoned out of their minds. And just wait before you call me hypocritical!

I'd done my fair share of the former and latter, but not once did I destroy my own place. I couldn't fathom how they did so much damage. It happened when I visited my dad and Ona in Napa one weekend. I drove to my job from their place, a two-and-a-half-hour drive. After school, I made the arduous, one-and-a-half-hour commute (if weather and traffic cooperated) from Palo Alto over the Dumbarton Bridge, up past Union City, and through to San Leandro.

I was exhausted and in no way ready for the sight that greeted me upon opening our apartment door. Our front door opened onto the kitchen and living room. We had one of those pass-through kitchens, where a short wall and bar was all that separated them. As I entered, to my left was a large hole in the living room wall. Our glass door that opened onto a small balcony was filthy. Our blinds were broken and lay in shambles in a heap on the living room floor. The pretty floral couch Ona lent me had taken a rough blow. One of its legs was broken off. They'd even broken the garbage disposal.

To make matters worse, the boyfriend snuck into my room later that night while I slept and clumsily tried to get with me. I managed to get him out of my room, but what if he tried to get back in? To prevent that from happening, I barricaded my door. I used my strength to move all my furniture against the door so Tuija's "gentleman" couldn't enter. I flew back to Napa the next morning. I moved out of the armpit of the world by the end of that week. I drove an oversized (but crammed) U-Haul over the Golden Gate Bridge. The crosswinds were fierce, and I was terrified I'd flip the truck. I'd felt safer when I went with three Egyptian strangers to the lagoon in the middle of the desert near Dahab.

In some way, the broken-down apartment in San Leandro was emblematic of my life in 1996 and 1997. They were rollercoaster years. I keenly felt the chaos in the wider world, including the sudden, violent deaths of Princess Diana and INXS frontman Michael Hutchence. And on a personal level, I moved across the country, chose teaching as a career, and ended up hating it. I moved at least three times within the Bay

198

Area and had multiple roommates. I drank and smoked pot daily. I turned into a woman I didn't recognize.

Hound Dog

I rang in New Year's 1998 with my new boyfriend Todd. We were exclusive after only two dates. He was smitten and lavished attention on me. I never had a man, especially someone who was seven years my senior and a working professional, think I was worth being with. I had always gravitated toward younger guys. If hindsight is 20/20, then I can see that I was overwhelmed by adulting. I thought Todd would take care of me and to his credit, he did the best he could. I moved in with him just as quickly as I had with Rick.

I loved "playing house." I didn't want to listen to Ona when she begged me not to give up my room in the house I shared with roommates in Mountain View. She warned me that I risked losing my autonomy by moving in with Todd. She added that I'd be without a place to call my own if things went south. Of course, I didn't listen to Ona's wisdom. I'm stubborn to a fault and I thought I was in love. I was totally in love—just not with Todd. I loved alcohol, marijuana, and sex. The order depended upon my mood on any given day.

I was happy to find someone who didn't make me feel ashamed of my vices after a long week of work. He liked to have fun the way I did. I envisioned living on Easy Street and believed that I had finally arrived at the "happily ever after" phase of my life. I envisioned teaching, making babies, moving into a home, and getting another dog. However, Todd dreamed of being provided for by a rich woman. He was tired of working like a dog to support himself and he was resentful that I only earned $12 an hour as a teacher.

I'd received a whopping 50-cent raise at the beginning of my second year at my school, but Todd didn't think that my teaching there was good for us. He urged me to get a better job, one that paid substantially more. He thought I needed improvement in other areas as well. He consistently compared my body to our neighbor across our second-story landing. She was taller, blonder, thinner, and more athletic than I was.

Todd pressured me to lose weight—not out of concern for my health, but because he wasn't happy with me as I was. He was also adamant about my going jet-skiing with him. He insisted that I wouldn't be afraid and would like it more if I went with him. He didn't know that I jet-skied in Jamaica. I wasn't afraid; I just didn't like things I wasn't in control of—especially if they went fast. I preferred activities that emphasized strength over speed, like rock climbing, hiking, and canoeing. Worse than the pressure to lose weight and enjoy sports was the unrelenting pressure from Todd to have sex every morning. I'm not a morning person and there's nothing worse than waking up to morning breath and having someone paw at you when your eyes haven't even focused yet. I repeatedly refused Todd, but some mornings, it was easier just to surrender. I just laid on my back and let him do his thing. He was in it for himself anyway.

I got a new teaching job that didn't pay much more than my last one, but we did get a dog together (a surprise from me to Todd. I adopted Digger knowing full well that our apartment complex didn't allow dogs. I've been known for not being a rule follower, believing that rules and regulations don't apply to me; I was (and sometimes still do) ignore them when I believe I have valid reasons for not doing so.

Digger was a beagle puppy who howled at all hours and upon hearing the slightest sound or sensing a hint of movement. When we gave him to my dad and Ona, Ona banished him to an outdoor pen on the side of the house. Within a day, he wormed his way inside. Within a few days, he slept in bed with them. By the end of the second week, Digger ruled the roost. He was supposed to be a miniature beagle, but when I got him from the breeder in the Santa Cruz mountains, I was dubious about his mini status. All puppies start out small, but his paws were huge. Despite that, I was surprised by how much he grew; he was like Clifford! He ended up clocking in at around a hefty 40 pounds.

Digger roamed free and was notorious for his outdoor shenanigans. He stole work gloves from the Mexican vineyard laborers and begged them for food, then stole it when they wouldn't give him any. Sometimes, he robbed them of their lunches and other times their ball caps. He also chased large jackrabbits from sun-up till sun-down. I thought it was hilarious that Digger always started his chase from the originating point of smell so that by the time he finally saw them and gave chase, the rabbits were too far ahead for him to catch.

Juke Box Hero

I left my position at the private Montessori school for an opportunity to teach at one of San Jose's public Montessori schools. I enrolled in a second teacher training program through Campbell University. I didn't want to go to more schooling but needed to obtain state licensure. I was only hired because I possessed Montessori teaching experience and the principal believed I could obtain my license within a year. I was paid on a per diem basis at a rate of $100 per day (only about $4 dollars more per hour than my previous position).

I would need to complete California's rigorous teaching credentialing process and pass the CBEST exam before I could be licensed. Only then would I be eligible to garner better pay and have summers to recharge. My new school didn't utilize team teaching, so I was on my own as a lead teacher in a mixed-age, first-through-third-grade classroom. I had just established rapport with my class when I was plucked out of it and was tossed into a Spanish-English immersion class.

I spoke just enough Spanish to give basic commands and answer simple questions unless I was drunk. Under the influence, I spoke Spanish and Hebrew better than I did when sober. I knew how to speak Spanish passably, but alcohol loosened my inhibitions. Without it, I was too nervous to speak Spanish around native speakers and I understood more than I could articulate. I wasn't proficient enough to answer parents' questions after school or at parent-teacher conferences. Most of the parents were Mexican immigrants who couldn't converse with me in English even if they understood me on a basic level.

I empathized with them and wished we could communicate. It took me a month to figure out what one child asked me at the close of every day. In front of his father he earnestly asked, "¿Maestra? ¿Cómo me porta Maestra?" In response, I shrugged my shoulders. Upon seeing our exchange, the father shook his son by his shoulders and gave him what sounded like a stern sermon. Seeing this upset me, but I didn't know what to do about it. Then, one day, it hit me: the dad was asking how his son's behavior was. From then on, I always answered, "Bien. Bien." The father never shook his son in my presence again.

The school didn't provide any guidance or mentoring to its first-year teachers. My students ran wild in my classroom. They didn't listen to me, even when I was confident that I'd delivered clear instructions in Spanish. There was no one to turn to for guidance. My coworkers intimidated me because they had better control over their classrooms and my insecurity hindered my desire to enlist their support. And it didn't help that I only ever saw my peers in passing. We only saw one another when we covered lunch duty on the playground and our purpose then was to ensure everyone's safety.

Most of us didn't have the luxury of a lunch break. I used every spare moment I had preparing for the next day's lessons. I thought if I were more prepared to teach my students, I'd gain confidence and then maybe some of it would spill over into interactions with other teachers. Others in my position might've joined a club like Toastmasters to further hone their communication skills. I, on the other hand, tried to overcome my social anxiety by singing karaoke in front of a bar full of nameless faces.

I went out every Tuesday night determined to overcome my fears. Sometimes, I went out on Thursday nights as well. Sometimes, Todd came along. I usually didn't want him to come with me because I needed something to call my own. In retrospect, I engaged in exposure therapy. I made myself go solo so I would be forced to interact with random strangers. The Karaoke Experiment involved drinking a glass of wine or a beer to loosen my nerves. I chose my seat with care. I'd look desperate and trashy if I sat at the bar alone. I therefore sat at a table next to the DJ to seem less conspicuous. I could always say I was waiting for friends if there were any empty seats at my table.

I was so nervous the first time I sang karaoke, but after the first few times, I recognized people. The DJ was friendly, and I felt secure near him. He looked out for me and sometimes, his girlfriend joined me at my table. I always sounded as shaky as I felt during the first song of the night, but the alcohol kicked in by my second turn on stage. I sang clearly and stronger and by my third time on the mic, the alcohol made me feel like a bonafide siren.

I sang songs with brazen lyrics like *You Oughta Know* by Alanis Morissette or *Damn, Wish I was Your Lover* by Sophie B. Hawkins—both of which gave me street cred among the women. Among the men, my song choices raised eyebrows and some belt buckles. Alcohol not only calmed my nerves but removed my anxiety and made me feel like I was a part of something. I made "friends" and found a home of sorts in the competitive and mobile California karaoke scene. In doing so, I all but forgot the real reason I started singing karaoke.

Love on the Rocks

I felt like Clark Kent: teacher by day, student-cum-rock star by night. I loved being a student since it brought me closer to my goal of being a public-school teacher and served as an outlet for social interaction. I didn't have any friends of my own since I gave up to spend all my time with Todd.

I was intrigued by a guy in my class named Joe and I wasn't alone in thinking he was hot. There were attractive women in my class and I'm sure more than half of them were into him as well. I was surprised and flattered that Joe befriended me instead of women I considered to be prettier. He was a rock climber and a single dad to two young girls. I climbed a few times and enjoyed it. I had just read *Into Thin Air* by Jon Krakauer and had begun following the careers of professional climbers. I especially admired anyone who'd climbed Everest. I froze in temperatures below 50° *above* zero, so anyone who braved extreme cold was heroic to me.

I've always been intrigued by people who risked their lives in pursuit of their passions. Rock climbing was easy subject matter for talking to Joe, who was both a skilled conversationalist and a flirt. He was more than just eye candy though. He was bright and passionate about the environment. When he offered to take me climbing with him after I floated the suggestion past him one day, I leapt at the chance. It hadn't dawned on me that I was an easy mark.

I was newly single as I had recently broken up with Todd, in large part because of my feelings for Joe. I wasn't under any illusion that Joe would fall in love with me; he was simply a catalyst for extricating myself from my relationship. My attraction to Joe on both spiritual and intellectual planes convinced me that I didn't need to settle just because someone was available and into me.

After befriending Joe, I knew I wasn't in love with Todd. I didn't want to be with him anymore. One morning before my eyes were fully opened, Todd casually said, "Good morning. Our neighbors just got en-gaged. Isn't that great?" I replied, "Oh? That's nice. I'm moving out." Todd was kind and let me stay with him until I figured out my next move (literally and figuratively). He was likely relieved that I had initiated our breakup. I knew he wanted someone different for himself and didn't want to be the bad guy.

Joe introduced me to Whole Foods and nag champak. He took me climbing a few times and got me good and high afterward. The lack of pretense between us was exciting. We weren't romantic. Our relationship was purely physical. He was in complete control and told me exactly what he was going to do with me. I didn't need to think about anything which was freeing.

I thought that being in control was overrated. I was helplessly flail-ing in my life no matter how much effort I exerted. I couldn't gain con-trol of my classroom and had no clue how to create tailored homework assignments for 24 students at different grade levels and with varied in-tellectual abilities and limited conversational English skills. Additional-ly, I couldn't pass the CBEST exam. I'd taken it three times and failed the math portion each time. I was just three points shy of passing on my last attempt. Without a passing score, I couldn't become a certified pub-lic-school teacher.

The fact that I was with some hot man who was well-versed in sex and knew what to do with me was wholly fulfilling. He said dumb things like "Daddy's gonna give it to you really good. Can you take all of me? Ooh yeah. That's a good little girl." But he had moves and the sex was electric. All I had to do was let him have his way with me. I knew our fun would come to an end, but for once I was okay with that.

Stupidly, I let it slip to Todd that I had slept with Joe. I thought we were buds because of how amicably our relationship ended. He told me many times before that he found skinnier women more attractive than me. We weren't together anymore, so I was caught off guard when he railed at me and showed me the door.

I couldn't give Ona the satisfaction of saying she was right about my having sacrificed my independence and I couldn't ask my mom and DP to help me out financially. My pride wouldn't let me, and I knew money was tight for them.

For the first time in my life, I was without a place to live. I spent a couple months staying with friends of Todd's. I ended up finding a room for rent in the home of a 40-year-old single mom who made ends meet by dancing at strip clubs and modeling lingerie in sleazy bars.

I gladly bounced from there a few months later after I found my roommate's kids' escaped pet mouse. I was awoken one night by a pesky noise coming from behind my bed. I flipped the light on and peeked under the top of my bed to discover the rodent happily munching pretzel remnants. I couldn't even handle that on my own. I called my mom in Maryland at 4 a.m. in the morning to ask for her advice; I love mice, but I didn't want one for a bedfellow.

I moved into a nice apartment with a sweet roommate in Sunnyvale. I finally liked my living situation and was prepared to nest and stop partying so much. But on January 25, 1999, I received a provisional diagnosis that sent my mind reeling and my life spiraling even more out of control. I needed to know why I couldn't figure out how to stay on top of my job. Why couldn't I remember spelling tests? I missed administering them even on the days when I wasn't out recreating the night before. Why could I never get out of my classroom before 6 p.m.?

CHAPTER 15 – ADD

I completed batches of tests just like the ones I'd taken at the ages of five and 13. I was given the same diagnosis as I was given back then, but in step with the times, my disorder had been "upgraded." The rebooted name for Minimal Brain Dysfunction was Attention Deficit Hyperactivity Disorder (ADHD), or ADD It's called the latter when someone has the disorder without the physical manifestation of hyperactivity or if hyperactivity presents itself as never-ending mind chatter. I prefer to use ADD because most people refer to it this way—especially when speaking about it negatively.

Not much was known about this neurological brain disorder when I was first diagnosed with it in the early 1970s. It was assumed to be a brain dysfunction when, in fact, it's a matter of someone's brain being wired differently than most of the population rather than it not working properly.

Imagine everyone without ADD living in houses and those with it in apartments. House dwellers have electrical systems that can be powered with smart technology like Alexa. With one word, the lights go on consistently—all of them. But for apartment dwellers, their electrical systems were installed before the smart device era: they require manual operation and sometimes, the lights don't go on unless you flick the switches a few times. Individuals with ADD have smaller brains than those without it. Non-ADDers' prefrontal cortexes, the portion of the brain behind the forehead, are more fully developed than in individuals with ADD.

But this "disorder" isn't solely a deficit. There are so many "ADvantages", and I intentionally use this spelling because of it. The benefits of ADD weren't well known in the 1970s. It wasn't yet known that individuals with ADD wouldn't outgrow their disability (or different ability). No one knew for sure if and how adults would be impacted as they matured. Many of those who were born as females were either misdiagnosed or went undiagnosed because they didn't present as being physically hyperactive. Countless more—especially women like me—appear dreamy and sloth-like. If "regular" people only saw our insides, they'd know it's a different story. If you could see inside our minds, you'd see that while we look like glossy 12-inch records, we spin more like 45s.

When I was told that I had ADD, it felt like an anvil was dropped on me. I vividly remember thinking, *If this is what it is—if I'm not alone, then where is everyone else like me? Why don't I know one single adult who thinks like me or acts like I do?*

This rebranded diagnosis was blunt-force trauma. I felt betrayed and I didn't even know who to direct my anger toward. My parents? They'd done their best to advocate for me and to protect me. I knew it wasn't fair to be angry with them, but I was. The more I read and learned about ADD, the angrier I became. I learned why females were more likely to be underdiagnosed. Unlike boys who are expected by society to be rambunctious, most parents taught their daughters to be demure, to be good and not be disruptive at school.

I rationalized that the unseen handicap I struggled gave me license to shirk the last vestige of responsibility for myself. I wasn't looking for help. I wanted empathy and validation. Everything suddenly made sense in terms of why I was so easily overwhelmed by life. I didn't know if there were medications for adults with ADD because I had only seen kids in my classes who were on medication for it. If meds were available and I took them, would I be forever dependent upon them if I wanted to function at my full potential? There were national support groups such as CHADD (Children and Adults with Attention Deficit Disorder) and ADDA (Attention Deficit Disorder Association), but I was in the anger stage of grief.

I felt justified in my self-destruction via alcohol, marijuana, and men. There had been something wrong with me my entire life and I finally knew what it was. I was inherently flawed, and it wasn't ever my fault, but I mistakenly believed it was.

If I were born defective and I couldn't blame my parents and society at large for the way I was, what choice did I have? Why didn't anyone intervene on my behalf in school besides my mom? She wasn't a trained professional, yet she was the only one who insisted I receive accommodations. Why did I struggle in isolation when something was wrong with me? Why wasn't I medicated as a child? Why didn't my parents make me go to therapy? I now had a name for my brain "deformity," but instead of feeling relieved, I felt more alone than ever.

Once I had abdicated responsibility, there was no stopping the self-loathing havoc I wrought on myself. I can't even read most of my journal entries from the winter of 1999. I was stoned or drunk or both when I wrote. I increased the number of nights I sang karaoke to three or four times a week. I started bringing home strangers or went home with them. I was the "promiscuous girl" Nelly Furtado and Timbaland sang about nine years early. I was a smart woman who made dumb decisions.

I didn't have a desire to catch a sexually transmitted infection or to be mistreated during consensual sex, but both of those things happened as a direct result of my relinquishing personal accountability. I was 27 and regularly brought home guys that were significantly (enough) younger than I was, which had less to do with me being a "cougar" and more to do with my inability to relate to men my own age. It didn't matter whether I was drunk or high at the time.

Once, I brought a guy home from one of my favorite karaoke bars who, despite being clearly more intoxicated, told me I was the dumb one for drinking so much. He uttered the same words as the Egyptian guy in the desert did: "You don't know me. I could kill you if I wanted to." Instead of harmlessly massaging my back as the guy in Dahab had, this guy bit my neck so hard I bore bite marks the next day. My breasts were bruised yellow, black, and blue. It hurt badly, but the experience was so intense that I didn't ask him to stop.

Another guy I brought home was a sexy Portuguese man who looked like my rock g—d, Chris Cornell. He wore form fitting red and green plaid pants with suspenders that hung loosely from one shoulder. He had an impressive vocal range and long, curly hair, which I've always been nuts about. He gave me one night of pleasure plus something more to remember him by. He didn't want to use a condom and I stupidly believed him when I drunkenly inquired about whether I should be worried. He assured me he was fine. He was fine alright, but not safe. He gave me the only STI I've ever had.

I befriended one baby-faced man named Dan, who looked like he was fresh out of college. He was sweet and treated me with respect. I enjoyed the nights I stayed at his place. We laughed and had sex into the early hours of the morning. The downside of staying at Dan's was that it coincided with my need to leave early for work. I started leaving a grab-and-go bag in my car because I never knew when I might need an extra change of clothes.

By springtime, I was weary of everything. California no longer felt like home because I wasn't tethered to anyone. I had no friends or self-respect. I never gained control of my classroom and I wasn't any further along in making peace with the fact that I had ADD since I was diagnosed. Like The Clash song, "Should I Stay or Should I Go," I agonized for months over whether to go back home. All four of my parents were tired of my waffling between the two coasts. Ultimately, I decided I was better off in Maryland with my mom and DP, so I resigned from my job and moved cross-country.

Just Like a Pill

I got a no-pressure job as a lead barista at a cafe, and I finally began to sort out who I was as an adult with ADD. I worked with a therapist whose specialty was working with adults with ADD. I also saw an osteopath who prescribed stimulant medication to better manage my negative symptoms. I experienced yet another metamorphosis.

I wish I could say that I blossomed during this epic period, but I didn't. In fact, I nosedived into the depths of despair. I didn't recognize myself before I moved back home, but after taking prescribed amphetamines for focusing, I truly became a stranger to myself.

Initially, Ritalin and Dexedrine initially helped me to focus. For the first time in my life, I could sustain attention long enough to perform detail-oriented tasks. The meds had a short half-life, however, so in a relatively short period of time, I required larger and larger doses to get the same effect. And then there was the catastrophic mixture of stimulants with depressants: alcohol and marijuana.

Many Monday mornings following weekends full of indulgence, I declared, "This is it! I'm going to stop drinking." I made this promise repeatedly but broke my solemn vows without a moment's hesitation time after time. I didn't feel like myself unless I had at least two drinks in me come nighttime. Two drinks might not seem like a lot, but the amphetamines intensified the effects of alcohol. And since two drinks made me feel baseline normal, I really needed four drinks in me to feel good or even buzzed, but factoring in my stimulant meds, that's essentially eight drinks. Then add in the fact that I had never handled alcohol as well as others did. What unmanageability!

There was a fine line between being flirty and fun and sloppy and desperate. There was an equally thin line between being sexy and being sick. I never knew what I was going to be like when I drank. Not from my earliest days of college drinking had I known when to stop and cut myself off. I might be alright with four drinks in me, or I might be a hot mess. Sometimes, I became aggressive. I shoved around people way larger than me on the dance floor because I wanted more space to do my thing. Men were caught off guard when they saw how tiny I was. They were surprised enough that they didn't shove me back or hit me.

It dawned on me that my drinking and sexual promiscuity were intricately connected. Alcohol seductively whispered that it was okay for me to compromise my virtue. It gave me a false sense of security. Drinking alcohol made me feel like I was holding onto the lead rope rock climbing. The rope didn't make climbing safer, but whoever was below me holding onto it seemed like they were in control. I knew that I could still get badly hurt even if I didn't fall off a mountain; the tension on the rope made my fall seem less brutal.

Similarly, alcohol made me feel bolder and sexier than I felt when sober. I knew it didn't fundamentally change how others saw me, but it helped me to care less about how I was perceived under the influence. It was easy to believe sweet nothings murmured in darkness, but the next morning was always brutal the next morning—especially after I slept with someone I drank with the night before. I never met dateable men in bars. I met men who wanted women like me—easy and gullible:

When I can relate to Cruel Intentions and Drugstore Cowboy and The Doors even if I've barely skimmed the surface in comparison to others who drink and drug. I've lost a piece of myself that I can never get back. I don't regret it entirely but I'm angry. I never thought I could admit this, that I want out. I don't like who I've become. Who cares if I can't be my free-spirited self or have arms like Linda Hamilton from Terminator or have

Madonna's abs. I can't berate myself any longer ... So, it's cold turkey or maybe AA.

I need Depeche Mode. I know David Gahan understands more than most ever will. Until I can handle it, not another sip of alcohol will graze my lips and I'm afraid. And my body will not know another's until I know two things.

(1) That I'm not a hazard to anyone; and
(2) That I can face the mirror in the morning.

How I wish that those words were sincere enough to bring a halt to my antics.

I usually start writing in a new journal at the start of each new chapter of my life. It usually just happens this way. I opened a new journal at the beginning of May 1999 when I was dating a guy I met at a Jewish singles' event. We were nothing alike and I don't know what we saw in one another. As usual, I tried hard to convince myself that I could be in love. We only lasted two-and-a-half months.

It was, however, the first time in a long time that I didn't feel completely miserable. I didn't cut back on my drinking or go to AA. I wasn't ready to give up my crutch, my only means of escape. Alcohol was the only thing that brought me to a place of numbness. Music and writing had been like my appendages, they didn't give me a rush, make me feel empty inside, or allow me to forget myself like alcohol and drugs did.

I did one thing good for myself which lessened the urgency of my need for escape. I began to forgive myself for my past. I knew that no amount of self-loathing would lessen the damage I did to myself. I was beginning to heal.

I accepted that my having ADD made me different from others. I began to consider the fact that maybe I was okay just as I was. I was ready to connect with other misfits. I didn't want my ADD to alienate me anymore. I wanted to form meaningful relationships and develop healthy habits. Like Rupert Holmes sings in The Pina Colada song (one of my childhood favorites), I *returned to the personal ads seeking an escape.* I responded to an online post about a writers' group someone was looking to form. I met up with two women and a man at the fountain in Dupont Circle. The man quickly left the group because Sheila, Andrea, and I were instantly as thick as thieves. I had found my people at last.

Sheila was the first person I truly connected with on a soul level. She didn't have ADD, but she struggled with severe depression. It felt like we shared a brain. We often knew exactly what the other was thinking and when we talked it wasn't unusual for us to say "Jinx!" multiple times.

We were like little kids on the school playground despite Sheila being more evolved in the professional sense. She had an inner knowledge about herself and an understanding of how the world worked. I'm forever grateful that the forces of nature brought us together.

Sheila is from New Jersey and is of Irish Catholic heritage. She's stereotypically very fair skinned and her face and arms are sprinkled with orange freckles. She has strawberry blond hair and extremely blue eyes. Whatever she says after a laugh is uttered in a languid, sexy way. She's not a goth, but black is her signature color. Dresses, skirts, and chunky shoes have always been part of her signature look. I've rarely seen her wear pants, and she didn't wear them back then. We had so many fun DC and New Jersey adventures together. I honestly believe if it wasn't for Sheila's friendship, the sky would've fallen on my back. She and Jessica, my longtime friend from Barrie, were my anchors during this part of my life.

At the end of June 1999, I got a job at one of the two major bookstore and cafe chains in the area. It started my true love affair with coffee and fed my dream of one day opening my own cafe. It also introduced me to people I have bittersweet memories of (but more of that in a minute). I ended up transferring locations but keeping the job as a second source of income after I was offered a more professional position.

I was brought on as a Recycling Specialist with a newly created division of Montgomery County's Division of Solid Waste Management. The program was called SORRT for "Smart Organizations Reduce and Recycle Tons," and I was its initial hire, being brought on to teach businesses how to implement and maintain recycling programs. It was the first time I experienced a panel interview. I thought they'd made a mistake when they hired me. I didn't think I was mature enough for the position. I was nervous about how my ADD would play out in a government work environment—especially one that wasn't all that structured.

I was expected to be out of the office and operate out of my car 60 percent of the time. My key task was to inspect trash and recycling facilities around a large portion of the large county; some of this meant rummaging through commercial trash and recyclable containers. My previous experience as an elementary school teacher contributed to me being assigned as a recycling liaison to the Montgomery County Public Schools. In this capacity, I educated administrative and custodial staff, as well as students, about the benefits and requirements of the county's 90% mandatory recycling regulation.

The same month I was offered this position, my parents decided that they were ready to sell the house that my sister Stacey and I grew up in. I still lived there with my parents at the time.

At the end of July, Stacey came back home to visit. We were now more friends than enemies, but I was still envious of her gracefulness, her beauty, and the easy way in which she interacted with our parents. I worked so hard to please them and I was barely acknowledged—at least it seemed this way to me at the time. When Stacey came home, our parents lavished her with attention and praise. I have a vivid memory of her making drinks before dinner one night. They were touched by her generosity, something she wasn't usually known for. Later, I was touched when Stacey remarked, "Your eyes are beautiful, Rach, and you look good!" I felt so ugly next to her.

The last thing I wanted to do was to go out to dinner with her and my parents. I didn't want to be a part of their conviviality. I was miserable and self-pitying. "I always offer to make drinks or pour wine for you guys, but all I receive is criticism," I fumed. My mom's retort stung, "You're an alcoholic. We don't want you making drinks for us. We don't want to see you drink in front of us." This and similar conversations about my drinking always stopped at, "Rach, why are you doing this to yourself? When are you going to stop? You obviously don't handle alcohol well. You're like your father."

My mom and DP never handed me a pamphlet about rehab or expressed their concern for me unless it was in the moment. In retrospect, I wanted to be saved by anyone other than myself, but I was resentful that they didn't try to intervene on my behalf. Even had they had done so, however, I don't think I'd have truly listened or consented to go to treatment because I didn't think that my drinking was that bad. This put the family in a Catch-22.

I began to contemplate suicide, but I knew I wouldn't do it. I was too afraid of pain and I abhorred blood. Besides, knowing me, I'd botch my own death and be severely hurt or disabled and that scared me even more.

Even still, I was a walking contradiction. I had been taking ADD stimulants for about three months at the time of my sister's visit. In addition to feeling focused and confident, I experienced what it was like to be able to eat all the sugar I wanted with impunity. With all the amphetamine in my system, I was rarely hungry for meals. That's why Stacey remarked on how good I looked. I was thin. For the first time, I knew what it was like to inhabit the body of someone like hers. I never sat still. I was in perpetual motion, a hummingbird flitting from one activity to the next without rest.

I was a stranger in my own skin, however. I was suddenly skinny on the outside, but I still felt chubby on the inside. I often wished that I could crawl out of my skin and molt like a snake. I had so much ADD medication in my system that I experienced all the negative side effects of being on them. The more I felt their ill effects, the more I turned to a dangerous combination of mixing my meds with alcohol and marijuana, which, of course, nearly always resulted in my sleeping with someone.

At the end of August 2001, my parents bought a condo in Arlington, Virginia. To make their move easier, they asked me to go through all my stuff that they stored in the attic. Purging my childhood of old relics, which I no longer needed, was unsettling. I couldn't go back to yesterday and I didn't care for my present.

My recycling job required too much self-structuring. It was proving to be too challenging for me to maintain. I was too overwhelmed. Not to mention that I was totally hooked on prescribed stimulants. I believed that I would fail at life without them but longed to rid myself of their effects. The attic purge filled me with a combination of longing and loathing. I tossed out pictures from school trips, the last few letters Bono sent me, and the pink Chuck Taylors he drew on which I swore I'd never throw away.

I packed up 10 boxes full of stuff to keep, including old photos of my mom when she was model thin and married to my dad. There were photos of both grandmas and Aunt Carolyn, all of whom were now dead, all from different forms of cancer.

I desperately wanted to escape the sad, nostalgic feelings that purging my past brought up. Without thinking, I blurted to no one "I need a drink right now." I felt claustrophobic within our big, open house devoid of furniture and full of trash and boxes.

CHAPTER 16 – DIRTY TUBS

I was originally going to change the title of this chapter because it's a silly one, but the more I thought about it, the more I realized how apropos it is. I loved No Doubt and their song "Bathwater," the lyrics to which are about accepting an old flame's poorer characteristics. I used to blame everyone but myself for the way I was and where I was (or wasn't) in life. It was like blaming my exes for their poor housekeeping skills when I should've been looking at my own.

Beaux, who I worked with at my bookstore job, was an example of "dirty bathwater" and my "grimy tub." He was one of a handful of cool individuals I interacted with at the bookstore cafe. He was one of the store's departmental managers and was tight with a crew of guys and a few women (including me) who hung out together after work some nights and most weekends. My nickname for him was Gruff because he was as grouchy as a tired bear.

There was sexual tension between us from the moment we met. Beaux wasn't good-looking in the classic sense, but I was insanely attracted to him, nonetheless. He had small green eyes and a mop of thick, brown hair. He wore big glasses and had a wide gap between his front teeth. He was in the Army Reserves and he comported himself like a soldier, with swagger. He was built like a tank: beer belly, strong arms, muscled thighs, barrel chest, and hairy back in need of some manscaping. He also possessed a low, throaty voice that turned my insides to mush—especially when his quick wit rose to the surface.

Beaux put his friends and comrades above all else, worked hard, and played even harder, but was an enigma to me because while brilliant, he had no professional ambition whatsoever. He was an avid reader, had eclectic musical tastes, and had a breadth of knowledge about world history and movies. I was addicted.

Beaux was often unavailable which, back then, made someone more desirable to me. There was a huntress in me that loved the thrill of the chase. Whenever he couldn't hang out, I craved him even more. Beaux's gruff manner made me fiercely determined to reach his softer side. I knew he too, had been rejected and felt as wounded as I did. Beaux was physically drawn to me, but he didn't want to be my boyfriend—or maybe he did but knew I wanted more from him emotionally than he either wanted to or could give to me.

He wasn't deeply religious, but he had grown up in a home that was devoutly Catholic. Crosses hung everywhere on the walls of his house, the inside of which I only saw a few times and only once during the daytime. When I was there, we were drunk, and he quietly and hurriedly ushered us upstairs to his bedroom so we wouldn't wake his parents.

Beaux wasn't wrong about my wanting it all. I wanted a real boyfriend—not just a "friend with benefits." I wouldn't have been content hanging with the guys, chugging beer, and playing darts forever, but that's all he did. I knew this deep down, but I didn't accept it. I was still big on seeing the "potential" in a potential mate. I was deluded in thinking that I was his path to enlightenment.

It would've been much easier had I wanted to date our mutual friend, Dan. We were more compatible. I was attracted to him but not in the same way I was to Beaux. Dan was softhearted, brilliant, and quirky. He was a good guy and a good friend. He knew I was barking up the wrong tree with Beaux, but he never lorded it over me.

In hindsight, I can see that Beaux was a version of my father. They had similar mannerisms and they both had avoidant personalities. The more aloof or misleading Beaux was (I liked to think he acted this way because he didn't want to hurt my feelings), the more I tried to attract and maintain his attention. Similarly, the more abandoned I felt by him, the harder I tried to connect with him. And how could I connect to him? As I had to connect with my dad: by drinking with him.

There was always that part of me that wanted to revel in the shared desire for reckless abandon that I could only obtain through alcohol. In one journal entry, I wrote:

At Beaux's house drinking. I want oblivion. From my pain; Dad's pain; Aunt Carolyn's pain, and Grandma Harriett's pain. They're all dying. Aunt Carolyn is dying from breast cancer that has spread to her ovaries. Grandma Harriett is dying from leukemia. And Dad is unintentionally trying to kill himself by drowning himself with alcohol.

My ability to put on blinders to my own reality was sad. I viewed the truth as an obstacle to overcome, to outstubborn. I cherry-picked my reality, believing some of it and ignoring the rest. Every time I began to let go of Beaux, he did something to draw me back and to make me want to win him over. Like Bono, he had said that he just wanted to be my friend. I was a plastic fish affixed to a toy fishing pole, and Beaux tossed me out into deep water then reeled me back in whenever it suited him. His mixed messages were confusing:

> *Beaux invited me to his party. He walked me to my car afterward even though I didn't ask him to. My only fault is that when he kissed me (always with chew in his mouth when he's stressed), I asked for more. He told me in that gruff voice of his that he liked my hair. He heard that I was coming back to the bookstore, and I asked if he could handle that?*

Unbeknownst to me, Beaux often hung out with the bookstore crew on the same weekends he told me that he was too busy. I heard about the gang's weekend fun secondhand, and from the few women in the bunch no less. I was surprised to find out that he talked to them about our sexual exploits behind my back. I wanted to be like the other women in the group, to be included all the time or, at least, whenever I wanted to be. But I wasn't like them. I didn't want to spend all my time drinking and hanging out in either Beaux's garage or at someone else's apartment. I didn't see anything wrong with how they spent their time. It just wasn't my thing. I liked hanging out and drinking with them, but I preferred to go to movies or a concert.

When I did hang and drink with the gang, I had an insatiable desire to prove that I could drink like a dude. I, too, could play darts, be tough, and be cool. I wanted to be one of the guys yet be treated like a woman. I didn't know I had become "*that* woman," the one people gossiped about and excluded because she was "too much."

Do you know what it's like to be "*that* woman" and not know it? To unwittingly find this out and pretend like it didn't matter when, in fact, it cut you to the core? Do you know what it felt like to put on an act of being a "modern woman" who went for what she wanted and flaunted it, but was secretly mortified when she did so? Do you know what it's like to feel mortified yet ignore the feeling because you were too desperate for connection? Have you ever longed for true intimacy yet settled for sex because your desire for it was stronger than your own moral fiber? I do. I was "that woman." My brother-in-law Jim urged me to write Beaux off. I needed to hear it from a man, that he wasn't worth wasting my energy on. But more than that, I needed to hear that from a man I respected.

I resolved to set my obsession with Beaux aside. I was gaining more confidence in myself because I moved out of my parents' home and into an apartment with Jessica. I continued to work my full-time recycling oriented "career" job, as well as my bookstore gig. My professional growth helped me grow my self-confidence and sense of self-worth. "Jim was right: I deserve someone who is equally into me as I am to them." However, I struggled not to give in to my primal craving for Beaux:

> *I need to be strong! I will not sleep with him when he's confused. I will not be someone to fill in his time with. I will go out with Mel who has been hanging around me at the bookstore and finally mustered up the nerve to ask me out on a real date. I swore I would never be convenient for any man again! And again, I told Beaux that I'll never call him—and again—I won't. You know that I caved again too since I'm intensifying my resolve here on this page. I'm on overdrive. I'm so amazed at how well I'm functioning for drinking and smoking pot last night and sleeping with Gruff and maybe getting four hours of sleep.*

Hey Man, Nice Shot

That was close to the end of September 1999. The combination of drinking, smoking pot, and taking Ritalin or Dexedrine was beginning to take a toll on me. The drugs, as well as the days and nights, all bled together.

I enlisted in an adventure that marked my first attempt at trying to control my drinking and marijuana use. I started working out at Mooney's

Boxing Gym in Rockville. I thought if I trained to box, I'd naturally be healthier and want to abstain from drinking. I didn't understand that it was the way alcohol affected me and why I drank that was problematic versus alcohol in and of itself.

I still took prescribed speed for my ADD and was boxing a lot, but my good intentions to lead a healthier lifestyle didn't manifest because I continued to party with the bookstore crew. We hung out and played darts either at Buffalo Billiards or in Beaux's garage. Often, it was still just me and the guys hanging out. I don't know why the other women in the gang hung out with Beaux and the dudes when I wasn't around.

One evening, Sheila gave me solicited insight into her take on relationships. It was better than any session I had with either my therapist or the osteopath who prescribed my meds. The latter had just switched me from Ritalin to Dexedrine when the half-life of the former grew too short and no longer was viable.

I had asked Sheila if she thought it was possible to have both a satisfying emotional and sexual connection with the same person. In my experiences, I had great sex with the men I was the least emotionally connected to and I had unfulfilling sex with men I was in committed relationships with. She said, "You can work with a man to be a better lover, but you can't make a man a better person. It's better to wear casual clothes most of the time because they're comfortable and make us feel safe."

But what she said next blew my mind. "Every so often, it's fun to dress up because it's exciting and different. It's more fulfilling to dress up with a good man and experience new circumstances with him than stay on the rollercoaster with someone who isn't worthy of you."

I resolved to heed Sheila's words and find a good man. Like I did on countless occasions where alcohol was concerned, I swore that this time around with dating, things would be different and in some ways they were.

One Fine Day

I put Beaux aside and only looked for love on JDate, the preeminent Jewish dating website. I didn't find a pair of Levi's in a man, per se, more like a pair of Hilfiger's. Enter Wesley.

Wesley was quirky and vibrant, which was a stark contrast to Beaux. He was also lanky and there was something panther-like versus soldier-like about him. Wesley had brown eyes and hair and was clean shaven. The only way in which Beaux and Wesley were alike was that they had both felt trapped in their jobs and didn't know what else they wanted to do. Where Beaux had worked for a prominent book merchandiser, Wesley worked for a renowned music retailer.

On our first date, Wesley told me that he was a drummer at heart and played gigs here and there. He played with a band a few times during the time we dated, but indicated that he aspired to be a full-time musician. The only time I ever saw him play, however, was on a play drum kit on the boardwalk in Ocean City, Maryland.

Wesley was interested in a relationship and was the one who found my profile on JDate and sought me out. He even came to meet me at the bookstore one night to introduce himself to me, which won him major brownie points. When we started dating, I promised myself that I wouldn't write about him. I was afraid to put his name on paper.

Bono only wanted "a whore in bed"; Rick lacked conviction and thought I was going to Hell; Todd convinced me that I was a scatterbrain; and Beaux was unattainable. But Wesley—he was soul mate material.

Plus, he also had ADD. He didn't take medication for it but did take meds to help manage his anxiety. This made me feel like it was okay to be my real self with him. I knew I wouldn't make his life miserable when I forgot my keys or wanted something spontaneously, spaced out, and acted silly. We were both a bit left of center. Wesley was brooding but wasn't as mercurial as Beaux. He was, however, every bit as sexy. I was amazed that he was attracted to me which pains me to write. It demonstrates how little I thought of myself, which was thankfully more than I had thought of myself when I had sought Beaux's affection.

Wesley hugged me versus kissed me goodbye on our first date, where he drew all over my takeout box from Houston's. I wondered to myself if that meant he wasn't into me. *What if I'm re-opening Pandora's Box? I don't want to be hurt again. I don't want to deceive myself and I don't want to lose.*

It turned out, however, that everything was groovy between Wesley and me. He was truly as into me as I was into him. For the first time in a long time, my affection wasn't unrequited. He asked me to read my poetry without me foisting it upon him. We were mutually relieved to share the dysfunction of ADD and we genuinely got one another. No one else had seen me and accepted me just as I was before, a first for me in the dating arena.

Another first—a man's asking my permission to kiss me. Wesley waited until our third date to kiss me. And I was sober for our first kiss. I didn't feel pressured to drink because he didn't drink at all. The only thing that was not a first with Wesley was that I prayed to G—d about him. I'd done this countless times before—especially when alcohol was involved.

G-d, if this can last for some time, I'll work out a lot and never want to be drunk again.

I'm profusely grateful to you and I will try not to screw this up, go too fast, push too hard, want too much. But I'm jumping feet first into deep water. Will I think of nothing else? My medicine is wearing off and I need sleep, only it rarely comes when I want it to. I didn't get to sleep until 2 a.m. or later.

You know, the usual combo of prescribed speed, caffeine, and sexual arousal (minus alcohol). I am drained from my phone argument with Mom. I am through with repentance and martyrdom. I am forever admitting my mistakes and she never says she's sorry. She expects me to learn at her speed. I am so hard on myself, and I always feel so horrible about my mistakes. I don't need her rubbing my nose in my piss like a dog. They're generally small mistakes, but she overreacts like I'm ruining my life! I am listening and I am learning, just at the same slow pace I've always gone at.

I wonder if she is aware that she sets me up and I fall. She wipes her hands and says, "I told you so." Then, she lingers in the shadows and lunges to drag me away from the fire again and again, only to say what a savior she is. Only to say how stupid

I'm being. Only to insinuate that I won't be able to make it in life without her. I know she's trying to have patience, but she doesn't. I will always fail her.

The fight was about my newfound relationship and happiness. I know she was only trying to protect me from harm and heartache, but my journal entry is a perfect example of how codependent we still were. We immediately reverted to our old ways of interacting with each other upon my return home. I still desperately wanted her approval in all aspects of my life, and I was miserable whenever she was disappointed in me. I resorted to drinking at her and *over* myself.

Wesley lived in the basement apartment of a townhome in North Bethesda. His upstairs roommate was a female which surprised me. He invited me over in the second week of December. I marveled at how accurately his place reflected his personality and values. He had Play-Doh, toys, and KISS and Rush memorabilia all over. I kept waiting for him to kick me out, yet he didn't. I wasn't *"that* woman" anymore! I couldn't believe that the sexy man standing in front of me saying, "Shit yeah, Rach," as I kissed him, didn't rush me into sleeping with him. I wondered, *what do I do now?* I drove home that night feeling like a virgin. I was giddy with anticipation for what came next: SEX!

He said he wanted to spoil me, only I didn't know what that meant. True to his word, he made me feel precious and safe. He didn't demand but softly whispered for me to roll onto my stomach. I didn't like to be in that position because it made me feel awkward and vulnerable. But Wesley kissed me, caressed, and supported me. I'd never felt anything more erotic than feeling him hard against my back.

I distinctly recall that we were listening to Marillion's song "One Fine Day" while we made love. The following week, he gave me his entire Marillion CD collection to listen to. He wanted me to know what was important to him and he made me many mixtapes.

We had only been dating for a month-and-a-half when things started to disintegrate. He got migraines more and more frequently. He told me that he even had one on the night we first made love. I didn't understand the source of his headaches, nor did I understand why he showed up at my place hours after he promised he'd be there. And then one night,

Wesley called me disoriented, saying he was on his way to my place. He ended up at Seneca Creek State Park, which wasn't at all near where I lived. He had driven in a foggy state. I was concerned and worried when he first called and frantic when he never showed.

I drank often but hadn't experienced withdrawal. Surprisingly, I didn't know much about addiction even though IDDIOP, I was addicted to substances, too. I had no clue that Wesley was addicted to benzos - Xanax, Klonopin, Ativan, and Valium.

December 26, 1999

One week till the next century, 2000. Everyone is preparing for the end of existence, Armageddon. I'm just focusing on next week. I'm packing the office that has been a hell hole. Once I clean it out, it will hold three other employees besides me. How on Earth will that work? Transition. As usual, everything is changing, always changing. It's winter and we've only had one snow but I'm already ready for warmth. I can't live with Jessica anymore. She's always miserable.

I didn't think the world would end, but it did feel as if the world were closing in on me. The one change I wasn't prepared for was Wesley's. I didn't understand why G—d dropped a beautiful mess at my feet. Why couldn't he just stay beautiful? I tried to drink less. I exercised more and harder. I didn't understand that Wesley's sudden change in behavior had nothing to do with me. Be codependent some more—it was what I knew. I allowed Wesley's misery to wash over me. I just wanted to make him and everyone else happy so that they'd never be angry with me.

I always tried to please everyone—all the time and sometimes, all at once. I now know this stems from growing up in a dysfunctional household. I associated my dad's anger and my mom's disappointment as rejection. And there's nothing worse than feeling (notice that I didn't say "being") rejected and thinking that it's somehow your own fault.

Ironically, on New Year's Eve heading into Y2K, the night that the world was supposed to end, I rejected Jessica and Sheila. I stood them up because they both wanted to spend time with me, but not with Wesley and me together. They didn't think Wesley was good for me, and I didn't want to be without my boyfriend at the dawn of a new millennium.

January 2, 2000

It is strange to be writing 2000. The world is still intact. No Armageddon. I was amazed by how many people truly worried about terrorism, missiles falling on us, power outages, etc. I didn't worry at all because I know there's nothing I could've done should anything have happened. But I worry about every-thing else!

Between the dawn of a new era and the day the skies exploded on 9/11, Wesley and I went around and around on an emotional hamster wheel. We made plans; he broke them. I ranted and raved; he deflected or projected. I drank him away in my bedroom alone at night, while he saw ex-girlfriends who rejected him and only reached out to him because they knew he was dating someone new.

I didn't understand that Wesley and I were both re-enacting patterns of behavior endemic in individuals engaged in emotionally abusive relationships. Wesley's mentality reminded me of lyrics from Garbage's "Only Happy When It Rains": "You know I love it when the news is bad. | Why it feels so good to feel so sad? | I'm only happy when it rains ... Pour your misery down on me."

Over the course of the next year, it sank in that whoever Wesley was when we first met and who I'd fallen in love with, he wasn't that person now. And I did love him. Despite the brevity of our courtship, he made me feel cherished and alive in a way I hadn't been before.

I didn't end things with Wesley when I should've because when they were good, they were exceptionally good. He made me feel higher than alcohol or marijuana ever had. I never knew anyone who was as un-abashedly goofy as him. One day in the grocery store, he asked me if a loaf of French bread felt soft, but instead of having me feel it with my hands, he whacked me over the head with it. Other times, he imitated Animal from The Muppets or told me dumb jokes. He always gave me little trinkets like the mix CDs he made me, a blacklight to better see the glow-in-the-dark stars I put on my ceiling, and royal blue slime in a Lu-cite canister. They were small tokens of affection, but I cherished them.

Sadly, there were many more times he left me with little energy. I didn't know yet that Wesley was abusing benzos. Even as I wrote about his use in my journals, I didn't understand or know what the side effects of benzos were or what the symptoms of withdrawal were.

January 6

I thought Wesley would feel better after a while, but he woke up at 4 a.m. sick as a dog again. He had a fever of 103. He told me his body aches all over. Why is he always sick?

January 9

I am so exhausted. Wesley sapped all my energy. I felt like I couldn't give anymore or cry anymore. He has put me last so many times. He tells me he doesn't deserve happiness. Well, I do. He used again and didn't show up last night.

January 14

I understand fully now how not present Wesley is and how often he's distracted. I hope when he goes off the Xanax, he won't be so flat and will be able to experience extremes.

January 25

I will go out and date, but there is no way I'm bailing on Wesley. He OD'd last night—took 20 pills. He's on suicide watch. He said he's happy I'm not embracing his horror so much anymore. He is just walking dead right now, and he doesn't believe that "good" people get addicted to substances. I can't stop crying. I feel like Wesley's so far away and lost. I feel like he's gone and I'm mourning what will never be: us.

January 28

Last night was incredibly sad and scary for me, but it propelled me to do the healthiest thing for myself and for Wesley. I told him he absolutely can't call me until he is off Xanax. I am ready to deal with me.

Sadly, Wesley and I were mirror images of each other. I coped with his benzo addiction by drinking more and more often. I couldn't imagine dealing with my problems without alcohol. I didn't believe that good people could be addicts. By this point, I was not just drinking at or over hurt caused by others; I was also drinking to do boring tasks like putting away laundry and doing the dishes. Then, drinking helped me cope with the reality of needing to sever ties with Wesley. I couldn't accept that he chose his addiction to Xanax over his relationship with me. I finally let him be and I began to date again.

I reconnected with Jessica and started going out again with other friends. I occasionally got together with Wesley, but I knew that we wouldn't ever get back together. He had told me as much several times; I just hadn't been listening. I was too focused on seeing his potential and playing the "if only" game: *If only he'd change, my life would be perfect. If only I drank less, I'd be able to set better boundaries and garner his respect. If only he got a different job, we'd be happy together.* That's an unfair and dangerous one to play because it blinds you to the reality of the present and being present in it.

Groundhog Day

January 2000 through July 2002 was mostly a Dexedrine, alcohol, marijuana, and male-storm (as opposed to "maelstrom" [although it was that as well]). Day after day after day for two years, each seemed to be the same: wake up, eat breakfast with coffee, take stimulants for ADD, go to a job, quit a job, look for a job, get stoned, get drunk, take Trazadone to help me fall asleep, wash, rinse, repeat.

I was a voluptuous size 14 in 1999, when I began taking medication to manage my ADD. By July the end of 2001, I was a gaunt size four. I exercised a lot, but not enough to affect that kind of bodily transformation. I was emboldened by all the attention I got from being skinny, but I felt like a fraud. Boxing gave me muscles and trimmed some of the fat, but the stimulants squelched my appetite and made it so I couldn't sit still long enough to prepare a meal. I lived in fear of what would happen when I went off the meds. I didn't want to go back to being chubby.

I took a job writing for a rabbi who promoted a form of basketball that was more inclusive of individuals with disabilities, as it could be played by individuals who use wheelchairs. I wasn't prepared for a rabbi to lack patience, so I was stunned when this rabbi snapped at me mid-conversation and told me to shut up. I told him off in return and quit on the spot. The only good thing about working for him was that he helped me to get an article I wrote about his game published in a parks-and-recreation magazine.

I was beginning to lose faith that I'd find meaningful employment again. I had no confidence whatsoever in my ability to keep a job anymore. I cajoled my landlord Randy into letting me do some landscaping work for him. I loved engaging in manual tasks such as building, refinishing furniture, and yard work—and I especially loved gardening. He accepted my pleas.

My stint as a landscaper lasted all of two days because he took every opportunity to ogle me.

He made sure I was undressed comfortably enough to work in the heat. Randy had me outside working on the hottest and most humid day of a Maryland summer. I dug trenches when it was 99° and dug them all day long. I worked so hard that I got sick and threw up. He was as dogged as a drill sergeant. We had talked about him being a Vietnam vet so when I quit, I sassily said, "I'm sorry, but it's too damned hot and I'm not cut out to be a soldier."

If I wasn't quitting my job, I would paint my room in cornflower blue, lemon yellow and sunset pink hues. I did anything and everything I could think of to make myself feel emotionally lighter because my life was becoming a waking nightmare. Sleep eluded me and haunted me. I heard sounds that didn't exist. I had no clue at the time that I was experiencing auditory hallucinations. I mistook the sound of my female roommate using her blow dryer late at night for the sounds of her having wild sex.

I was convinced that she and her boyfriend were having all-nighters every night. I was desperate to sleep. I didn't want to be the roommate who masturbated to her roommates having sex in the room above, but I couldn't help it. My roommate was a hot, Latina young woman who walked around in shorts that barely covered her rear. Her boyfriend was equally as sexy. Be it Dexedrine, alcohol, or my feminine cycles, I was always turned on.

If I was lucky enough to drift off into sleep, I dreamt (and, over time, became convinced) that Mystery, my black long-haired cat, was trying to suffocate me. I didn't have a clue as to what her history was, and I don't even remember how I came to adopt her. Sometimes, Mystery slept on my chest, and she was a big girl like me (or like I used to be before taking stimulants). I sometimes woke myself up screaming.

I was relieved whenever I found Mystery meowing at my window to be let in. Other times when I woke up, I'd want her to comfort me, so I opened my window a crack and whistled for her. She ran to me whenever she heard me summoning her, but instead of comforting me, she scared me. Mystery would attack my ankles without provocation, and she wasn't playing. She'd suddenly morph into a demon cat who forgot that she loved her human.

Even if my cat weren't trying to kill me, my dreams were so vivid and disturbing that I couldn't breathe. My heart beat an out-of-rhythm paradiddle. I'd bolt upright and crying and the whole cycle of trying to fall asleep repeated itself. I would finally fall back asleep in the wee hours of the morning until 5 a.m. came around. Then it was the birds that roused me—those motherfucking birds! I loved birds, but in the pre-dawn hours they pissed me the fuck off.

Like the songbirds that innocently enraged me, I inadvertently upset my roommates by smoking pot in the house at all hours. And if it wasn't the wacky weed, it was my constant need to rearrange things in our kitchen. I tried to be sensitive to their needs, but I felt like they didn't hear mine. I wanted to be included in their camaraderie, but they excluded me from the cool club. I was an outsider in my own house. I locked myself in my room, smoked marijuana, and listened to my music all the time because I didn't know what else to do.

My weed, wine, and tunes were my boon companions. I thought it was my right to smoke marijuana in my bathroom and in the oversized crawl space in our basement that I'd taken the initiative to turn into my private stoner's den. I paid just as much rent as they did; I'd lived in the house longer than they had; and, regarding the den, I was the only one small enough to enter it without being stooped over. (I'd finally found a room I could reach the ceiling of!)

One day, my male roommate Eric invited a friend over. He gave me a warning that his friend was conservative. *What do I care? He isn't coming over to see me,* I thought. I was smoking marijuana in my half-bath sanctuary and blasting Shawn Mullins' *Soul's Core* CD. I listened to it ad nauseum. How was I supposed to know that my roommate's "conservative" friend was a cop? He wasn't on duty when he came over, so what was he going to do, arrest me? Eric was furious with me. He ranted at me at the top of his lungs later that evening.

Another time, I thought that he, Jessica, and I agreed about repainting and redecorating the kitchen. I asked if it was okay for me to repaint it. I had nothing else better to do at the time. I swore they gave me their consent, but it was just another instance of my misreading or mishearing what they said. I didn't realize that they wanted to be present and help me paint. I thought that I was doing them a favor by taking it upon myself to do the job.

I took all the doors off the cabinets, so that our Fiestaware-like plates and bowls were displayed. It was a look I'd seen in Real Simple Magazine and loved because it was cottagey. I painted the cabinet trim in royal blue and the rest of the kitchen lemon yellow. I taped down all the baseboards and tried my hardest to be neat in my efforts. I still got paint everywhere. Thick, yellow stalactites of it were suspended from the ceiling. Our grainy wooden baseboards were smudged in lemon and navy. I even managed to get paint on the kitchen's light sockets, door jambs, and tiled floor. Eric and Jessica demanded that I pay a professional contractor to repaint.

I was under constant scrutiny by roommates, employers, family and even friends. No matter what I did, those I loved only viewed me as impulsive and immature. I didn't measure up to their standards for me. They regarded me as abnormal. I was acutely aware that my ADD made me different from them and others. I reveled in my uniqueness, but I didn't want to be judged or found lacking by anyone. A poem I wrote exemplified this:

ADD Wildflower

If I was a field of wildflowers,
You'd marvel at my beauty,

Soundtrack of a Misfit

At the sheer wonder of my incongruity.

In fact, you'd be disappointed if I revealed a hint of organization.
In the Springtime, you'd eagerly await my unpredictable bloom.
Hell, you'd be entranced by my display of diverse colors.

When Summer rains blessed me, you'd be grateful for my seasoned growth, my maturation.
I am a wildflower garden obscured by rampant structure.
My splendor is overshadowed by your uniform thought processes.

My spontaneous displays of creation are thwarted by your need for linear consistency.
I am a wildflower garden.
I am ADD.

The combination of my impulsivity and the misapplication of my creative energies got me into a lot of trouble and contributed to my being consistently judged by others. I lacked this insight at the time. Back then, I only knew that I was going off the rails. I didn't know how to stop the train.

Long before I derailed, I asked the osteopath if there was any possibility that the amphetamines were negatively interacting with my birth control. He assured me there was no reason for concern. I asked if perhaps I was prescribed too high of a dosage of Dexedrine. Again, I was told "no." I informed him of an odd sensation I experienced with increasing regularity, that it felt like I was talking with a mouth full of mashed potatoes. When that happened, my words sounded slurred and garbled. He again assured me that Dexedrine didn't cause such severe side effects.

These side effects were happening to me, however, and they were terrifying. My parents witnessed my aphasia (forgetting words), circle talking, and slurred words, but insisted my partying too much was the reason I experienced these side effects. I was partying too much, but so were my friends, some of whom also took stimulants and psychiatric medications, but none of them experienced the array of negative symptoms that I did.

I was scared shitless and my parents, who I could always turn to for help, didn't believe that I was in trouble. They casually dismissed my fears which hurt my feelings. I was miserable and out of my mind, but no one was there for me. My drinking and marijuana use, when mixed with my medication, did contribute to some of the extreme side effects, but it turned out that my suspicion about the contraindications between Dexedrine and my birth control pills was well-founded. My dad, of all people, listened to me when I told him everything I experienced. It was he who took it upon himself to solicit the support of scientists who poked holes in what my osteopath and therapist told me.

I never understood what my dad does for work from one day to the next, nor have I been able to keep track of how many different businesses he started up or worked. It made no sense to me why someone who used to be in the recycling industry was working with Pfizer scientists to try to reverse heart disease. What mattered was that my dad believed that I was in a true crisis. The scientists my dad knew researched the effects when Dexedrine and estradiol were taken and determined that not only was I on way too high a dosage of Dexedrine, but that the cocktail of amphetamine and estradiol had in fact, contributed to the horrific side effects I experienced.

The cocktail of stimulants, birth control, and recreational substances caused the mania, as well as the auditory and nocturnal hallucinations. I never saw the actual research findings. If my dad ever gave them to me, they would be lost in one of my many moves. And the PubMed articles I found during research for this book only provided information from studies conducted on rats. But my online research on infrequent yet severe side effects of Dexedrine Spansule included:

- Hallucinations
- Feelings of dissatisfaction
- Significant and unexplained weight loss
- Mood swings and restlessness
- Aggression
- Insomnia
- Muscle twitching or shaking
- Teeth grinding.

• Depression; and
• Suicidal thoughts

I don't know why I didn't seek a second opinion when the osteopath didn't believe me or why I didn't stop taking Dexedrine or why I didn't research potential side effects before I began taking medication for my ADD. I think it's because society teaches us that medical professionals know our own bodies better than we do.

(A significant sidebar: I didn't tell the doctor the extent to which I was drinking and smoking marijuana while I took Dexedrine because I knew he'd tell me to stop. I wasn't about to do that. I always read the warnings on prescription bottles and all they said was "Consumption of alcohol may intensify the effects." Effects of what? I drank plenty of times on antibiotics and nothing bad ever happened. I wasn't ready to give up my sources of recreation and escape.)

I thought a lot about my drinking again and how it negatively affected me. My journaling became a research project on alcoholism, and I was the test subject.

I read, highlighted, and copied paragraphs and entire pages from Caroline Knapp's memoir, *Drinking: A Love Story*. I knew people who drank to excess, but nobody I knew—not even my hard-drinking and partying friends—drank to do their laundry or to do the dishes as I did. Now, as I read Knapp's book, for the first time, I heard another woman describe how she loved alcohol because it allowed her to deal with the mundane. Never had I read anyone else compare their relationship with alcohol to relationships with men that were no good for her.

I documented how I felt whenever I drank: overwhelmed, bored, scared, depressed, angry. I changed my drinking habits. I swore off shots altogether. I stopped drinking vodka because I was convinced it made me aggressive. I swore I'd be a social drinker only; no more drinking alone George Thorogood-style for me.

I was severely depressed and suicidal. I found and tossed a tiny gun I stumbled upon in a closet of a family friend I was housesitting for. I was tired of living in my own skin. My body rebelled against me and betrayed me. I didn't want to experience vivid hallucinations anymore. I craved eternal sleep because I was exhausted.

Fortunately, the ultimate escape for me was the "geographical cure," something many people who are chemically dependent resort to escape themselves. I beseeched my dad and Ona to take me out to California again. I don't know that they were thrilled to foot the bill for my move out west a second time, but they also didn't want to lose me to suicide.

CHAPTER 17 – CALIFORNIA LOVE

I flew back to California on July 4, 2002. I'd never been happier to be embraced by my dad and Ona. I breathed in my dad's stale cigar-smelling shirt and breathed out my first sigh of relief in years. I knew they'd protect me from myself.

They had moved to a new area of Napa since I was last there. They resided on a large estate overlooking the cow pastures and vineyards beyond Brown's Valley. I was shocked to see Steven, who was 16, sitting on a couch like he owned the place. I was even more surprised to learn that he now lived with my parents.

They introduced me to him two years earlier. At the time, he lived in a state-run group home for boys. Befriending young boys who lived there was one of the *tikkun olam* ("repair the world") projects undertaken by the synagogue my dad and Ona belonged to. Evidently, Steven had legally changed his Irish birth name to a German-Jewish one; he'd taken a Hebrew first name and my dad's (and my) last name; he was now Seth Marks. I was too floored to speak but internally screamed, *For fuck's sake, I need a drink!*

I expected to be shown to my bedroom in the house. I was totally unprepared to be ushered through the back door into the backyard. Ona, my dad, and Seth escorted me to my new abode: a tacky trailer parked in their backyard. How they thought I would be happy living in a mother trailer while their delinquent, "adopted" son lived in the biggest house I'd ever seen was beyond me.

To be fair, they thought I wanted privacy. I'll grant them that it was cute. I liked sitting at a tiny table and having my own tiny kitchen. It was funny that I could just about touch my bathroom if my feet were hanging off the side edge of the built-in queen-sized bed. However, I believe that my move into the trailer set off a chain reaction because four events happened in rapid succession that profoundly changed the trajectory of my life.

The first event gave me a degree of smug satisfaction, but it wasn't anything I should've been proud of. Ona, Seth, and I were driving from

Blockbuster Video. I was in the back seat of Ona's Mercedes and Seth was in front. I remember this day clearly because Seth checked out a horror movie. I loudly declared to anyone within earshot that I didn't want to watch it. It would give me nightmares if I even heard it.

Ona talked smack about my mom the entire car ride back through Brown's Valley. Seth had never met my mom and didn't know the first thing about her but listened intently. What gave Ona the right to bad-mouth her? My anger morphed into rage as I warned her that if she didn't stop talking about my mom, I'd hit her. I, who doesn't even kill spiders, threatened to slap someone. Ona either didn't hear me or didn't believe me because she kept up her conversation with Seth.

The next thing I knew, I drew back my left hand and brought it smack down on her left cheek. I repeated the same motion with the back of my hand. I was stunned by my own actions. I felt strangely detached from myself. *Did I just bitch-slap Ona?!*

I was lucky that Seth was caught off guard because he could've killed me. He was 6'3" and built like a linebacker. He had a notoriously dangerous temper and was uber-protective of Ona. (Years later, he was incarcerated in a maximum-security prison for the latest in a string of arrests fueled by his addiction to crystal meth and a lifetime's worth of trauma. He's still in prison today. My dad and Ona still speak to him regularly, but I haven't talked to him for years.)

Seth and I had a complicated relationship. We aren't related by blood, but we regarded one another as siblings and even engaged in sibling rivalry. However, our fights were anything but ordinary. They were fueled by intense feelings of jealousy and displacement on my end and the need to maintain control over Seth's. His status as only son and seemingly favored child of the household only added to my heightened emotions and reactions.

His need to bait me into retaliating was key to his remaining in Ona's good graces. I was nearly 14 years Seth's senior, but my emotional reactions were on par with his. Unfortunately, my emotional dysregulation served to safeguard his physical security. It was my inability to control my reactions that led to the second and third events in this confusing familial soap opera.

I was lucky they didn't press charges on me for assaulting Ona. They would've been within their rights to do so. Instead, my father gave me the choice to stop taking my ADD meds and birth control pills or be committed to a psych ward at Sonoma State Hospital. I chose the former.

I was desperate to feel like "me" again and hadn't had any marijuana for two weeks but was still experiencing violent hallucinations. I no longer had my cat but was now convinced that a mountain lion tried to get to me each night. I swore I heard it clawing at my trailer's door. I was certain that it would fall through the roof and land on my chest as I lay in bed. There was never a mountain lion. I don't even think that Marcus, the family cat, lurked outside.

I went to see a psychiatrist who helped me taper off the stimulants. By August 11, just over a month after my arrival in Napa, I was off ADD meds entirely. I ceased wanting to take my own life or cause anyone, including myself, bodily harm. I also stopped feeling inexplicably angry. I regained the ability to speak articulately again. I finally slept free of hallucinations and everyday sounds became normal again. I experienced happiness for the first time in years.

My slow crawl toward a new and improved version of myself was set in motion by the falling of the first and second dominoes. My bitch-slapping Ona made it clear that living with her and my dad wasn't viable. Even had I not slapped her, there was too much tension between Seth and me and between Ona and me. I couldn't live in a tiny trailer without working plumbing, nor could I live in the mansion with a 16-year-old boy with raging hormones. The only viable solution was my moving out. I needed a place to live. I also needed a means of supporting myself.

My dad and Ona wouldn't help me pay rent unless I attempted to support myself, which meant my applying for and using public assistance. I moved into a rented room off Jefferson Street with a nice, older woman named Bernadette. She had a large dog and worked nights at a nursing home up the valley. Her home boasted a narrow pool but was otherwise run down.

I discovered the source of our one and only issue within my first week of moving in. I saw what I thought were cute baby opossums in the mimosa tree on the night I moved in and even pointed them out to my dad. I thought it odd that he didn't say anything. Something didn't jibe. I knew that opossums could climb, but I didn't think they were social animals. Finally, I saw from their shadows as they scampered from roof-top to treetop that they weren't opossums... or mice (their tails were too long). We had rats!

They squealed and scratched into the wee hours. I drank copious amounts of wine to ignore their presence. I knew I should say some-thing to Bernadette, but I was too embarrassed to. Wasn't I "Wilderness Woman"? By week's end, I informed her that we had an infestation she needed to resolve, or I was moving out. Pest control came and laid down warfarin-laden traps all along the roof. When they came back to check on them, they informed us that the traps had killed not a few but hundreds of rodents.

For the first three months I lived with Bernadette, my dad and Ona paid the balance of rent that I couldn't cover with the wages I earned from administrative temp gigs. The $150 per month I received in food stamps covered my groceries but not toiletries. This baffled me. I under-stood the logic behind the federal government not allowing me to use food stamps to buy alcohol (I reserved some of my work money to feed my habit), but soap? I didn't understand why individuals like myself who were genuinely trying to find permanent employment weren't allowed to put assistance toward toiletries. *What were we supposed to do—go with-out deodorant and soap? That'd go over well for interviewing.* Being even partially dependent upon government subsidies was an eye-opening experience. It made me realize how difficult it was for those without fam-ily support to make a living.

On September 11, 2002, the final domino toppled. I was at my dad's and Ona's sipping a couple glasses of sparkling wine and watching coverage honoring the victims of the previous year's terrorist attacks. We drank to forget the lives that were lost, the lives that were forever changed, and the New York City skyline that used to be. I was sad and buzzed, but I wasn't drunk. I was angry at something Seth said to me and decided that it was time to make my exit. I got into my red Dodge Neon, which was parked on the side of the road, at the top of the very steep hill. I wanted to listen to a cassette so badly that in my haste, I decided my music was more important than my safety. In the few seconds I took my eyes off the road to snatch the mixtape from the passenger-side floor, I slammed into a parked couture car.

I'd inadvertently turned my steering wheel to the right, while bending down going 25 mph. I wasn't prepared for the impact since I didn't think 25 mph was fast. Surprisingly, the jolt was enough to bruise my jaw and the entire right side of my body. The passenger side fender was crushed, and its front tire busted. I was going to leave the scene of the accident because I was scared and tipsy. I beckoned a few teenage boys to come to my aid in the hopes that they could take the destroyed tire off and put on the spare so I could make my getaway. Call it Murphy's Law or fate but they couldn't get my tire off. I was stuck.

I remember being "cute" with the police officers who arrived on scene when they insisted I perform a field sobriety test. "I can't walk a straight line of the best of days; I have poor eye-hand coordination." My attempt at humor was a fail. They didn't think I was cute. Never in a million years did I think this "Jewish princess" would be arrested, handcuffed, and shoved into the back of a cop car. Metal handcuffs applied by a not-hot policeman in uniform is not sexy. Neither is being chained to a hospital bed. Least sexy of all is having to call your father to pick you up from jail.

Even an almost-hit-and-run wasn't enough for me to stop drinking, but it did serve as a wakeup call. I almost fled the scene of an accident, which would have resulted in a felony conviction. Luckily, I was charged with misdemeanor DUI for which my driving privileges were suspended, except for when I drove to and from work. By the time I went to court, I had a full-time job as a barista and Spice Islands Marketplace employee at the Culinary Institute of America (I call it "the other CIA"). I hated that I had to have my employer see that I was convicted of a DUI, but my new boss told me that nearly everyone in the Valley got one at some point, which made me feel somewhat better. Still, I would have to indicate my conviction on job applications for the next seven years, and even now, 19 years later, if an application asks, "Have you ever been arrested?" I'm obligated to answer in the affirmative.

The only thing that didn't suck about being arrested was attending mandatory classes on drunk driving. I'm forever grateful to the female instructor who informed me that she had once walked in my shoes. She caught my attention when she told the class that most women who drink to excess didn't usually die from alcohol itself, but from consequences associated with their drinking. She described how drunk women most often died from accidents: falling and hitting their heads in the shower, unintentionally burning houses down because they'd forgotten to blow out a candle, or electrocution because of blow-drying their hair too close to their sinks. This hit home; I'd already fallen in the shower and had nearly set Bernadette's home on fire.

I began paying more attention to my drinking yet again. Even so, there were many more drunken nights and just as many hungover mornings. I prepared a latte for a customer once and blurted out, "Excuse me," as I walked speedily to the bathroom to throw up.

Once, Grandma Harriett saw me in the throes of alcohol poisoning. I was green in the face. I scared both her and my dad, who encouraged me to go to the hospital, but I refused to. I chose to tough it out in isolation instead of bringing shame to myself in public again. After that incident, I succeeded in being more responsible than I ever was before. I never called out of work, no matter how hungover I was.

I also worked two other jobs on weekends and special occasions to provide for myself. Napa Valley had no shortage of catering gigs, and I loved my work. It was fun to observe parties and to be sober while working (and thereby attending) weddings and other functions. I usually got to take scrumptious food, flowers, and fine wine home.

I joined a social civic service club called the Napa Twenty-Thirty Club. It reminded me of Keyettes, the club I'd once been president of while at Barrie. I became good friends with a few people through The Club, including Cheryl and Darlene. Cheryl was the youngest member. She was bright, spacey, beautiful, and model-thin. She didn't have a mean bone in her body. We became roommates for a while in the nicest apartment I'd lived in for many years.

Our friend Darlene was a tall, thin drink of water. She lovingly and jokingly referred to us as "the long and short of things." She was a single mom who loved her speedy red car, doing Patron shots, and partying on the weekends when she didn't have her five-year-old son (who was nearly as tall as I was). I spent the night at her place often as she lived within walking distance of Downtown Joe's, one of the only bars in Napa at the time. Sleepovers allowed us to party into the wee hours and I didn't have to worry about getting behind the wheel intoxicated.

I felt like an imposter in this group of successful young adults. Most of them were lawyers, doctors, and realtors. Then there was me. I worked three jobs in the culinary field and not as a chef. I worked in catering and food related sales. I was filled with self-pity and resentment. I didn't belong. To combat my feelings of inadequacy, I drank, and I drank, and I drank. Besides, that's all anyone that I knew did. I don't even know that The Club truly benefited the local community. I'm sure we did some good, but I hated my experience. I was different from everyone else and felt like I didn't belong.

Behind the Wheel

My full driving privileges were restored six months after my DUI. My license still bore a sticker on the back of it that flagged me as having had a previous offense. I didn't want another conviction, so I either (a) didn't drive if I was going to be drinking; or (b) drove but referred to the Blood Alcohol Content chart the female DUI class instructor gave us as a parting gift for completing the course.

The day that I traded in my plastic, restricted driver's license for a temporary unrestricted, paper, hole-punched one (to indicate my prior offense), I went out with my friend Sherrie to Anna's Cantina in St. Helena near where I worked. I was the designated driver) that night, so I only had one glass of wine immediately upon entering the bar and followed that with a shot of Patron Silver. Then I stopped drinking, except for water, and danced my tush off. I had so much fun dancing sober, having forgotten my pre-alcohol days in college.

I bumped into a coworker from one of my side catering gigs, a "friend with benefits." I felt awkward when he spotted me dancing and asked me to step away from my friend and go outside with him. He was a volunteer firefighter on the side and his cronies openly razzed him for walking away with me. It dawned on me that his firefighting cronies had heard of me or deduced the nature of our relationship from observing us together. It wouldn't have bothered me if I were okay with our relationship, but I wanted to be more than someone's side piece again and I was crazy about my coworker.

I rejoined Sherrie and we hung out, drank soda, and danced for another three hours before clambering back into my dad's prized old AF

silver Mercedes convertible. The relic was temporarily mine since I'd
turned in my red Neon after it was fixed post-DUI. Everyone but me
loved my car. I hated it because I sat too low in it to look over the dash-
board. I couldn't see the dividing line, it had no pick-up, it rattled whenever it accelerated, and there was also always something wrong with it.
On this fateful night, the car had a broken taillight.

It's a 20-minute drive down Highway 29 from St. Helena to the border of Brown's Valley, where my apartment was. Halfway down the dim-
ly lit road, discreetly tucked into a cozy nook, an officer of the law lay
in wait. He pulled me over and it dawned on him as soon as he asked for
my ID that he was the one who'd arrested me before.

Napa was a "one-horse" town back then, so it wasn't surprising that
he remembered me. Officer Nasty asked me to get out of the car after
I answered all his questions about drinking honestly. My friend hadn't
been drinking either that night even though I was DD. She informed the
officer with certainty that I'd told him the truth: I'd had a shot and a glass
of wine and then stopped drinking altogether. I stepped out of the Mercedes and complied with blowing hard on the breathalyzer three times.

I blew a .07, which is one point below California's legal limit. The
officer was quick to inform me that *any* alcohol registered by the breathalyzer constituted a violation of my probation. I never thought to read the
terms of my probation. I simply folded the yellow sheet up and shoved it
in a folder with my other DUI-related documents. I assumed, like other
people in my drunk driving class, that I could have alcohol in moderation. I thought that as long as I wasn't above .08, I was safe from the law.
Turns out I wasn't even supposed to use mouthwash with alcohol and get
behind the wheel.

I was handcuffed for the second time that year. The officer instructed
Sherrie to drive my car to the station while he shoved me into the back
seat of the cop car. This time, I was stunned to learn that I might be sen-
tenced to a month in jail for violating my probation. Another court date
was set. I was an .08 when I had my DUI and jail wasn't a consequence
then. I couldn't afford to spend a month in jail. No way I was going to
go to jail! I had interviews lined up and being locked up would seriously
put a damper on my job search. Besides, Jewish women didn't go to jail.
And I know they didn't wear prison issued underwear!

Sadly, this is truly what I was the most worried about at the time. That and the fact that I was a peace-loving hippie chick. How would I survive jail when I wasn't even five feet tall? There was nothing hardened about me. I didn't have a poker face and I wore my heart on my sleeve. I'd be eaten alive if I went to jail for a month.

The public defender assigned to me got the charge reduced to 90 hours of community service. I was so relieved. I spent that entire summer in a neon, orange vest and white construction hat picking up trash alongside Silverado Trail. I didn't see being on the "road crew" as a punishment. I had a blast meeting new people and performing manual labor, but it also reinforced a valuable lesson; I never got into trouble with the law again nor did I ever drink any alcohol and get behind the wheel.

That experience did convince me to change my drinking. I stopped doing shots (again) since I never felt their effects until I was hammered and by then, it was too late. I had a fine line between having fun and being drunk and sick. I also stopped drinking vodka (again) as I believed that some brands (I didn't know which ones, though) were more likely to flip my aggression switch and turn me into Scrappy Doo. I knew I either couldn't drink at all or if I had even one drink, I had to stay at a friend's place.

This is where my coworker/volunteer firefighter Sam came into play. Napa has its share of overachievers, but to me he was The Man. He could do everything and anything from firefighter to beekeeping. It didn't hurt that he was hot in a Clark Kent kind of way. He was ordinary and even conservative when he wasn't in his firefighter get-up, but there was something about him that I found incredibly sexy. Sam made my belly do flip-flops on a constant basis and I was genuinely interested in him. I followed his every move for over a year but didn't think he had a clue. Hoping he'd see me; I did kind little gestures and invented reasons to interact with him daily.

Sam had the sexiest, huskiest voice. I called over to his workstation while he was in the middle of something just to hear him when he picked up the phone. I spent idle work hours undressing him in my mind. I imagined what he looked like under his buttoned-up plaid work shirts, corduroy pants, and oxfords. Then, one day, Sam flipped the script. He started paying attention to me. He found reasons to be around my workstation.

Once I became capable of speaking intelligently to him, we talked about books, music, movies, and cooking.

When he finally asked me out, I wasn't sure I heard him correctly. I thought I was attractive, but since I'd stopped boxing and taking prescribed amphetamines, I'd put weight back on. I was neither fat nor thin, but since I knew at least one of his previous girlfriends, I was sure I knew Sam's type: Barbie doll-shaped women who were a bit frosty.

One night, I met Sam at his house at the agreed-upon time. I wanted him to take me seriously, so for that reason, I didn't wear anything too revealing. I managed to put together a sensible outfit that maximized my assets without being too in your face. He greeted me with a hug and a peck on the cheek and then showed me around his place. I was impressed by his music, movies, and cookbook collections. He asked if I wanted anything to drink and I replied, "I drove, so I'll just have one beer." We went outside and I learned that he kept bees. I wanted an apiary. I never knew anyone who had one.

We went back inside, listened to some music, and talked for a bit. He complimented me on my outfit, which brought on a fresh case of camp stomach. *We'll probably get going soon and go to dinner,* I thought.

But then he kissed me, and I reciprocated. I wasn't disappointed. I still believed we'd leave for our date at any moment. Without warning, Sam pinned me down with one hand and stripped my clothes off with his other. I asked myself how he pulled that off. I wasn't even tipsy, but I didn't see it coming. My mind said, *this has nothing to do with me. I didn't do anything wrong. I guess he wants me, too, but this isn't how I pictured this going down.*

I looked up at Sam and stammered, "Um … I'm naked." He replied kindly but pointedly, "You can leave if you want, if you're not okay with it." That's when I knew he never intended for us to go on a proper date. He had one thing in mind only, and I couldn't drive because I had just pounded my beer.

I didn't want this to be the end. Was it consensual? I didn't say "yes," but I also didn't say "no." I felt manipulated because I wasn't given a choice about being suddenly naked before him. However, he'd given out and I didn't take it. Things could've been equitable had I volunteered to serve him as a sub in a consensual bondage type of relationship, but *Fifty*

Shades of Grey hadn't come out yet. I didn't know how that stuff worked and I didn't know that I could've been the one in control without needing to exert any control at all.

I caved and said "yes" then, the next time, the time after that, etc. I demanded that Sam make a proper meal for me once and he did. I also managed to assert myself and tell him I needed him to be more sexually generous. He complied but remained the one in control. I naively thought I'd figure out a way to win his heart.

My experiences with Sam were always exciting and fun, yet it wasn't the type of relationship I longed for. There were vineyard shenanigans and even a strip tease *Magic Mike* style with him in full firefighter garb. That was every bit as titillating as in the movies, but I knew I was always going to be *"that* woman" with him. I thought I was past that. I wasn't going to be the woman Sam took to meet his mother. I'd never know what kept him up at night or what dreams lay in his heart, and I wouldn't ever know what he really thought of me.

Like other vampires I'd succumbed to, I knew I'd never see Sam in the light of day apart from work. I felt sexy and desired by Sam because I was given insight into the narrowest slice of his world. For all his bedroom bravado, he wasn't as sexually free as I was. I wanted to know what else he was naive about. It killed me that I'd never know, but I lived in fear that he'd turn a cold shoulder if I pried even the slightest. Had I had a stronger sense of self and self-worth, I might've had a chance at a real relationship with Sam—or with other men I met and was interested in. My previous relationships were characterized by my use of alcohol, marijuana, and sex. I didn't have the faintest idea of what a real relationship even looked like.

Closing Time

During the three years I lived in Napa, I was always on a quest to find what would satisfy my soul. For a while, I thought my happiness was tied to the land. I thought I'd work at one of the family-owned vineyards and get involved in public outreach. I envisioned myself educating visitors about terroir and viticulture. I was passionate about wine, and by that point, I knew a good deal about the industry. I loved that the growing of grapes dated back to biblical times and was surprised to learn

that there were even three Jewish-owned, kosher wineries in the Valley. I thought there might be a way to combine my love of my heritage with two of my other loves, the environment and wine. I was unsuccessful in securing a winery related job. Next idea? Become a chef.

I worked for a couple of the Valley's most successful catering companies and worked full-time at the CIA. Working in the field opened my eyes to how intricately connected culinary arts are to the land and different ecosystems. I discovered that chefs take the sourcing of their ingredients seriously, and that a refined palette can deduce where one olive or pepper or another key ingredient was grown. I was intrigued further by the way a chef can employ all the senses to accomplish this.

I'd always loved being in the kitchen. My earliest memories involved stirring ingredients with my mom to make dinner and being a sous chef for my dad when he made my favorite breakfast: ham, eggs, and pancakes. When I was seven, I wrote down instructions for my mom on how to make hamburgers. I put them on an index card and filed it in the index-card recipe holder box that my mom kept on our kitchen counter. I even added a drawing of hands shaping full-sized patties. More than any other place, the kitchen has represented safety to me. Nothing bad ever happened to me in the kitchen (save for when my mom accidentally dropped a large Pyrex bowl that gashed my foot when I was five). Both my East and West Coast families regard the kitchen as the center of family life. We've always gathered around the kitchen to enjoy good cuisine and company.

It wasn't a pie in the sky notion for me (pun intended) to want to explore cooking and baking as a career, but my nemesis math dashed that dream. I was surprised to learn how much math and science is required to become a chef. Cooking can be futzed around with—a dash of this and that or a substitution here and there. But the same can't be said for baking.

Baking involves precise measurements and a fundamental understanding of chemistry to ascertain what the mystery is. I argued that I could chef just like I played piano: by intuition. There are plenty of musicians out there that don't know how to read music but are brilliant musicians. Why couldn't I cook and bake using a calculator and cheat sheets instead of relying on memorized complex mathematical conversions?

When I proposed this to the CIA's education directors, my suggestion was met with a resounding "no."

It seemed that no matter what I tried to fill the hole in my heart with—alcohol, a new career, a man—nothing did the trick. I felt like a misfit no matter what I did. In fact, it seemed that my whole life had been the soundtrack of a misfit. All the musicians I loved belted out songs wrought with the agony of unrequited love, loss, heartbreak, and sorrow. And many of my favorite singers waged wars with substance abuse just as I did. My life's soundtrack's baker's dozen looked like this:

- "Still Haven't Found What I'm Looking For" by U2 (Gospel version)
- "Walking In My Shoes" by Depeche Mode
- "Rebel Rebel" by David Bowie
- "1,000 Julys" by Third Eye Blind
- "What's My Name Again" by Blink 182
- "Don't Let Me Get Me" by P!nk
- "Flutter Girl" by Chris Cornell
- "Haunted" by Poe
- "Lock and Load" by Bob Seger
- "Sometimes" by Erasure
- "The Twist Inside" by Everclear
- "Rain" by Patty Griffin
- "Solsbury Hill" by Peter Gabriel

My career aspirations in Napa had dwindled. I was tired of living in my most recent living quarters, a 300-square-foot Hobbit hole addition to my elderly landlord's garage. My tiny abode consisted of a built-in armoire/closet and drawers, a galley kitchenette, a toilet, and a shower. Not having the luxury of a tub to soak in was made more tolerable by the fact that I did have plenty of kitchen storage space. And while teeny, the place was awfully cozy. From my kitchen counter, I could watch TV on my queen-size bed.

However, the table and bed were the only pieces of furniture that fit into the place. I also no longer had a vehicle; the lease expired on my candy-apple Neon. Waking up at 4 a.m. to walk two miles to my bakery job was miserable. I briefly fled Napa for Santa Cruz but returned after three months because I couldn't find administrative work there.

CHAPTER 18 – LOCK & LOAD

The title of this chapter is a nod to Bob Seger and one of my dad's and my favorite songs. It was time to get moving again. I said a sad farewell to my dad and Ona and moved back east. As usual, I had no game plan except to flee my present and to improve my future.

I stayed with my parents in Arlington for six months while I settled back into the faster-paced life of the East Coast. I worked on a few long-term temp gigs, and one even led to a full-time job with an association based in Old Town, Alexandria. Sadly, just as I became comfortable with my responsibilities, the organization decided to cut my department.

I made a friend through a Meetup dinner group who worked at the National Geographic Society. She told me NatGeo was hiring an administrative assistant in their Creative Marketing department. I had always wanted to work for NatGeo. I wanted to be Jacques Cousteau up until the time I began college. And I'd gone to the hippie-esque traveling graduate school program in hopes of becoming an environmental journalist a la those that worked for and with NatGeo.

The NatGeo building's entrance at 16th and M Streets in downtown DC housed an S-Bus stop, where a mammoth magnolia tree reigned. I viewed this tree every time I took the bus down 16th. I often wondered who sat in the window near its canopy. It turned out that my interview was held in a large corner office on the third floor that overlooked *my* tree.

Mary, the head of the department, was a savvy career businesswoman who learned to take charge in a male-dominated arena. Her office was decorated with artifacts and photos and intricately woven rugs; this was a well-traveled woman who sat before me. I felt smaller than I had in a long time.

Mary quietly reviewed my resume and casually remarked that it appeared that I didn't know where my train stopped. I knew what she meant; I knew that I had held numerous jobs in my short-lived professional life. I answered her with what I hoped was an equal amount of candor.

"I don't believe that progress is linear. I recently learned that I have

ADD and that makes some jobs too difficult for me." I quickly added that the job she was hiring for seemed perfect for me and expressed my deepest desire to work for NatGeo ever since I was a young girl. (Never mind that I thought it would be in the capacity of an explorer and not an administrative assistant.) Mary nodded and smiled politely and concluded our interview.

I was stunned to receive a call a week later informing me that the position was mine if I wanted it.

Hell yes! I was ecstatic. I finally found my work home and was closer to my life's purpose. I envisioned retiring happily after a long and successful career spent rubbing shoulders with photojournalists. I imagined going off on vacations of my own led by fellow associates in the African bush, the Alaskan tundra, the forests of Borneo. I didn't plan on staying in DC.

In my role, I helped the Creative Marketing department organize special events, which was great because, by then, I had experience with caterers and sophisticated menus. I also learned all about blow-in mail pieces, the renting and selling of marketing lists, and ever-changing consumer trends. I wanted to prove to Karen, the second-in-command under Mary, that I was worthy of remaining on her team because she and Mary were the first bosses to treat me with the respect of an equal.

Plus, I viewed Karen as a mentor. She put up with my asking her a million questions a day about different aspects of marketing. She also regaled me with stories of her travels and the daily lives of her young children. Karen also introduced me to new music, including Ben Folds Five and Ben Harper. I thought that this was so cool, given that she was considerably older than I was but was *très* hip. I wanted to be like her when I matured. I wanted to step up a rung on the corporate ladder. I tried teaching myself the basics of using a Mac and working with InDesign, which I thought would help me attain my goal, but the learning curve was too steep, and I lacked the patience and passion for creating mailing pieces.

When I reached the year mark of employment at NatGeo, I saw an opportunity to transfer to Missions Programs. The shift was technically a lateral move, but it was a promotion to me. It was a step in the direction I genuinely wanted to go. Missions Programs was a now-six-person department that funded Young Explorers, housed The Genographic Project, and sponsored the organization's cultural events, including the All Roads Film Project. The project and its film festival was multi-city indigenous film, photography, and arts happening.

I was excited to be part of a racially and ethnically diverse team composed of individuals of Native American, African American, Latinx, and Croatian descent. I wondered if they'd acknowledge and understand that despite being white, I also had an ethnic culture I was deeply connected to. It turned out that I was, in fact, accepted—not so much for my cultural inheritance but for who I was as an individual.

My team embraced my quirky personality, creativity, and laid-back attitude. While everyone else stressed and literally ran between buildings to meet project deadlines, I slowly and calmly dealt with festival participants. I thrived on dealing with difficult personalities. I loved winning people over. It was a skill I honed over years of customer service experience. I prided myself on being able to talk to anyone and gaining their respect through kindness and compassion. I learned that a few of the benefits of being an individual with ADD in this job were being able to think quickly on my feet while remaining calm and combining stubbornness with hyperfocus. This enabled me to stay the course and not give up on difficult tasks (assuming I had enough interest in them). Additionally, my spontaneous nature helped me to quickly change tactics based on my intuition.

I also possessed another hallmark trait of many individuals with ADD: creativity. I never shied away from thinking "outside the box" because I never felt like I belonged in a box. I loved being tasked with planning parties and special events, such as the premiere parties our department co-developed with the Academy of Motion Pictures Arts and Sciences (the people who put on the Oscars [!]).

It was thrilling to design events and bring them to life. With the help of my teammates and Marriott's in-house catering team, we turned Nat-Geo's cafeteria into an elegant ballroom worthy of hosting Oscar-nominated foreign-language filmmakers. I dug up large, discarded film reels from the basement that we strung up on wires and suspended from the ceiling. We also used the reels as centerpieces holding votive candles. AMPAS provided miniature Oscar statuettes and full-size film posters that featured all the nominees. It was thrilling to provide support, even if only in a small way, in highlighting and advocating for the careers of Native filmmakers and artists.

Less glamorous was my daily struggle to accomplish complex administrative tasks independently. My position with All Roads required close attention to detail and constant updating of and attending to many moving parts simultaneously. It wasn't that I couldn't perform these tasks but doing so was draining. I needed to be able to sustain focus on minutiae for hours on end, but my mind didn't "do" details well for long; it thrived on creation versus maintenance.

Unfortunately, the part of my job that was creative or right brain oriented constituted fully one- third of my overall responsibilities. It took all my mental energy to stay focused and perform complex, left-brained tasks. For example, most of our film festival participants lived overseas where they made films about their cultures. As a result, I was responsible for coordinating multi-leg travel plans with in-house travel agents and keeping track of where participants were at all the time and at all hours of the day and night. I maintained multiple calendars, including a department-wide production calendar; a travel calendar; a hotel rooming matrix; and a ground transportation schedule.

I was given sole responsibility for determining how much reimbursement to request in cash per participant. And worst of all, I, and I alone, had to withdraw, distribute, and record how much cash I gave to each filmmaker or artist. This wouldn't have been so difficult if I only had to do this while we were in the office. I would have had easy access to computers, printers, and my coworkers if I needed their help.

But we also took the film festival to LA and Santa Fe. I was terrified to fly with large wads of cash. Do you know how many books, sunglasses, headphones, and winter coats I've left behind in airport terminals? I couldn't even balance my personal checkbook correctly, but I was now responsible for hanging onto large amounts of money, remembering who I gave it to, and how much I gave them. Try as I might to stay organized with all the systems I created, I couldn't. I either short-changed attendees or gave them too much money.

I worked 17-hour days when we were on location and was the one who my teammates called to put out fires. I ran from hotel room to hotel room handing out money; herded participants; and ran supplies back and forth between venues—and did all this lugging around my purse, a laptop, and multiple welcome packets and envelopes full of cash.

It was a grueling routine to uphold for several days in a row, with a day or two of travel in between cities. I imagined that this was how touring musicians felt, overstimulated, and depleted at the same time. Unlike musicians who go on tour, however, I was spending $600 of their hard-earned tax refunds repaying their managers for money they accidentally lost. They are rock stars after all.

Our All Roads manager, Francene, had ties to the Smithsonian and was part of the Native media industry. She was also deeply connected to her Diné Navajo and Sioux communities. She shared her knowledge of the Navajo matrilineal and matriarchal culture. In doing so, she taught our team about the true importance of All Roads: to serve as a platform for indigenous cultures to share their heritage and strengths with all who would come to learn at our festivals.

Francene honored us all as individuals, but she taught me a lot about the value of teamwork. I had been a part of a team on several occasions during my lifetime and I thrived on being a part of a community, but I had grown used to feeling like an outsider in recent years. I had all but forgotten how good inclusion it felt.

Under Francene's leadership, inclusion and teamwork were my saving graces that first year with All Roads. We were highly capable in our own rights, but we operated best when we harmonized logistically. Lenny was a cool cat who had knowledge of the music industry. He moved to the beat of his own drum and seemed proud of it. I respected him for that as well as for his ability to set music to our marketing festival trailer. And man, did that guy know how to network with all kinds of people.

Then there was Ari. I've never seen someone so "on" as she was. The coolest thing about her was how real she was with everyone. She made no apologies for being unpolished in an industry known for its snootiness. She had worked on stage productions in New York City and befriended everyone, including Baryshnikov, whom she referred to as Misha. I doubted that she knew him as intimately as she implied but was humbled when she proved me wrong. We went to New York one weekend to help a mutual friend who was a filmmaker with a premiere. She showed me around her old place of work and who leapt into our elevator but Baryshnikov. Ari affectionately gave him her wide, gap-toothed grin and beamed, "Hi Misha," while I looked like a dumbass, with my mouth agape.

We were a team that worked hard and partied harder. I embraced the entertainment aspect of my duties with All Roads, which required me to be both personal concierge and chaperone. I was dizzy with the novelty of meeting and briefly working alongside talented, and sometimes famous, individuals. I felt privileged to be among them.

A close-knit team was something I hadn't experienced before. We ventured out everywhere together while we were in L.A. and Santa Fe. I didn't know anyone else that went to parties, bars, and dance clubs with their coworkers and bosses. In Santa Fe, we even went to a spa together. It took a lot of courage to wear my bathing suit amongst my coworkers but drinking sparkling wine and doing bong hits with them helped to ease my self-consciousness. I still chuckle when I remember all of us "grownups" playing with plastic toy goldfish in the Zen pool.

Sober

As my favorite recording artist P!nk sings in her song "Sober," it's basically all good until it's not anymore. My third year at NatGeo and my second year with All Roads was all about sobering up. At the same time this was underway, other unexpected changes occurred. They were jarring, but ultimately auspicious both personally and professionally.

It started with going to the Sundance Film Festival, which I lobbied hard to attend, accompanying Francene. I was an independent movie buff long before I worked with All Roads and it was this festival's founder, Robert Redford, who had first turned me onto indie films.

The first indie film I saw was one he produced, *Incident at Oglala*. Apart from a winter's trip to Lake Tahoe, I'd never seen so much real snow; the town was truly a winter wonderland. I didn't meet many famous actors, but I wasn't disappointed. It was enough for me to be introduced to Wes Studi since *The Last of the Mohicans* is one of my favorite movies, and Studi's portrayal of Magwa was bone-chillingly good.

I attended film screenings, premiere parties for indigenous films, and went dancing at night with Francene and our festival's production duo.

Park City, Utah is a tented party city, so, of course, I was surrounded by alcohol. Surprisingly, I didn't drink much. It dawned on me that I had a good time at all the after-parties with only a drink or two in me. I even managed to get out of my comfort zone and talk to strangers. For the first time, I thought that maybe—just maybe—I could have fun without alcohol.

I'd been binge drinking for a decade and in that time, I did many things I swore I'd never do. I got a DUI and violated my probation; I slept with people without knowing their names; and I'd begun to black out for brief spans of time. I would wake up bruised and piece together that I must've fallen and hurt myself. Most times, I clearly remembered stumbling into things. Once, I gave myself a nasty concussion when I tripped over my own skirt and fell on the thinly carpeted concrete of my apartment complex. I also fell on my right elbow so badly that it took years before it healed.

I was a young adult in the '90s when River Phoenix overdosed on drugs and Kurt Cobain took his life by shooting himself in the head. And by this time, I was actively grieving the startling death of one of my favorite actors, Heath Ledger, who had died after taking a mixture of pills, some of which were supposed to help him fight off pneumonia. His death might've been accidental, but he had lived life in the fast lane, drinking and drugging to lessen his emotional pain.

Maybe it wasn't a coincidence that seeing his performance in the movie *Candy* influenced my decision to quit abusing my vices. I saw myself in both his and his girlfriend's characters—and they were both heroin addicts. I didn't want to die because of my addiction.

Once again, my dad played a part in rescuing me from myself. He called me one day and nonchalantly said, "Yo, Rach. So, I've been doing this non-drinking thing for about six months now. I'm going to these meetings, and I'll be damned, it's a good thing. Who knew? I thought I was the life of the party, but it turns out I'm reserved and depressed when I drink. You should think about stopping too, kid—especially since it's not good for ADD."

I was floored. *He did what? Got sober? My dad?* Alcohol was music that warped and united us from my earliest memories. It was my father who gave me my first sip of frothy beer when I was only a toddler. He railed at me in a hard, alcohol-induced fury or spoke in rhapsody under the gauzy, mellowness of wine. I despised him because of his drinking yet understood and connected to him through my own. The moment my dad uttered the magic words, "I quit," I knew I, too, wanted to be free.

My worst fear had been that he'd mock me if I were the one to stop. In my adulthood, our times together was a montage of drinking: vineyards, restaurants, multiple homes, backyards, and special occasions. Now, my dad's sobriety was the catalyst for my own. I was safe. He wouldn't tease me for wanting something he didn't or wouldn't care about.

I didn't remember it until looking back through my journals, but I was preparing myself to stop a full year almost to the date before I did stop drinking for what I hope will be for good. In the rooms of recovery, however, you learn to never say "never."

January 13, 2007

This will be like a breakup with a passive-aggressive lover. You stay clear away from him despite weak moments of wanting, all the while knowing there's no way this will work fine except occasionally; you will allow yourself to forget and taste it/him all over again. I can't do this when it gets me nowhere. Now I'll call myself the "special event" sipper. This will be the only way I will be safe (and happy). So begins the experiment of alcohol abstinence. No sex and no alcohol. Where is pot anymore? It's like a long-lost friend I remember fondly and miss. At least this time, this parting is easy. There's no throwing up, just numbness.

A year and two weeks later:

January 27, 2008

Nothing monumental happened last night. I went to Rumberos restaurant in Columbia Heights where I always felt cozy and safe. I had dinner and two glasses of wine (Pinot noir and Merlot) over the course of two hours. Then, Alberto [an intern] picked me up and we went back to my place and proceeded to talk over a bottle of Sangiovese and two Valium each. And then he asked me to change into something sexy and I complied as usual, desperate for physical attention. There was no chemistry, and I felt every bit my 12 years older than him. And that was it. I couldn't go through with it anymore. I was thankful that the blood from my last period killed the moment. Out the door he went, and I was thankful that we'd only slept together twice before because it was like saying goodbye to a friend.

My behavior wasn't professional or sophisticated. I prided myself on being both. I went into my bathroom and was disgusted with the woman who stared back at me. I didn't recognize her. That woman's eyes were red, and her face was blotchy. The happy, scrappy woman I once was had been replaced with a duller, jaded version of myself. I'm tired of playing Mrs. Robinson. Being a cougar was a role I prided myself on, but I couldn't do it any longer.

I wasn't tipsy or high; I was defeated.

Early Recovery (A Year in Review)

"Whatever you put before your recovery you stand to lose."
—12-Step recovery axiom

January 29, 2008

Two days ago, I did something I honestly wasn't sure I'd ever do. I walked in dry-mouthed and foggy-headed to my first recovery meeting. I looked around the packed room (on Sunday) and saw "normal" men and women who were all seemingly functional. I knew I had literally opened a new door into a portal. Goodbye alcohol and good riddance! Safe travels somewhere else, somewhere outside of me. I called my dad to tell him that I stopped drinking.

January 30, 2008

I have my doubts. I wonder if I will ever pick up a glass of wine or champagne or beer again. I know it would be my downfall. So here I am today —just today, just now. In three days of going to meetings, I have felt such a connection. I know I am not alone. There are rooms full of people like me who can't afford to flirt with alcohol. It is a feeling of solidarity, support, and strength.

February 18, 2007
Twenty-three days. I can't believe it hasn't been 30 yet. It feels like I haven't had a drink in forever. And right now, a nice cool glass of buttery chardonnay to go with this couscous would be divine. But I feel so much better without alcohol. My quality of life already feels better. I'm exhausted though because I've met so many new people. I am beginning to make new friends within the rooms. I am still cautious and not trusting of "sudden" friendships. I had a good holiday weekend with Hilary and Claire and Sarah. But I was beginning to feel too hungry and frantic, and I just needed quiet to go get chocolate with them from Whole Foods. It was hard for me to say no because I really like them, and I want them to like me too.

Hilary, Claire, Sarah and Allen, and Erin were among my closest friends in my first year of recovery. Our bonds, despite being new, were stronger than any I'd had before. I could talk to them about anything, including my deepest fears and anxiety. Hilary was poised and beautiful, yet she was as unaware of her beauty as my roommate and dear friend Janis was. She was also a bit spacey, which made her even more endearing. Despite being geographically close, Maryland and Northern Virginia tend to be worlds away and our paths diverged once we both were sober for a few years. I am connected to her today through social media and have fond memories of our friendship.

Claire was striking. She was leggy as a colt, with auburn hair and freckles and a pert nose. She was a dynamo who drew everyone in. Like the Sting song about a woman being "all four seasons in one day," Claire was alternately cerebral, whimsical, nostalgic, or crass. She is the closest I've had to a best friend since I was besties with Nonnie when I was five. And to think that I was initially a little afraid of her makes me laugh. We've been through a lot of life's ups-and-downs together, and after 13 years of friendship, she might know me better than anyone, except for my family and sponsor.

Sarah, was a SoCal beach beauty who had the snarkiest wit, paired with a sexy drawl. She lived by the law, as in she defined herself by her work as a lawyer. I adored that despite being highly intellectual, she devoured gossip magazines and binged-watched reality TV shows. She is like family to me in that I don't see her as much as I used to, but she always has a space in my heart.

And Erin. Think of a blond hippie chick dressed in the camouflage of someone preppie a la Ann Taylor. She had a magnetism that drew others in, but she only let precious few into her inner circle. She had a fierce determination to take over the world with her therapy practice but couldn't settle on a shade of paint for her office if her life depended upon it. In her ADD-fueled nonlinear way of thinking, her life did depend upon it. I totally understood and related to her quandary. She couldn't move past the paint dilemma because a therapy office is intended to be a sacred space and how can you design a website or move forward with planning out a private practice if you haven't been able to wholly envision yourself in that space.

Like most of my other recovery friends, Erin was a year ahead of me in her recovery journey. I believe she was put into my life to show me the way when I was lost and to model for me that it was okay for me to be wholly me as a sober individual with ADD and have it all. I, too, could be zany and earth loving, and music loving and still claim my seat in the echelon of professional therapists. She isn't in these journal entries, but she was a huge presence in my life, and I am grateful we trudged a shared path for many years.

February 20, 2008

Twenty-five days. I can't wait to get to 30 because I've never gone 30 days without drinking since I can remember. Last night I couldn't stop thinking about "my story." I went to a meeting recently and this woman came up to me and said in a way too bubbly voice, "Hi. I'm X. What's your story?" And I was like, "Huh? I don't know what you mean." And she said, "Well, I used to go to bars and talk to all these guys and they'd pat me on my head and then I'd pull my pants down." I fell out laughing. I might've bent forward over my knees laughing. I blithely replied, "That's my story, too." And it was.

February 26, 2008

Twenty-nine days. Incredible! Now I notice how dusty my stuff is and how white my bathroom ceiling is. I play more with my cats. I don't fall asleep without popping a Kirkland-brand sleep aid yet. My mind is abuzz at night. I watched the film Candy tonight, with Heath Ledger in it. I can't believe he's gone! It's not like I knew him, but still! I could resonate with the bleakness in the movie. Thank G —d I'm terrified of needles or I'm sure I would've tried heroin like he was into in the movie. I never wanted to tempt fate. Wait. That is stupid! I'm in recovery now. I tempted fate so many times with alcohol, huh?

I wasn't perfect about my recovery early on. And some would argue that my taking over-the-counter medication to fall asleep at night wouldn't count as being sober, but I wasn't drinking. Early on, I also drank non-alcoholic beer a few times before talking about it with Sarah's boyfriend (and later, husband) Allen, who had a very long-term recovery at the time. My sponsor (also named Sarah) didn't make me change my sobriety date, but some sponsors would've. I was still struggling to deal with people and situations that overwhelmed me.

February 27, 2008 (one month sober)

Today was 100% overwhelming. After my meeting and meeting with my sponsor, Sarah M., I realize I am sad and I mean it quite literally, drinking O'Doul's non-alcoholic beer knowing full well that there's no miracle to be found in it. I know it will not make me feel one iota less sad or helpless. Long story short, I was verbally abused by a Sallie Mae collections representative. I'm only 72 days into the 270 allotted before my wages can be legally garnished and end life as I know it. I am trying to pray for the bitch that made me cry and panic. (Fifteen minutes later) Me again. I'm crushed that my father isn't com-

ing to Philly this weekend. Tears. Stopping. (Twenty minutes after that) Me again. I love Mom. She made me feel better. And the best part of my day is I know that Shayna [my niece] is excited that I'm coming up to see them. She and Noah [my nephew] are angels whom I would do anything in the world for.

March 30, 2008

Sixty-three days sober. It feels good. I'm going back to Napa to visit Dad and Ona and Seth in two weeks .... I'm very excited. It will give me a sense of closure to be back in a place where I did a lot of drinking. My only hang up is Sam. I think it will be very hard for me to be there and not call him or see him.

Two days later ...

April 1, 2008

I had an intense craving to drink tonight. In my meeting I couldn't identify what it was. But now that I'm home and in my kitchen—looking out and into my neighbor's windows it occurs to me that the triggers are loneliness and hunger. Hunger for food but also for touch and intimacy. Even if it was fleeting, the texted sexual flirtations with Sam last night were great for the hole —the gulf of need.

May 10, 2008 [a few months sober now]

Who ever thought I'd be on a retreat with sober people? Surely not me. But here I am. I snuck away to the woods for some "me time." It is awesome to just sit against a tree with crushed acorns all around. There's little traffic to be heard near Camp David (almost a stone's throw away), and there's more birdsong. And best of all—no one is talking right now. It is chilly and damp but glorious, I am extremely tired but peaceful. I miss the woods a lot, even though I live right on top of them. But I won't explore by myself in Rock Creek Park anymore. I miss the smell of damp earth. A squirrel just came to check me out. I think we scared one another. I am too cold to stay out here but it was great for half an hour or so.

June 2, 2008

I went against my usual nature and practiced resistance. I didn't want to spew impulsively while I spent time on a hike walking next to scruffy Patrick. I didn't want to make my time next to him seem less important or grander than it was. I admit I am a sucker for scruff and green eyes, but I wasn't thinking of boyfriend material. I was for once, simply enjoying what I felt with him—synergy. I rarely feel this with others and rarely have I experienced it with a male. It just felt nice to know someone felt the same way as I did—that it was great to be outdoors and feel the vibrance of the rainfall. I love that feeling of welcoming in the rain. That is all. Nothing more.

July 18th, 2008

This is exactly what I needed! I'm out of the city and its hustle and bustle. I'm at the shore in Stone Harbor, NJ. I've never been here before, and it is perfect. It's like Calistoga on the Atlantic. And I am surprised by how at ease I feel with [my friend] Sarah and Claire and her friends. It's great to be with other alcoholics and amazingly, I feel like I belong. As soon as we got here, we went into the bay and in an instant, I reverted to my childhood self —at home in brackish water. I love swimming below the water's surface. The quiet is beautiful, a calm exhilaration if that makes sense. It's like coming home. The salty air reminds me so much of being at Camp Tockwogh. The fish must be deep in the water now because the terns and gulls are not diving into the water. I am happy I stayed behind while everyone else went to a meeting. I love the tranquility as much as I love the camaraderie of my new friends. I love it when the cotton candy blue sky is striated with its cotton candy pink counterpart.

August 21, 2008 [almost seven months sober, or as my friend Jim E. says, "That'd be six months"]

It was so nice to share my story tonight with people I care about and open myself up to. It was great to feel confident about how much I have gained emotionally by giving up alcohol. I'll have seven months on the 27th. Dad will have 10 months on the 5th of September, which is two days before his 66th birthday. It has been great to share sobriety with him. It was also special having Irene there. She saw me through some of my "finer" moments. Last night, I learned how unnecessary it is to waste time obsessing over an outcome I can't change. I honestly felt all the forces of the universe protected me or provide a better outcome for me than I could've anticipated. I recognized that I would've overwhelmed Mark too much if he had agreed to come to Stone Harbor with me and my friends. It was selfish of me, even though my intentions were good. I am happy that I didn't totally fuck things up by being too impulsive or not respecting Mark's boundaries. (I introduce Mark much more fully farther along in this chapter, but he is who I started dating at seven months sober.)

September 13, 2008
I hope by putting Mark down on paper that I am not jinxing myself. We've been dating for a couple of weeks now. I am crazy about him. He is unlike anyone I have dated. He is very considerate and affectionate and easy to talk to. I think we can relate more fully to one another because we are both in recovery and both in the same month of recovery. I'm less afraid to be around him than I have been with anyone for a while. It might be because I was single for seven years. I already know he is not perfect, and I accept that. He loves music like I do, as well as learning and trying new things, like museum exhibits and different types of food. We are also complete opposites. He loves baseball, but I prefer basketball. He likes cool weather, and I prefer hot. He plays drums too. Not that I do, but I seem to be innately attracted to drummers. Mark likes history and nonfiction, whereas I like English language (as a subject) and reading novels.

October 14, 2008

Tonight's musing: how do I know if I am in love? How bizarre that I don't know how to answer —me who has always fallen fast and furious and, I add, rather faultily. I love Mark. I love how he treats me and how he gets me. I love his witty and quirky humor, his curiosity for random things like pop trivia and politics .... I love how readily he has embraced my family and friends, and how accepting he is of my religion. I just feel so "normal" with him, and I'm not used to someone being in love with me. My three previous actual relationships were largely unrequited, unhealthy, and drama laden. I felt like I'd die without them for even a day and that my happiness and life depended upon them. It was up and down all the time, like being on a rollercoaster. This relationship is not intense, but I sense that this is good and shows I am finally, mostly mature. I also see Mark's flaws and I never wanted to notice or accept my other partner's flaws even though theirs were large red flags and his are more minor.

November 11, 2008

Veterans Day. I realized sitting in the bath just a few minutes ago that what I said in the meeting tonight wasn't entirely true. I don't love drama; I am just so used to it. I do miss having extreme emotions only because I don't know how to feel or what to feel after long stretches of calm. It makes me feel like I am missing something. Then, when drama does happen, I feel totally unsettled and unbalanced. Tonight, I feel lonely. I haven't felt this way recently as intensely as I do now. Irene [my friend who got me the job at NatGeo] used to be my go-to friend for everything, but as of today, we are no longer friends. I don't know why. She said she wasn't sure about our friendship in an email and that's it. She asked for space from me. I decided that I am not going to go through another make-up round with Irene. Not again. I have never lived up to her unstated expectations of me.

Before getting sober, I was extremely attracted to drama. It didn't matter if it was with boyfriends, friends, or family. I'd never admit that I was at the time, but I thought a life worth living meant it had to be filled with intense highs and lows. Blame it on my dad's moodiness; my mom's moods running hot or cold dependent upon what I was or wasn't perceived to be doing to please or disappoint her; my sister's relationship dramas of the past; my own hormones; social media and media in general; or the shifts in the weather from day to day. Once I put the drink down, I experienced true happiness for the first time since I was a camper at Tockwogh.

But it was also a bit of true culture shock. I struggled to figure out who I was without the drama. I stopped writing so much because of it. It was the depths or heights of emotions that had fueled my journaling and poetry.

December 9, 2008

[My sponsor] Sarah had me write out a multiple page fear inventory. She reviewed it with me and showed me how close to a drink I could've been even though I had no desire to drink during my recent drama with my relationship. She also pointed out where I cherry-picked the parts of my recovery program that I wanted to work on. She pointed out how this is something I've been doing consistently since she started working with me. I wanted to shout, "Fuck you! At least I've been consistent about something." But I didn't. I am trying to change my behavior and not be resistant or unduly creative or undermining. Sarah also pointed out where I have been potentially codependent. I don't want that. Been there. Done that. Oh, joyous character defects.

January 27, 2009
(9 AM)

I have a year of sobriety as of today. Yesterday I felt ecstatic. Today I feel low. I really want to feel euphoric, and I can't get that feeling; not even with exercise, listening to music or being in nature. I even felt panicky in my stomach on the bus.

(9:52 PM)

Today and tonight turned out to be a gift from G —d, Shai in Hebrew. It reaffirmed for me why a sober life is so good for me. I went to the gym at lunch and from inside my locker, my phone rang. I had an intuition to open the locker and return the call. It was Aida, a woman with a month of sobriety who need- ed to talk. It felt so good to be there for her and get outside my self-manufactured drama. I felt that G—d or the force put her in my life exactly when I needed her to be. Then I went to the Tuesday Night Beginners meeting to get my one-year sobriety chip. So many people I have grown to love were there: Mark, Tony, Kirsten, Noelle, Hilary, Jim, and Ame [my newly minted sponsor]. Oh yeah, my old sponsor told me, "You're still sick, as evidenced by the fact that you won't commit to going to one meeting every day." I think it's a miracle I haven't had a drink in a year. I'll take that.

I did have two separate one-day interludes with marijuana four years apart from one another (2012 and 2016). On both occasions, I called my sponsor Jennifer nearly immediately afterwards and jumped right back into my program. She is adorable and as tall and thin as I am short and round. She has a cute reverse bob that she has worn in the same style since we started working together 12 years ago. I love her, and don't know where I'd be without her support and patience, and sometimes firm-but-honest feedback.

I am glad Jennifer is so consistent because she reminds me of safety. She constantly reminds me that I don't have to be a squirrel running up and down a tree. I can hang out on a branch and just rest sometimes and not decide to do or be anything. She gets me. She is part of the "Wolf Pack," a term I came up with for the sober people—especially the wom- en I share my daily gratitude lists with via email. It's the most consistent practice I've ever had. I've been doing it on a nearly daily basis for 12 years, and I get to read my friends' lists all throughout the day or once a day in digest form. It helps to keep me sane and grounded. I am not a misfit when I remind myself that I do gel with others and that I belong.

When I had my "slips" on those two separate occasions with marijuana, my dad and some others close to me insisted that I could consider these hiccups or blips. They didn't think that my doing a few bong hits or eating a pot brownie the size of my face warranted my resetting my sobriety date. But I knew that I used marijuana for the exact same reasons I used to drink alcohol: I couldn't stand to sit with my feelings of fear and discomfort.

I used the oft-heard contention that substances in any form had allowed me to be more creative. I was an overwrought creative empath. Wine-fueled nights were fodder for writing in my journal. Drinking was anesthesia for my emotional pain. Before I got sober, I thought substances defined me. I was a wine connoisseur, then I was a wino, and I was always a pothead. I embraced these labels. I used them to relate to others who identified with my vices, but I was really viewing myself through distorted lenses.

My beliefs about myself and the way I treated myself blurred the real me. Alcohol and marijuana were curtains I kept drawn at all hours to cloak the true me. I kept myself hidden in a dark, walled-off room. It was my inability to allow myself to feel my feelings and then walk through them with grace that prevented me from being the woman I aspired to be. I didn't realize that the sky wouldn't fall, nor would I implode if I waited for my larger-than-life feelings to pass.

Early into my second year of recovery, I heard a woman named Rosia, who was new to the DC area but not new to recovery exclaim in a meeting. "Feelings are meant to be felt and not acted upon." That was novel to me. My friend Noelle said that at four years sober, she was "getting used to letting go of living crisis to crisis." That, too, deeply resonated with me because I connected to the sentiment on a soul level.

I learned that "early recovery" is considered your first five years "in the rooms" or anywhere else that supports the adoption of working a spiritual program of some type. Initially, this was daunting for me to process, but I've now been "around" for 13 years, and I feel like I learn new things about the recovery journey and myself all the time. This is especially true when it comes to my relationship with mom.

I discovered that if I slowed myself down and wasn't too quick to react, I was able to see my mom's true versus misunderstood motives. I became more forgiving of her imperfections and realized that like me, she too, was quick to react out of fear. Like Sia's song "Fire Meet Gas-oline," it was our opposite ways of handling our fears that made our reactions so explosive.

I began to apply some of the recovery slogans I heard in the Rooms when I got triggered by stinging remarks my mom made which seemed out of proportion to whatever it was, I said. One such statement is "If you get resentful during a holiday meal – you can always do the dishes." I have a long list of helpful recovery jargon that I keep in Evernote on my phone. It's like a recovery kaleidoscope. Instead of holding my phone to the light, I scroll through and see beautiful tidbits of wisdom I've gleaned from meetings.

The kaleidoscope is always accessible if I'm in need of comfort or feel like a drink would solve all my problems. I use these recovery slogans to remind myself not only "what my party looked like" (thanks for that one, Sarah K.), but why the adventure I'm still on is the best one I've embarked upon and why I literally stand to lose anything I make more sacred than my sobriety.

I've learned that my fight-or-flight tendencies stemmed from trauma I experienced in both childhood and young adulthood. Trauma blunts our true connection to ourselves and teaches us to distrust even those who try to protect us. Profound changes took place in my life, and they all began with my willingness to explore my role in those traumas (which is in no way an implication of blame) and begin to let go.

I'm not good with percentages but I believe that it's only because I "put the drink down" and have learned to "Drop the Rock" (this is both a recovery slogan and book for working steps six and seven of a 12-Step program) that our relationship has improved by 75%. We still get into it from time to time but our funny text chains with Stacey, our frequent comforting phone check-ins, and her praise over my continued growth leads me to believe that we've successfully rewritten our shared narra-tive. Goodbye Mrs. Codependent.

I was exhausted from holding onto my hurts for so long. I clung to the unfounded belief that I was fundamentally flawed because I expe-rienced traumas which included my being made to feel exceptionally different from everyone else, I knew. But something powerful happened that Sunday morning in January of 2008 when I climbed those 12 stairs and began a new way of living with myself.

Pre-recovery, I blamed everyone else for the way I was and everything that happened to me, and I numbed any pain with alcohol and marijuana. When I put substances aside, I was suddenly faced with the fact that I have agency to act, react, or respond. Once I got over the initial shock that life did get instantly brighter but was not always roses, I decided that I was powerless over everything really except how I move through life.

Once I was honest, open, and willing enough to turn my attention inwards in terms of how I acted, I was stunned to discover that I was more resilient than I ever imagined I was or could be. I could feel multiple emotions at once and not act out chemically over them. More importantly, I learned that it is possible to choose how I wanted to act before I reacted. I am still not great at doing this but before getting sober, I was just so angry that the world was seemingly against me.

My friend Tony H. floored me one day when he said these words, "The way you do anything is the way you do everything." I interpreted this to mean being intentional in choosing how you will behave and then apply that same energy and intention to everything.

Anyone Else

If you know The Moldy Peaches or have seen the movie Juno, you'll get the reasoning for this subheading title. I met a guy named Mark during my second or third week in the rooms, who I thought was cute in a bookish way. Part of my attraction to him was that he introduced himself by means of asking me what book I was reading. He had somewhat oversized round glasses and a goatee. He was tall, broad shouldered, and very pale. He didn't fully open his eyes when he shared, which I found off putting. Still, I thought he was cute. A bit later, we bonded over our mutual distrust and discomfort during the silent part of a guided meditation meeting we both attended.

I saw him during the first couple months of early recovery but then didn't see him again until around the seven-month mark when a mutual friend invited us both to a DC United match at the dilapidated RFK Stadium. I couldn't maneuver the crowd enough to get a seat next to him. I figured that if our paths crossed again, I'd find a way to talk to him.

Shortly afterward, I spied him at a large meeting in Georgetown. The vibe more closely resembled the DC bar scene than it did a 12-Step meeting. I felt out of place but couldn't leave. Sponsor Sarah insisted that I put my hand up and share my desire to sing karaoke alone at Fast Eddie's. I used to go there religiously on Tuesday nights by myself to sing. I didn't know anyone else that liked karaoke, and I craved the adventure of going alone. It replaced the high I got from drinking. I had gone there to sing a few times since I got sober and felt safe there because Jade, the female bartender, had also decided to stop drinking and respected the fact that I was sober.

I dutifully shared at the meeting and made a beeline for the exit. I still felt extremely anxious and overwhelmed in large, loud crowds; because of my ADD, all I generally hear is something like the adults in *Charlie Brown* specials. Just before I reached the door, Mark came up to me and told me that he liked to sing karaoke too. I bravely seized my chance and gave him my number. I told him I'd let him know when I was going to sing the next time. Mark and I began dating maybe a week after I gave him my number.

In retrospect, I understand why people in the rooms caution against dating in early recovery. I'm not sure either Mark or myself were emotionally sober enough to handle dating. One of the patients I'd end up working with when I became a mental health counselor (spoiler alert) shared his decision to date two people simultaneously since he was at the year mark in his recovery. He explained that dating more than one person is part of his strategic relapse prevention plan. He believes that spreading himself emotionally will prevent him from diving too deep, too fast into a serious relationship. This patient's plan might be the sagest insight I've heard regarding dating in early sobriety yet.

Neither Mark nor I was sure if we were on a date or not the first time we went out. I asked if he wanted to see *The Dark Knight* (there's that Heath Ledger again) with me. We grabbed sushi before the movie. It was hard to concentrate on our dinner because I had a full-on conversation with myself inside my head while having an actual conversation with him. *Does this count as a real date? What if he wants to hold my hand? What if he doesn't? Should I offer to pay for myself? Am I talking too much? Does he think I'm smart enough?* We agreed that the movie was like a pre-date.

Our first real date was when he invited me to dinner. We went to an Italian restaurant and talked all about our mutual love of music. I was still attracted to him but wondered if we'd make it to a second date, because I wasn't sure I could date someone younger than me who listened to "noodly" Steely Dan. Months later, he confided to me that he wasn't sure he could date someone so short and who had multiple tattoos.

Mark was a perfect gentleman, something I'd never experienced during my drinking years. We had so much fun that we hopped a cab to another restaurant to have dessert and listen to jazz. He scored major brownie points by walking me all the way home after midnight, a two-mile walk-up steep 16th St.

Our second date was the following Tuesday, when we went to karaoke together at Fast Eddie's. I knew then I could date him because he sang a song by INXS. And our third date was that weekend when we went to the National Portrait Gallery. We went on more than three dates together before having sex, something I hadn't done for years. I wanted to wait until we'd been dating for a month, something I'd never done—and I didn't make it this time either. (Mark concurred that we made it to our fourth date.)

Mark was the first person I had sober sex with, and the first time was good. It had been a while since I'd had sex and it had been many years since the last time Mark had been intimate with anyone. He had considerably less experience in that department than I did. This has sadly been the greatest source of angst in our relationship. For some reason, the closer we became emotionally, the more frightened he became of disappointing me in the bedroom. This contributed to making me feel like a misfit even in my own partnership.

I had had my sexual adventures, which were a mixed bag of pleasurable and emotionally painful experiences. It allowed me to grow confident in who I was as a sexual being. I'm confident and outspoken in what I like, and this unintentionally added to the pressure Mark felt to please me. And the one thing neither of us had was a desire to employ the two things that always worked (at least for me) before: alcohol and drugs. Without them, I found sex to be an awkward production. I was conscious of my weight in a way I wasn't before I got sober and I was conscious that without a partner who knew some moves, I became less confident that I knew what I was doing.

I was used to being with men who were vocal about what they wanted and what felt good. Mark was his own person, and I didn't yet know his love language. I initially mistook his quietness for a sign that I wasn't pleasing him. This was a new experience for me, and it rocked my confidence. *What if I only know what I'm doing when I'm drunk or high? What if our sexual relations don't improve?*

But beyond that, between the six- to eight-month mark of our relationship, I noticed that Mark had more things on the shelf I gave him in my closet. He stopped going back to his place as frequently. I knew this meant that we were headed for living together. I knew this meant that we were serious about each other, but I wasn't going to play "House" again. If he was moving in, it was with the understanding that we were headed towards marriage. Could I marry someone that I loved but didn't connect with on a physical level?

Mark and I had a heated fight just before he left on a week-long business trip. When he returned, his first words to me upon letting him into our apartment was, "We need to talk." My heart sank to my feet. I was convinced he was going to break up with me. I started to cry and couldn't fathom why he was (a) so calm; and (b) opening his laptop while having The Conversation. But he surprised me by opening a Google Doc that displayed photos of three different styles of wedding rings and asked me which one was mine.

It wasn't the romantic proposal I envisioned—not by a longshot—but I couldn't remember feeling so happy. He proposed in a fashion so completely aligned with his character. Our differing ideas of proposing is a good example of how Mark and I are in some ways opposites. I expected something whimsical and romantic, and I got logical, timely, and thoughtful. This proposal story is also emblematic of how our differing communication styles have, at times, caused us both to feel like misfits in our own marriage.

Mark delivered a simple, organized presentation. There were four or five photos of engagement rings for me to choose from. In contrast, when

I plan something or want to talk to Mark about our planning something, it goes a little like this:

> **Me:** Babe, I was on Groupon and they have some good travel deals. We could go to Maine or Florida or Cancun or maybe Europe? Hotwire has cheap flights, and I can ask for time off. All we need is a backpack. I already called ...
>
> **Mark:** Babe, it's 2 p.m. I'm in the middle of work. It's going to cost a lot of money. Do you want to go somewhere warm or cold? I'm confused. Maine will be cold, and Florida will be hot and humid.

I flood Mark with options and ideas. I present wishes instead of facts and sometimes, I'm not sensitive to the timing of my delivery. Mark thinks my proposal is spontaneous and whimsical and that's because while I've been thinking about a vacation for weeks, I don't mention it beforehand and just blurt out my thoughts as "let's do this" versus "I've been thinking about this for a while and here is what I've researched."

What results from many of our interactions is misunderstanding, hurt feelings, and feelings of rejection. Mark's M.O. is to shut down and mine is fight-or-flight. In fact, in the beginning of our courtship, my instincts were so strong that I threatened to break up with Mark every other week and twice on Tuesdays. Even now, I'm not great at keeping my emotions "right-sized." This is just one of an infinite number of 12-Step phrases or slogans we try to live by.

We jokingly refer to ourselves as The Bickersons because our usual pastime is arguing. Neither one of us loves the constant strain this puts on our marriage, but I think we're becoming more accepting that it's just how we are. I'm usually even-tempered but when I'm mad, I'm FURIOUS. Similarly, when I'm upset, I'm not just sort of hurt; I'm tragically wounded. Instead of shrugging things off, I often overreact, yell, or snarl.

I'm notorious for mumbling and Mark is a LOUD talker. I used to think he had a hearing problem, but he doesn't. He's just used to being loud because ... well, he's just loud. I have difficulty discerning if Mark speaks in a loud voice and, in fact, I can't stand it when anyone raises their voice near me or at me. One symptom of my having ADD is being extra sensitive to auditory stimulation. Plus, I reflexively associate it with my younger years when my dad lost his temper and verbally assaulted anyone in his path. My dad's raised voice was like thunder before lightning struck the ground near your feet. His voice was so booming that I became petrified with fear. I froze in place and tried to make myself smaller, to avoid confrontation.

Mark and I have completely different demeanors too. I am usually mellow and even keeled. I take a lot of things in stride and prefer peace above all else. I am often called a hippie. In contrast, Mark is more like Jack Lemmon in *Grumpy Old Men*. He's not what I would call curmudgeonly, but he often exudes a sense of angst and urgency that often baffles me.

Part of this is since he struggles with bipolar disorder without mania. Mark doesn't experience any of the "up" cycles, nor does he cycle frequently as many people with this type of bipolar disorder do. He is highly anxious and always has low-grade depression. But his razor-sharp wit, thirst for knowledge, intellect, and ability to remember all the things I forget and everything he ever learned is what drew me to him and what keeps me intrigued.

As for me, Mark is intrigued and perplexed by my impulsiveness and need for semi- frequent change. Even when it comes to things that I've thought of for a while, I'm spontaneous in my timing. Mark doesn't understand why I needed to suddenly color my hair sapphire blue at 10 p.m. or why I said I was going to the thrift store but came back with a new cat.

Mark doesn't have an impulsive bone in his body. He is the epitome of compulsiveness. I marvel that he can eat a whole pint of ice cream in one sitting (I can't make that commitment to anything cold) or always puts his clothes away the very first thing anytime we travel. We jokingly refer to the redundant arguments we have about the different results our actions have, as the Battle of the Wills.

Whenever we go for a drive to explore a new nature trail or dog park with our oldest four-legged son Elliott (the most adorable dachshund-beagle mix ever), Mark is ready and out the door at precisely the time we agreed upon. He gets ready immediately, then has a conniption that it takes me longer than five minutes to get out of the house. He is all about efficiency and arrival at our destination. I get excited by the adventure versus anxious over getting anywhere on time. My operative mode is non-harried. Sometimes, I stall just to piss him off, but it honestly takes me more time to get organized.

And I'm never out the door on the first try. I always forget something I need such as keys or sunglasses. I could care less about timing. I hate rushing adventures. They're meant to be savored. On our honeymoon to St. Maarten, Mark had all his clothes put away before he let himself enjoy the view from our balcony. I, on the other hand, ran into our time-share (a wedding gift from my parents) and threw the balcony doors wide open and shouted, "Hello, St. Maarten!"

Think of us as Kettle Corn: our contrasting qualities combine to form a pleasingly balanced taste. Or maybe we're more like melody and beat; we're strong enough to stand alone, but sound better when put together. Over time, we've learned how to communicate more fairly, more like a duet as opposed to demanding soloists. If I've learned one thing from being in long-term recovery, it's that rigorous honesty, when delivered with compassion, is the secret to maintaining integrity. Mark and I have had to compromise, but by being honest with one another, we haven't had to compromise the quality of our relationship.

It's taken a lot of self-work to be able to verbalize when I feel hurt, disappointed, or afraid. I didn't realize until now how Mark's steadfastness has allowed me to feel safe in our relationship. And it's only because I've felt safe that I've felt like I've had the upper hand any time I've threatened to leave. There are days I marvel why anyone would volunteer to take on another person's baggage, let alone the baggage of inheritance. My family is loving and kind but we're a LOT. It's like a symphony, where my family hits all the staccato, *fortissimo* notes and his family represents the legato, *pianissimo* notes.

Mark is an only child. His parents are warm, loving, and quiet. They have their own anxieties, which Mark's taken on and adopted, but his family is consistently calm and quiet. My family is predominantly extroverted, and nothing is ever consistent about us except for our inconsistency. My mom and David are funny, witty, and adored by their 55-and-over retirement community. And there's never a dull moment in my sister Stacey's household; it's always teeming with dogs and teenagers. Then, there are my West Coast parents who remind me of the cinematic Fockers, with their type-A personalities and shenanigans. As for me, I'm introverted and quiet, but I am also a handful.

In writing this, I bless my stars that Mark said, "I do" and that he's stayed by my side. And I've given him a few reasons to do so. Our stories as a married couple experiencing early and continued recovery together are numerous enough to write a separate book about. I will say that we've managed to do more than just survive our journeys in recovery side by side.

We've truly grown up and evolved together. We've individually worked on staying sober one day at a time and have as a couple endured more tribulations than either of us ever could've imagined. But we've also had our share of happy successes. We've both gone back to school for advanced degrees, we've begun new careers, and have improved our quality of living slowly—again, one day at a time. We've been able to weather such storms together because we've never stopped doing the heavy lifting of self-work in our 12-Step programs. We attend meetings both separately and together, see individual therapists, and engage in open and mostly loving communication with one another.

We're still both reactionary versus responsive. It's embarrassing to admit that after nearly 13 years together; we are just now in a place where we're both ready to focus on being more emotionally regulated. I am better at teaching this skill to my therapy clients than I am at practicing pausing before responding myself.

The recovery slogan that "pain [is] the touchstone of all spiritual progress" rings true for us. We needed to get to a point in our relationship where we were tired of hurting one another when we should be loving one another.

I believe that this is especially true given that we are a year-plus into a global pandemic and things are only now starting to look a bit brighter. I know that people die every day, but there's nothing like a shared crisis to make the beauty of life more evident. Life is too short.

CHAPTER 19 – COME TALK TO ME

In 2008, when our country went into a recession, many people found themselves out of work. NatGeo tried to stay afloat amid economic instability but ended up cutting costs to survive. Employees were let go in waves over the course of a year. I didn't relish the thought of being unemployed, but I was disillusioned with my duties with All Roads because they took every ounce of concentration and energy I had.

I was glad that budgetary crackdowns meant that the film festival component of our program would keep us in DC. I wouldn't have to coordinate logistics on a large scale any longer. It also meant that I could attend to my recovery, which was my main priority. Besides, getting sober was good for my personal life, it wasn't a boon workwise. I was considered un-fun by my coworkers. They still reveled in the party lifestyle: work late and drink until much later. I didn't have any problem going to happy hours with my team and ordering a soda, but they were more aware of the way in which they drank in my presence; I was buzzkill.

As a result, the coworker that I was closest to started palling around with another coworker, and I stopped being invited to hang out. I was hurt, but I realized that without the shared interest in alcohol, I didn't have much in common with a few of my teammates. My sobriety enhanced my self-esteem, which made it easier for me to speak my mind. I no longer meekly agree with every decision.

I also came to the realization that I only enjoyed my job because it was mission driven. I loved Nat Geo's programming, but I didn't want to support it in an administrative capacity. And despite my background in environmental science, I wasn't really a scientist. I didn't have the skills that transferred well to work in the field as an Explorer.

In March 2009, funding for the headquarters' portion of the festival was cut and I was out of work. I was ready to make a major career change. I knew I needed to redefine "success" for myself before I repeated past work mistakes, or worse, relapse on alcohol or marijuana.

I didn't know what I wanted to do, but I was confident that whatever I did it would involve helping both people and animals. My cubicle was decorated with posters of leopards and lions, some of which I took myself during the weekends that I volunteered as an animal behaviorist and educational interpreter at the National Zoo. I gave administrative non-profit work one more go, thinking that perhaps my role with All Roads simply wasn't the best fit for me.

I thought that in a different role, I might hit my stride, but I again struggled and ultimately failed when it came to performing detail-oriented tasks. I was fired from two different organizations in rapid succession because I messed up Excel spreadsheets and incorrectly processed credit card payments for conference registrations. One of my bosses took apart every box of conference folders I assembled because I hadn't realized that not all binders were supposed to receive different content.

Attention to intricate detail was a behemoth I couldn't conquer no matter how hard I tried. I decided that if I was going to succeed, it had to be on my own terms. I literally couldn't afford to make decisions based on what others—even my parents or Mark—thought were in my best interests. They didn't know the amount of intense focus it took for me just to be mediocre in a relatively low-end office job. They didn't have to re-experience the trauma of being told repeatedly, "You're kind and well-intentioned, but …." There was always a "but" and I couldn't handle one more. My self-esteem, which had taken sobriety and hard work to build back up, had taken a nosedive.

I knew from attending enough 12-Step meetings and working a program of recovery that giving up was not the same as defeat. Yes, it's quitting to throw in the towel, but it's also freeing. Surrendering allowed me to shift my focus from what I couldn't control and take ownership of what I could. I decided that it was time to be more like my father and to reinvent myself. I didn't want to work for anyone else and I wasn't going to work behind a desk. I decided to do something I loved: walk dogs.

I don't know how to go about things on a small scale because when I'm excited about an idea, it's full steam ahead, a hallmark of my ADD. I intentionally slowed my roll and methodically researched what was involved in starting up a full-fledged pet care business. I was notorious for my "ready, fire, aim" approach to things and I wanted to do things differently.

I've also never been one to shy away from taking a risk. It's a trait I share with my father, and it's saved my life before. I started RachelzPetz and used credit to pay for a website that I designed and wrote all the content for. It didn't take long before I had enough customers to cover the cost of the website and other self-promotion. It kept me busy, and I lost weight from all the walking. I became known in my neighborhood, and it felt good to be my own boss.

In many ways, running my own business was perfect for me. I worked harder because I knew my success depended solely upon my own efforts. RachelzPetz catered to my strengths, many of which are benefits of having ADD: risk-taking, creativity, spontaneity, hyperfocus, and acting calmly under pressure. Creating a website and marketing myself afforded me the opportunity to apply creativity, writing and interpersonal skills. Securing clients required a degree of organization that, as a one-woman show, was manageable enough. And client meetings depended upon my being personable, persuasive, and trustworthy.

I've learned that you can't be successful being in business for yourself if you're not honest and willing to own up to your mistakes. I made my share of innocent ones. I got trained in pet first aid and CPR. I purchased liability insurance and became both bonded and insured. But I couldn't foresee every possible faux paw (oh yes, I just went there).

Luckily for me, I didn't experience anything too awful. I had incidents where security systems were wonky, and I had to call a pet owner or two while they were out of the country. I couldn't get some keys to work properly, which meant that I wasn't able to get dogs out for walks. Once or twice, I accidentally left the owner's doors unlocked. I also forgot to feed the cat as scheduled and the owner was gone for a few days.

The worst thing that happened while working for myself wasn't my fault. I was dog and house sitting for a couple who failed to inform me that their golden retriever was a bonafide escape artist. Mason was super strong and sneaky, and he deftly slid past me while I tried to block him with a gate that hadn't even latched. He used his nose to wedge open the front door which I thought my tush blocked. He barreled out the door and gallivanted toward a park on Capitol Hill. Mark and I spent hours looking for him. I called the owners, who were in Europe, and they weren't phased by my call, and in fact, that's when they chose to tell me that he tended to emancipate himself. I called the Humane Society and Washington Animal Rescue League. I hardly slept that night because Mason didn't return. The next morning, Animal Control called to inform me that a neighbor had found him and had brought him inside their home late the previous night. They dropped him off minutes before I got the call. Unsurprisingly (and fortunately), Mason was unscathed (and likely unfazed) by his adventuring.

During the time that I ran my pet care business, I seriously contemplated becoming a zookeeper. I was in my seventh year of volunteering at the National Zoo. I went from being an outdoor behavior watcher at the free-ranging Golden Lion Tamarin exhibit to being an educational interpreter at the Great Cats exhibit. In 2009, zookeeper Rebecca Kregar Stites started a captive lion-breeding project. She and fellow Great Cat Keeper Kristen Clark Beatty needed volunteers to observe a newly forming lion pride and record behavioral data. I volunteered for the project before you could say "Rawwwr!"

The Zoo didn't skimp on volunteer education. They took it very seriously and made sure that all volunteers had hours of biology training. I previously learned all about cheetahs, maned wolves, and Grevy's zebras from lead keepers and biologists, including Craig Saffoe. He was so patient and affable with everyone, and I picked his brain every chance I could. Plus, he was now supervising Rebecca and Kristin. I got to learn from all three of them and it was literally awesome. Not many people have been able to get such hands-on training about lion identification and breeding behaviors.

Every weekend, rain, or shine, I walked a mile up 16th street and down Harvard Street into the Zoo's back entrance, and onto Lion and Tiger Hill. Some mornings, Luke was solo in his pride land. At other times, he was with one or both sister lionesses, Shera and Naba. Through my observations and the recording of data, I was able to help Zoo staff determine when Shera and Naba became comfortable enough with Luke to bow low to him, a behavior known as lordosis. This indicated that the sisters were ready to mate. Similarly, when Luke sprayed his scent everywhere (and I do mean everywhere) or when he opened his mouth in an absurd looking grimace known as flehmen, it indicated that he was ready to copulate and further his legacy.

A zoo's major focus is to preserve the existence of wildlife. Inherent in this is increasing the genetic diversity of its species. Animals bred from diverse gene pools, whether in the wild or captivity (including those who've been artificially inseminated), are healthier and therefore more valuable than species interbred throughout generations. Competition for genetically diverse species is fierce among zoos around the world. Therefore, most participate in an international Species Survival Plan (SSP).

Rebecca's vision in having Luke form a pride was the contribution of his genes. His offspring would enhance the genetic diversity of captive bred lions and enhance the overall lion gene pool. Luke's success in forming his harem would signify a huge win for science. Rebecca's project was no small affair, and I'm fortunate to have witnessed and played even a bit part in her endeavor. She inspired me in my desire to pursue becoming a zookeeper myself. I loved every day I spent completing routine tasks, but no two days were alike, which helped to curb my ADD-related trait of becoming easily bored with the same-old, same-old.

As a result, Rebecca offered me an internship with the Great Cats staff. I believed it would improve my chances of ultimately gaining employment at the Zoo. I got to go behind the scenes of the captive lion breeding project, as well as help tend to other animals housed within the Great Cats exhibits. I helped prepare food and clean out the enclosures of Andean bears, giant anteaters, coatis, and caracals. I also participated in enrichment activities, such as spreading scented oils around the caracal enclosure or putting a dead rabbit in the lion habitat. I consider myself to be a squeamish person but oddly, this didn't faze me. Hosing down caracal cages, however, freaked me out. I had to crawl into the narrow cement cages and pray that the giant, creepy sprickets (half spider-half cricket) didn't leap on me.

One day, I was cleaning interior enclosures in the lion and tiger area as Luke was outdoors sunning himself and flirting with Shera and Naba, and the tigers were in the opposing yard. They were likely hiding from observers. I walked down the narrow cement walkway toward the refrigerator that stored "sparkle poop" (glitter and frozen peas were often added to help identify one animal's output from another's) and other fecal samples. Suddenly, I heard a loud thunk on metal. I spun around to see two enormous, furry striped paws pressed against the metal gate of one of the cages. Günter had a good laugh at my expense; I nearly peed myself.

A year into my internship, I became a Keeper's Aide at the Kids' Farm. This involved helping to feed and groom livestock, including cows, rabbits, chickens, goats, donkeys, and alpacas. The only animal I didn't assist with there were the hogs because they were not known for their affability. I especially loved assisting with alpaca target training, as they gave nosey kisses on demand in exchange for treats. The training was an effort to help ease the alpacas' anxiety and to allow keepers and medical staff to operate safely around their powerful hind legs if they needed medical care. My other favorite chore was using a wet vac to vacuum up goat poop. I know I'm weird, but it was oddly gratifying to see a yard full of pellets and then make it spic-and-span by hoovering them all up. Loving up goats and donkeys and getting alpaca kisses was comforting and helped to ease my anxiety.

I applied to many zoo positions within the National Zoo, as well as with other zoos in different cities throughout the U.S. I cast a wide net and was dejected when all of them rejected me. I had a master's in environmental education, had been volunteering at the National Zoo for seven years, and was interning with the Smithsonian (the National Zoo operates under its aegis).

Like a record on repeat, I was either cut off or not cut out for what I loved most: animals and food. I couldn't be a marine biologist or a chef because those careers were too demanding in the math and sciences. Now, I wasn't accepted as a zookeeper, and I was struggling to stay afloat as a small business owner since not having access to a vehicle severely hindered my ability to succeed in DC's uber-competitive and highly saturated dog-walking industry.

I was cut yet again. Keeper Aides were required to volunteer at least nine hours per week. I spent at least three weekend days a month volunteering at the Zoo for the past seven years. I attended every mandatory training and stepped up to fill in for others as needed. I was whole-heartedly devoted to my volunteer obligations, but I also needed to make ends meet. I couldn't afford to turn down work. I sometimes needed to take last-minute opportunities if they arose on the weekends. I was upset that the lead keeper at the Kids' Farm couldn't work with me the few times I needed to adjust my volunteer hours. I was fired from my unpaid volunteer position without so much as a discussion after all the years of love and labor I'd given the Zoo.

I angrily wondered, *who else gets fired from a volunteer position?* It made me feel ashamed of myself. And as you might imagine, all my old feelings of feeling different and less than smacked me in the face. I still consider myself fortunate to have witnessed Rebecca's project result in the wildly successful endangered lion breeding. I saw Luke, Shera, and Naba parent two different sets of cubs. I got to observe the joy on Rebecca, Kristen, and Craig's faces when they held adorable lion cubs after they passed their swim tests, a rite of passage to spend time outside in enclosures with water filled moats.

School's Out Forever

At 41 years old, I thought my rite of passage would be world travel. Turns out the only traveling I did was from my home to dog walking gigs and from walking to night school. Never in a million years did I envision myself going back to yet more school.

I needed a career I could perform in any urban or suburban area in the country, one that would maximize my assets and downplay my shortcomings. I previously overwhelmed myself by applying to all kinds of positions, none of which maximized my strengths. I needed a win. I couldn't handle putting myself back into DC's power brigade. I'm not a starched suit. I'm a flowing maxi skirt.

I decided to focus on one that was narrow enough in scope yet broad enough in applications. I knew how to provide stellar customer service, but I couldn't survive as a career barista despite how much I loved the coffee/bakery industry. I got too bored and restless when business was slow and too frazzled when it was too fast paced. I was adept at operating cash registers but wasn't good at closing out at the end of my shifts. I had little interest in being a retail manager because what I craved was inter-action with customers and management is largely behind the scenes. It was time for me to conduct an internal inventory. My outstanding assets?

• A love of helping others.
• The ability to easily connect with people from all walks of life.
• Intimate knowledge of what it's like to struggle with a dis-

ability; and
• Finesse in creative marketing and public outreach.

Ideally, I wanted to work with people and animals. Being a farmer was a dream of mine, but it wasn't realistic this late in the game. I didn't major in agribusiness, and I didn't know a single farmer to network with. The only realistic and relatively easy career path I could foresee was becoming a mental health counselor. Who knew? Maybe I'd find a way to work in animal-assisted therapy. Plus, the mental health field is one of the few fields that respects seniors and doesn't force them into early retirement.

In his inspirational book *The Alchemist*, Paolo Coelho wrote, "When you want something, all the universe conspires in helping you to achieve it." On the other hand, the famous mythologist and author Joseph Campbell said, "If you can clearly see the path laid out before you; it's not your path." Whenever I've felt dismayed because I haven't had a clue which direction to go or which choice to make, these sayings have brought me peace of mind. They remind me that if I want something enough and put my faith in the invisible forces at work, I will be exactly where I'm supposed to be.

So it was that I found myself at the University of the District of Columbia's School of Counseling when I spotted a catalog that advertised the school's newest capacity-building grant, a graduate degree program in vocational rehabilitation counseling. I wasn't aware that this branch of counseling existed, but it made complete sense. I didn't predict this fork in the road, yet here it was. I knew in my gut, the house of intuition, that this was my golden egg.

I am an educator at heart—just not the classroom variety—so I wrote my entrance essay on my passion for experiential education. I incorporated my struggles as an individual with the invisible disability of ADD. I explained that it was a disability counselor who was the one who told me at a young age that I'd be lucky if I got into college. I asserted that I would be a better counselor than she was, and that I'd be sensitive to different learning styles and competencies. I admitted I had struggled with another invisible disability, addiction. I explained that with help and support from others, I learned positive coping techniques and had stopped playing the victim in my own life. I vowed that I'd use these experiences to connect with and to help others who have disabilities or different abilities.

I became a student again, pursuing certification as a vocational rehabilitation counselor and licensure as a Licensed Professional Counselor (LPC) in the first class of grant-funded students at UDC. I was surprised to find that half of the students were my age or older. I was even more surprised to learn that some of my classmates believed that my life was easy simply by virtue of my being born white. I knew that UDC was a Historically Black College, but I didn't think that others would perceive my life as being easier or my attendance as taking a spot reserved for "one of their own."

One of my introductory classes was Multicultural Education. I was embarrassed and literally schooled about white privilege. Yes, I played a part in systemic racism simply by virtue of my being white, but that didn't mean my life was easy. I spoke up about my struggles with ADD, my need to often work two jobs, and my experiences being marginalized by virtue of my Jewish ancestry. Standing up for myself helped my classmates to understand that I understood the concept of struggle. Similarly, my classmates' directness with me and the few other white students in our program opened my eyes to the reality of the many shades of prejudice, bias, racism, and classism.

Pathways to Success

UDC is in Northwest DC, the largest of the city's quadrants and considered the safest. It's referred to as the safest quadrant of the city. I'd lived, worked, and now studied in it for years and rarely ventured much outside of it, so the culture shock was palpable when I began my practicum at Pathways to Housing DC.

I exited the bus at Florida Avenue and Q Street, NE. This intersection was familiar to me only because I inevitably ended up lost on this exact corner anytime I drove from my childhood home in Gaithersburg to my friend Russ's apartment near Catholic University. It had long been a rough neighborhood and was only just beginning to improve (sadly) because of gentrification.

Most days, I didn't waste any time after getting off the bus, as I felt unsafe. I literally speed-walked from the bus stop to my practicum site because the only businesses at this intersection were a liquor store on one corner and a pizza shop catty-corner to it. I wasn't scared that I was one of the only white people around, but I was acutely aware that I was oftentimes the only female. Inside Pathways, the main lobby where my office was situated was a thinly walled box (possibly 10' x 10') without any soundproofing. I was convinced a consumer would fall through its walls and land in my lap.

I shared this "office" with my supervisor, David. He was the only employee who possessed the Certified Rehabilitation Counselor (CRC) credential I was working towards. I credit my boss with teaching me how to leverage humor to establish rapport with potential employers and community workers by walking right up to workers and managers cold turkey, initiating meaningful and informative conversation about their places of business. This usually led to being warmly welcomed to return for follow-up conversations and further rapport building. Such relationship building was paramount to addressing potential future employment placement for our consumers—all of whom needed workplace accommodations of some kind. (I learned that we referred to the individuals we tried to find employment for as consumers as opposed to clients because they consumed or utilized our core services.)

Almost all of Pathways' consumers were assigned to work with a cadre of Assertive Community Treatment (ACT) Team employees, consisting of a case manager, therapist, nurse, psychiatrist, and housing specialist. Our consumers lived at or below the poverty level and most lived for a time on the streets and in homeless tent communities and shelters.

Given all of that, imagine how hard it was for the individuals I worked with to find a job without having a home address, access to computers, or appropriate interview attire. It was hard to fathom that some consumers didn't possess the requisite social skills needed to engage in an interview. School had already opened my eyes to so much but working in the field taught me more than any classroom teacher or textbook ever could have. Everyone assigned to my caseload actively abused alcohol and/or street drugs and struggled with severe psychiatric disorders. Despite this or maybe because of it, they wanted to work. Despite all they endured, they wanted to work to escape the monotony of their daily lives.

I, too, was beginning to see how employment could be exactly the type of intervention they needed to escape their shared bondage of addiction. It helped that I understood this on an intimate (albeit not wholly equal) level. I wasn't homeless, but I understood the value of having a job. Oftentimes, working was the only thing that made me feel somewhat normal. Working gave me a source of connection to others. Work, even without pay, gave me a sense of purpose, value, and pride. I discovered that I wanted to work for the exact same reasons as those I worked to find employment for. While they lacked traditional work experience, they all possessed street smarts and survival skills. I believed that made them an asset to any potential employer.

I'm grateful for my experience at Pathways. I worked with people who wanted to help improve the lives of those who need housing and public assistance. But after a year of interning and almost a year as a paid staff member, it was time for me to move on.

Once my boss left, there was no one else qualified to provide me with the clinical supervision I needed to satisfy my CRC credentialing requirements. I took a pay cut by accepting a position as a Supported Employment Counselor at Community Connections in southeast DC. CC is another one of DC's Core Service Agencies (CSAs) supervised by the Department of Behavioral Health (DBH).

I had flown under the radar at Pathways because my role and services were vital, and I was their only Supported Employment Specialist. At CC, I was part of a team of similarly employed team members. We met regularly with our department head to discuss performance enhancement strategies, review our collective failures, and celebrate the successful job placements of consumers. We received free clinical team development and training. When I wasn't in the field, I sat in a cubicle (blech), but it was a nice and safe work environment.

CC also had ACT Teams, but I no longer worked with consumers who couldn't attend to the "activities of daily living" independently. I was relieved to work almost solely with individuals who could at least bathe, dress, and keep themselves clean. I was also relieved that I no longer had to drive around to the more dangerous neighborhoods as nearly all the consumers I now worked with could get themselves to CC's headquarters, which was located on top of a Metro stop and near multiple bus routes. Best of all, most consumers I provided support to had previous work experience. All these factors made it more realistic for me to place them in positions of competitive employment.

The downside to my transition to CC was that my performance was evaluated and measured using DBH's CSA criteria of providing five billable face-to-face contact hours with consumers per day. Sixty percent of our hours had to be conducted in the community. Suddenly, my worth was gauged by quantity over quality, which required me to keep a scrupulous accounting of my time.

I wasn't a fan of the fee-for-service model, but my purchase of a car after 11 years of navigating the city without one made the possibility of my meeting my field quota more likely. In fact, having my own vehicle was strongly suggested to me by my previous employer; it was that or be out of work. It didn't help that I dinged up not one but two company cars at Pathways. (Fun ADD trivia: Individuals with ADD are more likely to get in car accidents than those without it because we're easily distracted by things we see while driving, as well as things we're thinking about while driving. Additionally, our reflexes tend to be slower, which makes things like braking quickly more difficult.)

Despite the perks of car ownership, I found the fee-for-service structure to be inherently punitive. Imagine this hypothetical scenario:

- If my first consumer was a no-show, I was left with less than an hour to conduct job development talking with potential employers near the office.
- If I were supposed to go into the field with my second consumer, and she forgot her resume and I didn't have a copy of it, I could spend my next hour assisting her in creating a new one. I got to bill for that hour, but it detracted from my total field-time quota.
- If that day was especially cold and rainy and my third consumer canceled because of that, I could knock out an hour of administrative work but again, it detracted from my overall productivity quota.
- If the rain continued and my two remaining consumers canceled, I would wind up being left with four hours' worth of

work that I had to spend meeting with potential employers in the community.

All of this would leave me without a game plan or with no desire to go out in inclement weather to drum up potential business by acting as a placement specialist versus a soon-to-be clinical mental health counselor. The prospect of spending four hours in the field filled me with anxiety.

As an individual with ADD, I didn't know how to effectively structure my time. I struggle to be productive in an unstructured work environment. The need to unexpectedly self-structure was anxiety-producing and contributed to my feeling depressed and hopeless. It wasn't my fault that consumers canceled on me for a litany of reasons—many of which were valid.

I believe that the system of having billable hours for professionals who work with individual's dependent upon Medicaid and other forms of government support sets them up to fail and creates an ever-present sense of insecurity. My coworkers and I went to work each day worried we'd lose our jobs if we didn't make our productivity quota.

We only had two strikes before being terminated for lack of meeting the productivity requirements. It didn't matter whether it was two months in a row or twice within a period of two years we'd be terminated. I constantly feared that I was on the verge of being fired. Service providers under DBH monitoring can't afford to retain employees who don't meet its billable hours requirement, no matter how skilled they are clinically. I understood this logically but emotionally, it was hard to accept.

New Kid in Town

Less than a month after I began at CC, my boss was wooed by a better job opportunity. I was happy for her but upset that this marked the second time within a six-month period that I experienced a change in management. Plus, I had taken the job because of my affinity and respect for the previous manager. I was apprehensive about her replacement. Our team was tightly knit and the new hire, Navid, shook things up. It was disconcerting. We didn't know him or his operating style, but one thing was certain, he was all about change from the get-go.

I'll never understand why some people welcome change, while others oppose it. For me, change has always been like a bad boyfriend who suddenly sees the light. I'm initially intrigued by novelty in all its shininess. However, my intrigue soon gives way to fear of the unknown. I wonder, *what changes will happen next and when? Why are changes happening? Will they be good? Will I still like things?*

I react to change in one of two ways: I either embrace the new or I rebel. In the case of Navid, I embraced him and the changes that came about under his tutelage. He spent his early years in Teheran, where he was born, but he moved to Berkeley for college and never returned. He retained enough of an Iranian accent that when he says quintessential Californian things like "dude" and "totally," they are much more lilting and singsong than any SoCal stoner could possibly sound.

Navid has a West Coast, laid-back management style, but don't be fooled because he's a skilled mover and shaker. He knows how to get things done. And if you're not on board with his vision, he'll politely show you the door. I think this quality makes him a skilled manager. He knows how to unify and excite both those he works with and those that work for him.

When he was struck by the idea of creating a garden that would be planted and tended to by consumers, he went full throttle. He consulted with managers of group homes at CC and met with a neighboring restaurateur to see if he'd be willing to use free produce in exchange for training (and subsequently employing) CC consumers. He also met with local urban gardening entrepreneurs to design and begin planting. Navid was intuitive and big picture-oriented like me, but where I struggled to make theoretical concepts actionable, he envisioned and developed concepts quickly. He was able to act on all the steps between ideas and end results.

Some of my coworkers were put off by his management approach. They thought he was about change for change's sake, but that was only because he was new to us. I saw that Navid was about changing to create a true community. He is a true believer in the sanctity of the human spirit. He understood that all humans are social beings who derive our sense of self-worth from doing and belonging to something greater than ourselves. Without connection, we often fall prey to social isolation, depression, and addiction.

Soon, Navid lobbied successfully for our team to be dispersed and instead be embedded within CC's different departments. I initially wanted to work with veterans but was placed within the Dual Diagnosis team because of my empathy for individuals with co-occurring substance abuse and mental health problems. He knew this was my wheelhouse; I think he sometimes knew me better than I knew myself.

I still struggled to adapt to the way things were done regarding productivity, but I gave it my best shot for a while. I liked the Supported Employment department when we were housed together as a team. However, I loved the Dual Diagnosis team. Jordan and Maya were kind and welcoming team co-leads who made me feel right at home. I had a cubicle with a window view of Pennsylvania Avenue, which was refreshing. The sunlight helped me to feel more motivated. I hadn't felt so connected to a team or community in a long time.

I felt close to everyone and didn't want to make anyone feel left out or less than. But I had a special affinity for Chrystal. She was teeny like me but where I was plump, she was slight. Where I wore my heart on my sleeve, she appeared outwardly tough but was a softie underneath her cool-dude exterior. I got out of bed some days just to see her strut in her sagging jeans, t-shirt, vest and knit cap. Her clothing was a uniform that read, "Do not listen to me when I say 'Dude, stay away.' Hug me please." We took a lot of breaks together to walk around the community and gush over big dogs. She's going to throw up when she reads this, but she was my ride-or-die.

I had a team I loved, consumers I enjoyed working with, supervisors I was crazy about, but I was miserable. I wasn't a therapist and I desperately wanted to be one. I was so close to submitting my application for LPC status. It was a matter of months and Navid continued to work with me, teach me, and show me the remaining critical skills I needed to be a strong clinical therapist.

One of his gifts is knowing how to speak to individuals who wrestle with substance use and feel misunderstood and disenfranchised by society. I marveled at how calmly Navid spoke to consumers who didn't listen to anyone else. Once, he somehow cajoled more than a non-garbled insincere response from a consumer who cursed me out just minutes earlier. He looked everyone in the eyes and compassionately asked questions that allowed whomever he spoke with to answer as they saw fit. By comparison, I observed many case managers talk down to clients when they lost patience with the responses they received to their closed-ended, yes-no questions. I've unintentionally asked these types of questions myself in a sincere manner and was genuinely surprised to get noncommittal responses.

I didn't know it at the time, but Navid was introducing me to Motivational Interviewing; a technique often employed in the addiction field. It allows individuals to evaluate their circumstances, free of shame and judgment. This style of intervention also lends itself to individuals maintaining their autonomy.

Despite Navid's tutelage, however, I felt inauthentic "selling" potential employers on hiring CC's consumers. I experienced a combination of insouciance and low self-worth. I felt rebellion begin to rear her head again. She tried while I was at Pathways, but I managed to push her aside. Back then, I was new to the field, and I could reason with myself that I still had a lot to learn and needed to pay my dues. I never wanted to be a recruiter, which is how I saw my role. I thought I might change my mind once I worked more and completed my supervision hours.

Three years later and nearly licensed, however, I was still no closer embracing Supported Employment. The consumers I worked with at CC were higher functioning, but I still didn't know how to convince hiring managers that their new hires would be worth it in the long run. High functioning aside, they too wrestled with active addiction and had issues with time management and authority. More than that, they lacked conviction in their own abilities. The latter is something that takes a long time to cultivate. Most managers don't have unlimited time or patience.

I was in over my head. I didn't know how my fellow Supported Employment Specialists managed caseloads of 20 consumers, all of whom struggled with addiction and complex trauma and relied on multiple forms of government assistance. Most consumers couldn't afford to get to our office, and I didn't feel safe helping them gain employment in their neighborhoods. Besides, they didn't even want to work in their own neighborhoods. They were sick of being confined to dangerous areas due to financial limitations.

I appreciated Navid's mentoring, but rebellion trumped need. I couldn't give my all to a cause I didn't believe in. Having ADD makes it a struggle for me to force myself to do anything that I don't feel invested in or motivated by. Some people hate their careers but manage to perform well. I can't. I'm just not wired that way. I felt that even my best effort wasn't good enough for upper management. I was on probation six months prior and knew that my fear of being fired was likely becoming a fact.

There was no way around CC's 90-percent productivity requirement. There was no exception for almost making the cut. I could make the 60-percent field-time requirement and still be let go if my overall productivity rate fell below 90 percent. Navid let me air my grievances and chose to accept me for who I am. He met me where I was emotionally in the same way he did with consumers and everyone else he interacted with. He knew I would work as hard as I could out of respect for him.

Navid chose to invest his time and energy training me to be a successful mental health counselor, knowing I was out the door as soon as I completed my clinical supervision hours. My best was spending my field development and placement energies for industries I knew well and enjoyed frequenting: restaurants, cafes, and retail clothing stores.

I was sincere in wanting to give back to the community while trying to get consumers hired. Navid affectionately joked that I was his only team member who spent her paycheck trying to get others paid. His ability to laugh with me versus deride me for my quirks is merely one of the reasons why Navid was a great boss and mentor. He knew how to reach me by using his offbeat sense of humor to keep my spirits up and keep me motivated.

This was especially true whenever he needed me to correct detail-oriented mistakes I accidentally (and repeatedly) made. I didn't always make such mistakes out of carelessness. In addition to ADD, I also have dyscalculia, meaning I reverse numbers. This happens even when doing simple computations and even when I'm paying attention.

Keeping track of billable hours, being attentive to consumers, staying focused on driving safely with them in my car, and developing rapport with employers was exhausting for my coworkers, and they didn't have ADD. Burnout from the volume and pace of human services work is the main reason for the high turnover at core service agencies. By giving my all to the job, I sacrificed myself.

I couldn't give consumers my full attention and remember to record hours worked or document reimbursable mileage. At the end of the day, I often forgot how much actual time I spent in the field and how many miles I drove. I returned to the office exhausted because I'm introverted and spending so much face-to-face time with challenging consumers was mentally and emotionally draining. It killed me to have to spend the remainder of my time performing menial and soul-draining tasks that required attention to detail. And I lost income if I forgot to document or messed up recording my time.

Bless his heart, Navid never yelled at me. He pressed his hand to his head in mock disbelief on the daily, *Tsk*ed at me and chuckled, but he never made me feel less than. This is exactly how I felt about myself in my role, however. I unwittingly became like the frog in the ink sketch Navid taped to the back of his door. A frog is stuck inside a pelican's gullet. The frog is squeezing the pelican by its neck and exclaiming, "Don't give up!" Sometimes people say this as a platitude. Sometimes, we'd be better served to do exactly that: stop fighting and let go. Mixed martial arts fighters know that even the best fighters tap out to save face, avoid permanent damage, and live to fight another day.

In June 2016, Navid encouraged me to let go because it was time. There was no way I could realistically save myself and staying out of loyalty was akin to tapping out anyway. I'd earned my Certified Rehabilitation Counselor credential and was a newly minted Licensed Professional Counselor. I was able to leave the field of supported employment behind and enter the realm of clinical therapy.

I have fond memories of Community Connections despite not liking the rules. The problem wasn't the organization; it was me. I wanted what I always wanted when I was sure of myself and felt that my sense of justice was being impinged upon, that everyone else had to conform to my needs. I still had some growing to do, but more than that, I needed freedom and a clean start to be the therapist I knew I could be. I was miserable as a Supported Employment Specialist. It was never what I wanted to be. It wasn't who I was.

Never Going Back Again

I allowed myself to enjoy the summer of 2016 because I hadn't felt so emotionally depleted since I hit rock bottom in active addiction. But once summer ended, I felt squirrely. Mark and I were back to needing a joint income to make ends meet.

I proved myself to be a hard-working team player, had a solid clinical foundation and was confident in who I was as a counselor. I had four years of work experience under my belt and was adept at working with individuals with co-occurring addiction and mental health issues. I thought I was a shoo-in for an established private practice. I was an experienced counselor, but private practice owners saw me as an employment counselor and not a mental health clinician. I couldn't get my foot in the door to explain that I did have clinical counseling skills. No independent practices were willing to take me on without my having had previous experience providing one-on-one mental health therapy.

I vowed I would never work for another core service agency ever again, but they were the only agencies willing to take on newly licensed therapists. Despite my reservations, I took another job with a core service agency. The clinical directors swore that, as a therapist, I wouldn't have struggles with consumers canceling appointments at the last minute. They promised that I wouldn't have to hustle to make billable hours. The agency did place value on staff training and development, and I did earn more than I ever had before, but in the words of '80's heartthrob Richard Marx, *I should've known better* ....

In my interview, I was assured that I'd have an office. What happened, though, was that I was shuttled between three offices spread across the city and none of them were private. I was constantly moved in and out of different work rooms. It's difficult for someone with ADD to constantly shift workstations as it results in not having all the information you need when and where you need it. I couldn't lock any of the offices. I had no means of safely storing my laptop or personal things.

I commuted back and forth between opposing quadrants of DC, schlepping my personal 17-inch laptop with me. It weighed a ton and didn't even fit in a regular-sized backpack, so I rolled a shiny, silver Michael Kors rolling travel bag up and down the streets in one of DC's most dangerous areas.

I could've overlooked the office scenario had I been paid consistently. The company withheld pay from employees on several occasions, each time with no forewarning and making it especially difficult for Mark and me to pay our rent on time. Then, there were the consumer assignments. I was assigned evaluations with children as young as five years old. I had no clue how to assess a child. I addressed this with human resources and was told to "put my big girl pants on."

As for the promise of not needing to hustle for appointments. I was "strongly encouraged" to double-book consumers for intakes and to go up to random individuals to cajole them into therapy sessions with me.

The only thing the agency delivered was providing training on treatment plan writing, and the conduction of biopsychosocial intake interviews. The clinical directors were highly competent and passionate about their work. I'm grateful to them for teaching me the foundations of writing treatment plans and in-depth Interpretative Summaries.

In mid-March 2017, I was offered a part-time job with a government contractor that provided counseling services to the armed forces. It would allow me to provide vocational counseling to service men and women who were nearing the end of their military careers, regardless of their discharge statuses. I planned on keeping my other job but reducing my hours. If I cut my hours by half, I could work for the core services agency in the capacity of a contractor. I also planned on keeping my private practice, which I opened in September of 2016. I envisioned seeing clients in my private practice a few evenings a week and on the weekends. I thought that I'd cobble these three jobs together and slowly establish myself in private practice. According to my vision, I would be fully self-sufficient in private practice after a year. But ...

The agency I worked for full time informed me that shifting to a part-time, contractual position would require that 15 of my 16 billable hours be face-to-face. This was unrealistic, given that the consumers I worked with relied on Medicaid and Metro Access (a public transit program for the differently abled that is notoriously unreliable). And then ...

The military related career "counseling" turned out to be a farce. I knew up front that it wasn't a clinical counseling position, but in my interview, I was told that I would get to help connected service men and women in creating and revising resumes. I looked forward to processing their experiences of separating from the military and looking toward independent next steps. It's entirely possible that my joy in leaving a fee-for-service structure blinded me to purely administrative counseling. The fact that there was an insurmountable mountain of paperwork to be completed before I could even step foot onto the base should've given me insight into what my next adventure might look like, but I was idealistic and excited.

I was dismayed to discover my first task was to read and reread five thick three-ringed binders worth of material. I nodded off at my desk daily. I was overwhelmed and bored by the sheer volume of information I needed to absorb before I could perform "counseling" duties. I needed to be able to identify and differentiate the insignias and uniforms of Army and Navy officers, as well as the ranks and insignias of enlisted men and women. I was also expected to utilize two separate computer tracking software systems, which required me to memorize two distinctly different processes. Ugh.

(Multi-tasking or task-shifting isn't something individuals with ADD are good at doing. They require a higher amount of dopamine to fire neurotransmitters than individuals with ADD possess.)

I had to sit and watch a month's worth of training videos, some of which were hours long, before I even got to work with a connected service member. I lasted three months before letting go before being let go, which I'm convinced was just around the corner.

It was on a gloomy and rainy summer's day in 2017 that I found myself down two jobs. Mark had been let go from his job the previous December, we had to pay rent for both my private-practice therapy office and our apartment, and all my old feelings of inadequacy gurgled inside me like hot magma. I briefly consulted with my higher power, but I wasn't full of faith at the time. I questioned a g—d that would allow us to be unemployed and penniless.

I hadn't been smart about the way I started my private practice. I plunged Mark and I deep into debt to pay for what I thought were the necessities of operating my own business: an office, furniture and decor, a website, a Google AdWords campaign, a Yelp discount on therapy, and marketing materials like pens and business cards with my logo. Mark, my sister, my parents and my sponsor all questioned my thinking. They separately but similarly suggested that just maybe I was biting off more than I could chew. But I had a vision, as well as the tenacity and stubbornness of an individual with ADD. Come Hell or high water, I was going to have my own practice.

The plan was to ease into having a full-fledged practice. I enjoyed working insanely hard at all hours. Like many adults with ADD, I'm energized by creating and doing things I wholeheartedly believe in. I wrote my own marketing copy for my DIY website and, in the process, shared a bit of my personal story on my website about why I chose a dandelion as my logo: I saw them as deep-rooted, sunny-headed, and tenacious wildflowers (not pernicious weeds as most people see them). I applied for insurance credentialing with two different providers. I networked with other therapists as well as local medical centers to advertise and promote my practice.

Working for myself allowed me to morph from a fledgling counselor into a confident and competent business owner. I set and adhered to my own hours. I still hustled for business, but for my benefit alone. I still had to write clinical notes and perform administrative work, but it was within my capabilities and in my timeframe. I didn't lose money on clients that didn't show. I was paid my dues in full either at the time of service or at the end of the month when the insurance companies I was paneled with paid out. Most importantly, I wasn't put on probation if I had an off month resulting from being depressed or overwhelmed.

I was steadily making a name for myself in the mental health community, and I would've stayed in private practice had I been able to afford to, but finances forced me to accept an offer of full-time employment at the end of January 2018. And just when I was sure that nothing more could go wrong, things went farther south.

I was hired as an Intake Specialist for a startup that provided intensive outpatient drug and alcohol treatment to teens and young adults. I had a huge corner office with a real swiveling office chair and a stationary desktop computer. I was finally part of something that made complete sense to me. I connected to the population the company served. I too, had self-medicated with alcohol and other substances. And I knew what it was like to find myself back in my parents' nest.

I labeled our clients as "failure to land" versus "failure to launch" because like me, they struggled with aim. They didn't have a solid plan for their future and lacked the coping skills one needs in order not to plummet into despair and addiction. They were as misguided and misdi-rected as I was when I was in active addiction.

The number of intakes I received slowed to a trickle and I was re-positioned. I was assigned to help invigorate the business's unstructured vocational programming, but unlike working with adult consumers who desperately wanted to work but lacked education and skills, these were spoiled, unruly and sullen teenagers. They resented being sent to treat-ment after school ended for the day, and most of them weren't old enough to work without a work permit signed by their parents anyhow.

I didn't mind being asked to help develop a vocational study and counseling program, but I don't fare well without any structure at all. I had no desire to implement and oversee a supervised, makeshift study hall. I wanted nothing to do with teenage boys who mouthed off to me and then refused to answer me when I asked them questions, but I had no choice but to grin and bear it.

I was so over being uprooted and untethered. The last thing I antici-pated was being scattered like a field of marshy, milkweed pods. Evident-ly, there was no longer a place for me with the startup. They'd just hired me three months prior. I was confused. I hadn't done anything wrong except share my frustration with my coworkers and they all whispered behind leaderships' backs because there was too much uncertainty about our roles. Why was I the one being let go?

There was a misunderstanding about my ability to become a Li-censed Professional Counselor in the state of Maryland. I'd applied for licensure before accepting the offer with the startup but three months into my new job, my application was unexpectedly denied. I had the requisite 60 school credits needed to satisfy the state's requirements, but I was two requisite courses shy. I'd need to take these classes, as well as the National Counseling Exam. It would take me at least eight months to obtain licensure this way. My only other means of obtaining my LPC was to wait until June 2019 and reapply as an out-of-state applicant since I was already licensed in DC.

Neither the startup's clinical director nor I were prepared to find our-selves in this predicament. It was awful. I was resentful of her because she brought me on without knowing that I was ineligible to perform clin-ical work without my license. She was angry with me for not gracefully accepting the unfortunate impasse we found ourselves at. My gut told me that I shouldn't have just assumed that I could work under supervision of someone else with a counseling license.

I knew that sometimes things happen in our lives that we just can't predict. There's a saying in the rooms of recovery: "Rejection is G—d's protection." Sometimes, however, this is too much to swallow. I had no other choice but to suck up my self-righteous anger and hurt pride. I knew that I would be in danger of relapsing if I held onto my roiling resentment. I wasn't about to drink away my rejection even though the thought flitted in my mind. I knew a better opportunity would come my way whether it was just around the corner or miles down the unpaved road.

She's Got Her Ticket

I interviewed for a position as an Addictions Counselor with another intensive outpatient program. In fact, the cofounder of this company was the pioneer of the IOP approach to substance abuse treatment. Still, I wasn't sure I wanted my whole life to be centered around chemical dependency and recovery; I had spoken with other counselors in the field who were in long-term recovery themselves and many believed it made it more difficult for them to work on their own recovery programs.

Unfortunately, the company didn't have full-time employment available, and I either wanted another full-time opportunity or a solid enough part-time position that would allow me to run my skeleton private practice as well as contract for someone else's private practice. The latter was something I began to do immediately upon being terminated from the startup. I enjoyed the benefits of working as a contracted therapist, which included not having to deal with complicated insurance billing or drumming up my own clients.

However, not having my own office or the autonomy that afforded me was discouraging. I had two offices, but both were freezing and loud due to the building's ancient air conditioning system. One day, its pipes leaked, and the ceiling fell in. Wet plaster fell onto the bright colored paisley therapy chair I recently purchased.

I called my sponsor in tears. She suggested that I reach back out to the IOP program to see if they still had the part-time opportunity I was offered in May when my attitude had been "I'm doing private practice full-time or bust!" You might say I was floored, then, when they offered me a full-time job. As one of my previous coworkers was fond of saying, "Sweet Baby Jesus!" I called it quits with contracting and closed the doors of my private practice. I enjoyed both professional adventures, but they weren't feasible at that point in time.

Whenever I'm feeling low, it helps me to remember that life can make a turn for the better when I least expect it. I believe that humans created G—d in our own image because we didn't want the burden of figuring it all out. I believe that as far back as ancient days, long before my ancestors were slaves in Egypt, that we needed the benefit of hope to believe in something more powerful than we were that would quell our fears over weather, famine, persecution, and other forces we had no control over.

I had felt powerless for so long that I forgot what it was like to feel a part of something greater than myself and my daily drama. The opportunity to work for Kolmac was the sandbar I desperately needed. It was a relief to stop to get my footing and breathe again. I was treading water in crisis mode for so long that I was on the verge of collapse. It was as if a 45-rpm record was playing too slowly, and the sound was as warped as a bad acid trip. Then suddenly, the speed was adjusted, and the soundtrack sounded normal again. I no longer felt like a misfit.

I agree with a 12-Step approach in the development of individual rapport with a higher power of our own choosing. I liken it to a cassette single. Remember those teeny cassettes that were popular in the '90s, which contained a single song per side? (You might not, but this is my book after all!) The flip side is akin to the 12-Step belief that our common wellbeing is paramount to an individual's sustained recovery. It's the development of deep and meaningful rapport with others that allows us to truly listen to our inner selves while binding us to one another. In his book *Lost Connections*, Johann Hari posited that the opposite of addiction is connection.

Lack of direction and meaningful connection to others led to my last relapse on April 21, 2016, while on vacation in Jamaica. My relapse was premeditated. I couldn't stand being riddled with anxiety 24/7. I didn't know if I would find a work environment that felt safe and would allow me to leverage my assets. I didn't want to be known or judged because of my ADD. I wanted to be respected and accepted despite it. I had people in my corner, but I didn't reach out to them. I wallowed in my feelings of self-pity and aloneness. I lost sight of my primary purpose, which was to stay sober and hang on for two more months until I became an LPC in DC. Leaving the world of supported employment was supposed to be the light at the end of a dark hallway.

Nearly all individuals with ADD are impulsive and need instant gratification. Holding on to hope requires utilization of emotional regulation skills and sadly, the short-term fix is more powerful than playing the long game. I had been in recovery for eight years at that point, but I still struggled to slow myself down.

In this instance, my bright idea was to eat a marijuana brownie larger than the size of my face. I bought the brownie across from the famous Rick's Cafe in Negril. Mark tried talking sense into me, but I wouldn't listen. I rationalized that it wasn't any different for me than his smoking cigars is for him. It was a hot day and the sun beat down on us as we began the walk back to our rustic "resort," so Mark urged me to eat the damn $20 brownie before it melted, and all was for naught. It was the most dense and nasty pastry I've ever eaten.

When we got back to our, we decided to head down and cool off in the pool. For five minutes, I was like, *Well, that sucked. I don't feel anything*. This was followed by five minutes of blissful glee. I swam the width of the pool to Mark's arms, and it felt like I had crossed the Chesapeake.

And then the world was lifted onto a turntable and played backwards. I lost touch with reality. It was terrifying.

I didn't know if I had relapsed or if I imagined it. I asked Mark whether I was alive or dead. I managed to build a little fortress out of chaise lounge pillows, which quelled my fear a bit. Mark had to help me up the stairs that led back to our bungalow. He looked up the side effects of marijuana edibles and barked exasperatedly, "According to this site, you're gonna be comatose for, oh, another five hours so fuck you. I'm going out to dinner while you sleep it off." And I did. I also eliminated green, Mary Jane-smelling crud for days afterward.

My expedition with edibles was the kick in the tush I needed to remind me what losing connection feels like. I needed to re-engage with my sober community, and I desperately needed to feel productive. The feeling of worth we gain through being wholly engaged in something is another one of the nine basic commonalities Johann Hari argued that all humans share.

For better or worse, and perhaps nowhere more so than in the DC area, it is what we do versus who we are that defines us. I needed to know that my clinical skills as a therapist were of value, and that I was worthy as an individual in my own right.

During the two years I was at Kolmac, I discovered that I had value and that I belonged. I felt lucky that all that was expected of me was to show up and be my true self. I didn't need to pretend that I was a great administrator. My supervisors and coworkers knew that I wasn't their go-to for staff procedures and protocol, but that I was their go-to if they had a question about ethics or community resources. They knew that I knew how to remain empathetic yet firm enough to be able to set and adhere to boundaries with my patients. This latter skill is something that still doesn't come naturally to me.

I got to share my whole self—flaws and all—in a way that was productive and meaningful to myself and my employer. It's also through sharing my whole self that I was able to help patients with their adventures in abstinence and long-term recovery. It's taken me a lifetime to learn that our flaws don't make us failures; they make us human.

My employment as an LPC working within the field of substance use disorders was my opportunity to transplant my roots from the limiting container of a fee-for-service model into a roomier one. It didn't require me to be a bonsai when I'm more like a dandelion. Unlike the tenacious wildflower I admire, I can't thrive under a myriad of conditions. I pride myself on being flexible and accommodating to a certain extent, but I also need stability and some verbal warm fuzzies. I wilt in more extreme conditions.

On March 17, 2020, our office went 100-percent virtual due to the global pandemic we are still in the middle of. No one could foresee the impact this would have. For me, working remotely has largely been a blessing. Unfortunately, it also made it clear that it wasn't viable for me to remain at Kolmac.

The reasons for my resignation weren't due to anything my supervisors or coworkers intentionally did. The move to conducting business virtually came at a price for everyone, but it significantly impacted those in clinical roles. We suddenly found ourselves tasked with a slew of "administrivia,", my term for non-trivial but detail-oriented administrative work—work that was previously organized and maintained by our office manager and administrative staff, such as scheduling urine screenings, being more hands-on in coordinating intake interviews, uploading documents to multiple online platforms, etc.

All our digital communication became about work and most work became administrative versus clinical in nature. The volume of administrivia grew exponentially the longer we worked remotely. I became overwhelmed with the clerical demands of the job. I no longer had the checks and balances of our administrative team who were so good at making sure the "I" s were dotted, and "T" s crossed. Pre-COVID, if I got confused, all I had to do was check a whiteboard or ask for something to be rescheduled. Now, without those backstops, I began double-booking myself for appointments and saving documents in one online system, but not another. This brought back the emotional morass I experienced once before, in my short-lived career counseling adventure on a military installation. My coworkers used to be able to cover for me and vice versa, but this was more difficult remotely because everyone had added administrative tasks to perform.

Plus, once clinical staff lost personal physical contact and could no longer stop by one another's offices to informally chat and get clarity on patient issues or discuss work over walks to Compass Coffee, we lost our collective soul. Everyone's stress levels were higher, and we couldn't conveniently chat with one another because we now needed to have everyone's cell numbers saved in our phones. We also needed Zoom phone numbers for them and our patients to reach us on. I needed to buy a new computer since I couldn't use Zoom communications on my old laptop. My new, inexpensive Chromebook wasn't compatible with some of the scheduling features, so I was constantly searching through emails to find important links for team meetings and the group sessions I co-facilitated.

It was time for a new adventure. I needed to reclaim a degree of simplicity in terms of the demands of administrivia. It was time to return to better leverage my clinical counseling skills, to connect with and help others, and to return to what makes me useful and most productive – employing my passion and creativity to encourage others to listen to their inner knowing of themselves and to redefine their sense of success—especially with clients who. like me, struggle with ADD both in their workplace and in their relationships.

EPILOGUE

Before I got sober, having ADD made me believe I was useless and less than others. I was full of shame and remorse. My feelings of being inherently inadequate are what led me to my becoming dependent upon others and external substances to give me relief from myself. I'm embarrassed to admit how far into chronological adulthood I was before I understood that:

> 1. I don't need to ask people to do things for me (my usual fall-back approach when I fucked things up).
> 2. It's okay to ask for guidance before and during tasks that are difficult.
> 3. I'm not missing the rule book everyone else was given at birth.

Others might have more common sense than I do, but that doesn't mean they don't need to ask for help. I've spent most of my life assuming that I was inherently flawed and vastly different. I didn't think I fit in anywhere. I took many wrong turns, both literally and figuratively. I spent years drinking over myself. I convinced myself that I was drinking away the hurt caused by others. I not only lacked a sense of outward direction; I lacked an internal moral compass. I was lost and disconnected.

Now, I'm able to cut myself some slack. I jokingly refer to myself as a "rebel without a clue" because I have a strong inner knowing of who I am versus where I'm headed. I know that whenever I get stuck and don't know where to turn, I don't need to be too stubborn to refuse help. Asking for help is one of the ways we connect with others and it isn't the same thing as giving up or surrendering. That quirky, uncoordinated, introverted, bookish, tomboy, punk-ish, Jewish, hippie with ADD never left. I schlepped her with me everywhere I ever lived. She is I, and I'm still here.

I know that when I'm feeling terminally unique, I can talk to my husband or friends who know what it's like to "fall on black days" (RIP,

Chris Cornell). Often, I get stuck in moments or hours of turmoil on the inside versus days feeling adrift. I'm still making wrong turns (even with GPS) and I'm still guilty of making "ready, fire, aim" decisions, but I'm also one badass earth goddess who knows how to truly listen to others. Today, I no longer listen to the soundtrack of a misfit. Instead, I proudly dance to the beat of my own syncopated rhythm. The playlist I listen to on any given day is beautiful, no matter how I'm feeling on the inside.

The Greatest—A Call to Action

To all of you with ADD who doubt yourself and your abilities, you are wildflower taproots. Allow yourself to feel grounded and blossom. You are worth it! Weed out the haters because if this global pandemic has taught us anything, it is that life is too short not to savor and share with others.

Author Bio

Rachel Leigh Wills is a Washington, DC area native. She holds a Master of Arts in Vocational Rehabilitation Counseling from the University of the District of Columbia. She is a Licensed Professional Counselor, poetess, writer, and speaker. She has previous experience in the field of environmental education (MS from Lesley University/Audubon Expedition Institute).

The author spent eight years in the capacities of an Employment Specialist and therapist in the Washington, DC Core Service Agency arena and for Kolmac Outpatient Recovery Centers where she helped individuals struggling with mental health and chemical dependency. She founded ADDvantage Counseling, LLC. and has served as a private practice owner and therapy contractor (currently with DC VA Counseling and Psychotherapy).

Rachel Leigh Wills is passionate about helping clients to navigate career transitions, redefine their concept of success and grow their self-esteem. Rachel's core areas of focus include working with adults with Attention Deficit Hyperactivity Disorder (ADHD); alcohol use disorder and chemical dependency; anxiety; depression and mood disorders. She combines cognitive behavioral and dialectical behavioral therapy techniques to help individuals better cope with extreme emotions and reactions.

Rachel Leigh Wills wrote Soundtrack Of A Misfit: Adventures in ADD & Addiction (on pre-order through both Amazon.com and Smashwords as a means of reaching others who struggle with ADHD and/or co-occurring disorders, as well as for those who have an appreciation for the underdogs and late bloomers. She has been passionate about music since the age of two, when she bought her first LP by Paul McCartney and Wings because she loved the song Band on the Run. In her debut memoir, she weaves in her ardor for music throughout. Her eclectic musical influences include Chris Cornell; Duran Duran; PINK; Fleetwood Mac; Eminem; K'Naan; and the Foo Fighters. She has been active in the local long-term recovery community and is open about her struggles with alcohol (primarily) in her work as a mental health therapist. When she isn't seeing clients, the author is likely spending time with her husband Mark and their beloved pets Elliott and Larry Katz (beagle-dachshund mix and mischievous black cat); writing, reading, listening to music, or exploring nature.

ACKNOWLEDGEMENTS & FOOTNOTES

This book is dedicated to many, to all of you who have been a part of my life and have helped me spread my wings and sow my roots:

- My parents—all four of them. Mom, for giving me an ear for music. Mom and DP, you have loved me through each day unconditionally. You have emotionally stayed by my side, no matter how far apart we were geographically. You have talked me out of making many wrong turns along the way and held me close when I stumbled. If you have a collective fault, it is loving me too much to allow me to bleed much.
- Dad, thank you for being a run-amok philosopher; for listening to a lot of manic bullshit; for making me breakfasts and other scrumptious meals; for introducing me to the magic of Bob Seger; and saving me when I needed it most.
- Ona, for encouraging me to write even when I didn't feel like it.
- My amazing in-laws, Barbara, and Skip Wills, for all your love and support and honoring of my traditions. I love you both immensely.
- Stacey, for being the ying to my yang, or something like that, and for being a true friend. Your sense of humor is the lightness in my life.
- Bruce and Mark Tankleff, for all your love, support, humor, and stories of Lindy the Wonder Bassett. Our cousin's reunion was a blessing.
- The Wolf Pack and the WIT Pack around the U.S.—you know who you are. You've collectively gotten me through every day for over 13 years. You are spread out across the country, but you are with me in my heart.
- Cathy Alter, for introducing me to Laura Sturza and other passionate writers, as well as for your encouragement and connecting me with Billy Fox.

• Billy, for being brutally honest with me during the first round of edits and giving me valuable insight for how to restructure the book and add more music.

• Andrew Gifford, for reading my introductory email and writing sample and for compassionately informing me to reach back out once my manuscript was in its final state.

• Ken Wachsberger, for replying to my emails and sharing a bit of your *ruach* for the creative process with me. Thank you also for sharing your helpful book, *You've Got The Time: How to Write and Publish That Book in You.*

• Cal Sharp, Creative Director of Caligraphics, for getting my vision and bringing SOAM's book cover and artwork to life. It's more vibrant because of you.

• Ruth Roman, for second-round edits and proofreading, as well as the gift of friendship and many pep talks.

• Joe Genaro from The Dead Milkmen and Golf Pro Music, for graciously allowing me to reprint lyrics from "Punk Rock Girl."

• Casey Reznik and Paul Kremen from BMG, for assisting me with permission rights to include lyrics from Garbage's song "Only Happy When It Rains."

• Michael Lipman, for assisting me with contacting George Michael's estate.

• Shout outs to Yakita, St. Amand, Yvonne, and Joseph of CFS. Joseph, if you read this, know that you all helped me learn how to write thorough treatment plans. Thank you for your unwavering patience in teaching me the difference between goals, objectives, and interventions.

• Brian, Elaine, Jen, Brenda, Yolanda, Alvez, and the rest of the Kolmac crew, for supporting me and helping me to grow into the clinician I am today.

• Sarah Sax and Louisa Carl, for reading my memoir and providing constructive critique and love.

• Geoff Woliner, for taking a chance on me and agreeing to write a foreword before he even read page 1.

• Esther Nagle and Ana-Maria Ignat-Berget, for reading

and providing testimonials.

• Sade Adeeyo, Melissa Nicolaou, Anjali Budreski, and Juli Ford, for being part of my support system and community. You are blessings.

• Isabel Kirk and the clinicians affiliated with her therapy practice, DC VA Counseling and Psychotherapy, LLC. Isabel is a warm, wise woman who embraces cultural competency and creativity among her clinicians. I am grateful to have found a strong and supportive team.

• Amy Martin Darling, for being both a friend and website designer.

• To my deceased relatives who protect me from somewhere where they're all playing together: Grandma(s) Mary and Harriett, Aunt(s) Sister and Carolyn, Uncle Bobby, Rocky, Ho, Digger, Kea, and Squirt

• The Delaware Legacy community—especially Steve and Nadine. Thank you for supporting my work and looking out for my parents.

• Kickstarter contributors (dear friends and family among them, some of which are acknowledged elsewhere in these acknowledgements): The Creative Fund by Backerkick; Kirsten Hancock; Beaux Harkirk; Mike DiGiovanni; Kelley Kline; Eryca Kasse; Sheila Tracy; Alexia Ramos; Joan Brewer; Jodi Latner; Elise Miller; Hannah Hunt; Joan Brewer; Yasemin Kasim, Ronit Erez (*b'ahava achoti*); Jillian Villars and Elise Bowman (and Louie [woof woof]; David Straw, Joe George (thanks for backing me!)

• Shanna Landolt for help and support with her #1 Bestselling Author Campaign.

• Walter and his team at Social.Media for helping me promote my Kickstarter campaign.

• Prefundia for assistance promoting my Kickstarter campaign

• To the Lang-Ballantyne family both human and four-legged. I cherish our friendship more than you know.

• Elliott and Larry Katz: Your mommy loves you so much

and is so sorry she didn't play enough while writing this book.
• Last (by request) and in no way least - my husband Mark.
You've been there with me through thick and thin. We've
trudged together hand in hand. I love you with all my heart.

Footnotes

[1] Lyrics to "Punk Rock Girl" courtesy of The Dead Milkmen and
Golf Pro Music

[2] John Paul Garrison, clinical and forensic psychologist

[3] Sarah Cassidy Ph.D., Jackson Laboratory for Genomic Medicine,
Gregersen et.al (originally printed in the American Journal of Medical
Genetics)

[4] BMG and Garbage permission to reprint lyrics from "Only Happy
When It Rains" lyrics

RX List   https://www.rxlist.com/dexedrine-spansule-side-ef-
fects-drug-center.htm

Made in the USA
Middletown, DE
27 April 2025

74741841R00188